Pediatric Ophthalmology and Strabismus

Section 6

2015–2016

(Last major revision 2014–2015)

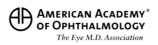

AMERICAN ACADEMY® OF OPHTHALMOLOGY
The Eye M.D. Association

Published after collaborative review with the European Board of Ophthalmology subcommittee

The American Academy of Ophthalmology is accredited by the Accreditation Council for Continuing Medical Education to provide continuing medical education for physicians.

The American Academy of Ophthalmology designates this enduring material for a maximum of 15 *AMA PRA Category 1 Credits*™. Physicians should claim only the credit commensurate with the extent of their participation in the activity.

CME expiration date: June 1, 2017. *AMA PRA Category 1 Credits*™ may be claimed only once between June 1, 2014, and the expiration date.

BCSC® volumes are designed to increase the physician's ophthalmic knowledge through study and review. Users of this activity are encouraged to read the text and then answer the study questions provided at the back of the book.

To claim *AMA PRA Category 1 Credits*™ upon completion of this activity, learners must demonstrate appropriate knowledge and participation in the activity by taking the posttest for Section 6 and achieving a score of 80% or higher. For further details, please see the instructions for requesting CME credit at the back of the book.

The Academy provides this material for educational purposes only. It is not intended to represent the only or best method or procedure in every case, nor to replace a physician's own judgment or give specific advice for case management. Including all indications, contraindications, side effects, and alternative agents for each drug or treatment is beyond the scope of this material. All information and recommendations should be verified, prior to use, with current information included in the manufacturers' package inserts or other independent sources, and considered in light of the patient's condition and history. Reference to certain drugs, instruments, and other products in this course is made for illustrative purposes only and is not intended to constitute an endorsement of such. Some material may include information on applications that are not considered community standard, that reflect indications not included in approved FDA labeling, or that are approved for use only in restricted research settings. **The FDA has stated that it is the responsibility of the physician to determine the FDA status of each drug or device he or she wishes to use, and to use them with appropriate, informed patient consent in compliance with applicable law.** The Academy specifically disclaims any and all liability for injury or other damages of any kind, from negligence or otherwise, for any and all claims that may arise from the use of any recommendations or other information contained herein.

AAO, AAOE, American Academy of Ophthalmology, Basic and Clinical Science Course, BCSC, EyeCare America, EyeNet, EyeSmart, EyeWiki, Focal Points, IRIS, ISRS, OKAP, ONE, Ophthalmic Technology Assessments, *Ophthalmology,* Preferred Practice Pattern, ProVision, SmartSight, The Ophthalmic News & Education Network, ⊕ and The Eye M.D. Association are, among other marks, the registered trademarks and trademarks of the American Academy of Ophthalmology.

Cover image: From BCSC Section 12, *Retina and Vitreous.* Ultra-wide-field fundus photograph from a patient with von Hippel–Lindau disease. *Courtesy of Colin A. McCannel, MD.*

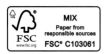

Basic and Clinical Science Course

Louis B. Cantor, MD, Indianapolis, Indiana, *Senior Secretary for Clinical Education*

Christopher J. Rapuano, MD, Philadelphia, Pennsylvania, *Secretary for Ophthalmic Knowledge*

George A. Cioffi, MD, New York, New York, *BCSC Course Chair*

Section 6

Faculty

Gregg T. Lueder, MD, *Chair,* St Louis, Missouri

Steven M. Archer, MD, Ann Arbor, Michigan

Robert W. Hered, MD, Maitland, Florida

Daniel J. Karr, MD, Portland, Oregon

Sylvia R. Kodsi, MD, Great Neck, New York

Stephen P. Kraft, MD, Toronto, Ontario, Canada

Evelyn A. Paysse, MD, Houston, Texas

Kanwal (Ken) Nischal, MD, *Consultant,* Pittsburgh, Pennsylvania

The Academy wishes to acknowledge the American Association for Pediatric Ophthalmology and Strabismus (AAPOS) and the American Academy of Pediatrics (AAP), Section on Ophthalmology, for recommending faculty members to the BCSC Section 6 committee.

The Academy also wishes to acknowledge the following committees for review of this edition:

Vision Rehabilitation Committee: Mary Lou Jackson, MD, Boston, Massachusetts

Practicing Ophthalmologists Advisory Committee for Education: Robert E. Wiggins Jr, MD, *Primary Reviewer,* Asheville, North Carolina; Edward K. Isbey III, MD, *Chair,* Asheville, North Carolina; Hardeep S. Dhindsa, MD, Reno, Nevada; Robert G. Fante, MD, Denver, Colorado; Bradley D. Fouraker, MD, Tampa, Florida; Dasa V. Gangadhar, MD, Wichita, Kansas; James M. Mitchell, MD, Edina, Minnesota; James A. Savage, MD, Memphis, Tennessee

European Board of Ophthalmology: Wagih Aclimandos, MB BCh, DO, FEBO, *EBO Chair and Liaison,* London, United Kingdom; Kirsten Baggesen, MD, PhD, FEBO, Aarhus, Denmark; Georges Caputo, MD, Paris, France; Rosario Gomez de Liano, MD, PhD, Madrid,

Spain; Peng Khaw, MD, PhD, London, United Kingdom; Birgit Lorenz, MD, PhD, FEBO, Giessen, Germany; Francis Munier, MD, Lausanne, Switzerland; Seyhan B. Özkan, MD, Aydin, Turkey; Nicoline E. Schalij-Delfos, MD, PhD, Leiden, the Netherlands

Financial Disclosures

Academy staff members who contributed to the development of this product state that within the past 12 months, they have had no financial interest in or other relationship with any entity discussed in this course that produces, markets, resells, or distributes ophthalmic health care goods or services consumed by or used in patients, or with any competing commercial product or service.

The authors and reviewers state that within the past 12 months, they have had the following financial relationships:*

Dr Fouraker: Addition Technology (C, L), Alcon Laboratories (C, L), KeraVision (C, L), Ophthalmic Mutual Insurance Company (C, L)

Dr Hered: MORIA (P)

Dr Isbey: Allscripts (C), Medflow (C)

Dr Jackson: HumanWare (C), *Reader's Digest* (S)

Dr Lorenz: Bausch + Lomb/Dr Gerhard Mann chem-pharm (C, L), Bayer Vital (C, L), Novartis Pharma (S), Optos (C), Pfizer (S)

Dr Nischal: Alcon Laboratories (S)

Dr Savage: Allergan (L)

Dr Wiggins: Medflow/Allscripts (C), Ophthalmic Mutual Insurance Company (C)

The other authors and reviewers state that within the past 12 months, they have had no financial interest in or other relationship with any entity discussed in this course that produces, markets, resells, or distributes ophthalmic health care goods or services consumed by or used in patients, or with any competing commercial product or service.

*C = consultant fees, paid advisory boards, or fees for attending a meeting; L = lecture fees (honoraria), travel fees, or reimbursements when speaking at the invitation of a commercial sponsor; O = equity ownership/stock options of publicly or privately traded firms (excluding mutual funds) with manufacturers of commercial ophthalmic products or commercial ophthalmic services; P = patents and/or royalties that might be viewed as creating a potential conflict of interest; S = grant support for the past year (all sources) and all sources used for a specific talk or manuscript with no time limitation

Recent Past Faculty

Aazy A. Aaby, MD
Jeffrey N. Bloom, MD *(deceased)*
Jane C. Edmond, MD
Scott E. Olitsky, MD
Paul H. Phillips, MD
Edward L. Raab, MD, JD

In addition, the Academy gratefully acknowledges the contributions of numerous past faculty and advisory committee members who have played an important role in the development of previous editions of the Basic and Clinical Science Course.

American Academy of Ophthalmology Staff

Richard A. Zorab, *Vice President, Ophthalmic Knowledge*

Christine A. Arturo, *Publishing Services Manager*

Stephanie Tanaka, *Publications Manager*

D. Jean Ray, *Production Manager*

Ann McGuire, *Medical Editor*

Crissa M. Williams, *Administrative Coordinator*

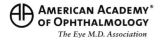

AMERICAN ACADEMY®
OF OPHTHALMOLOGY
The Eye M.D. Association

655 Beach Street
Box 7424
San Francisco, CA 94120-7424

Contents

7   Diagnostic Evaluation of Strabismus and Torticollis

8   Esodeviations

General Introduction

The Basic and Clinical Science Course (BCSC) is designed to meet the needs of residents and practitioners for a comprehensive yet concise curriculum of the field of ophthalmology. The BCSC has developed from its original brief outline format, which relied heavily on outside readings, to a more convenient and educationally useful self-contained text. The Academy updates and revises the course annually, with the goals of integrating the basic science and clinical practice of ophthalmology and of keeping ophthalmologists current with new developments in the various subspecialties.

The BCSC incorporates the effort and expertise of more than 80 ophthalmologists, organized into 13 Section faculties, working with Academy editorial staff. In addition, the course continues to benefit from many lasting contributions made by the faculties of previous editions. Members of the Academy's Practicing Ophthalmologists Advisory Committee for Education, Committee on Aging, and Vision Rehabilitation Committee review every volume before major revisions. Members of the European Board of Ophthalmology, organized into Section faculties, also review each volume before major revisions, focusing primarily on differences between American and European ophthalmology practice.

Organization of the Course

The Basic and Clinical Science Course comprises 13 volumes, incorporating fundamental ophthalmic knowledge, subspecialty areas, and special topics:

1 Update on General Medicine
2 Fundamentals and Principles of Ophthalmology
3 Clinical Optics
4 Ophthalmic Pathology and Intraocular Tumors
5 Neuro-Ophthalmology
6 Pediatric Ophthalmology and Strabismus
7 Orbit, Eyelids, and Lacrimal System
8 External Disease and Cornea
9 Intraocular Inflammation and Uveitis
10 Glaucoma
11 Lens and Cataract
12 Retina and Vitreous
13 Refractive Surgery

In addition, a comprehensive Master Index allows the reader to easily locate subjects throughout the entire series.

References

Readers who wish to explore specific topics in greater detail may consult the references cited within each chapter and listed in the Basic Texts section at the back of the book.

These references are intended to be selective rather than exhaustive, chosen by the BCSC faculty as being important, current, and readily available to residents and practitioners.

Videos

This edition of Section 6, *Pediatric Ophthalmology and Strabismus,* includes videos related to topics covered in the book (see the Related Videos section in Chapters 7, 11, and 14). The videos were selected by members of the BCSC faculty and are available to readers of the print and electronic versions of Section 6 (www.aao.org/bcscvideo). Mobile-device users can scan the QR code below (a QR-code reader must already be installed on the device) to access the video content.

Study Questions and CME Credit

Each volume of the BCSC is designed as an independent study activity for ophthalmology residents and practitioners. The learning objectives for this volume are given on page 1. The text, illustrations, and references provide the information necessary to achieve the objectives; the study questions allow readers to test their understanding of the material and their mastery of the objectives. Physicians who wish to claim CME credit for this educational activity may do so by following the instructions given at the end of the book.

Conclusion

The Basic and Clinical Science Course has expanded greatly over the years, with the addition of much new text and numerous illustrations. Recent editions have sought to place a greater emphasis on clinical applicability while maintaining a solid foundation in basic science. As with any educational program, it reflects the experience of its authors. As its faculties change and as medicine progresses, new viewpoints are always emerging on controversial subjects and techniques. Not all alternate approaches can be included in this series; as with any educational endeavor, the learner should seek additional sources, including such carefully balanced opinions as the Academy's Preferred Practice Patterns.

The BCSC faculty and staff are continually striving to improve the educational usefulness of the course; you, the reader, can contribute to this ongoing process. If you have any suggestions or questions about the series, please do not hesitate to contact the faculty or the editors.

The authors, editors, and reviewers hope that your study of the BCSC will be of lasting value and that each Section will serve as a practical resource for quality patient care.

Objectives

Upon completion of BCSC Section 6, *Pediatric Ophthalmology and Strabismus,* the reader should be able to

- describe evaluation techniques for young children that provide the maximum information gain with the least trauma and frustration

- describe the anatomy and physiology of the extraocular muscles

- explain the classification and diagnosis of amblyopia, as well as the treatment options

- describe the commonly used tests for the diagnosis and measurement of strabismus

- classify the various esodeviations and exodeviations, and describe the management of each type

- identify pattern and vertical strabismus, as well as special forms of strabismus, and formulate a treatment plan for each type

- describe the features of the various forms of nystagmus and understand their significance

- list the possible complications of strabismus surgery, and describe guidelines to minimize them

- design an approach to the diagnosis of decreased vision in children, and list resources available to these patients

- differentiate among various causes of congenital and acquired ocular infections in children, and formulate a logical plan for the diagnosis and management of each type

- list the most common lacrimal drainage system abnormalities seen in children and formulate a management plan

- list the most common diseases and malformations of the cornea, anterior segment, and iris seen in children

- describe the diagnostic findings and treatment options for childhood glaucoma

- identify common types of childhood cataract and other lens disorders

- construct a diagnostic and management plan for childhood cataracts

- identify appropriate diagnostic tests for pediatric uveitis

- differentiate among various vitreoretinal, optic disc, and metabolic diseases and disorders found in children

- list the characteristics of ocular tumors and phakomatoses seen in children

- describe the characteristic findings of accidental and nonaccidental ocular trauma in childhood

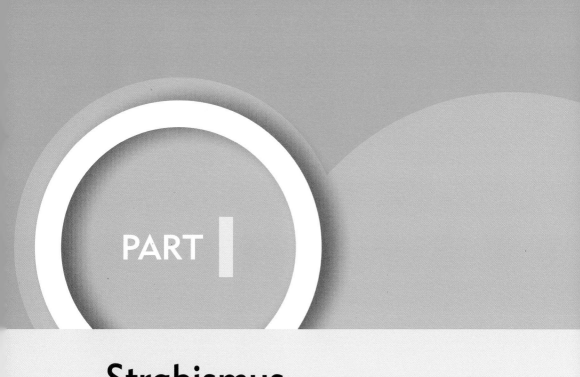

PART I

Strabismus

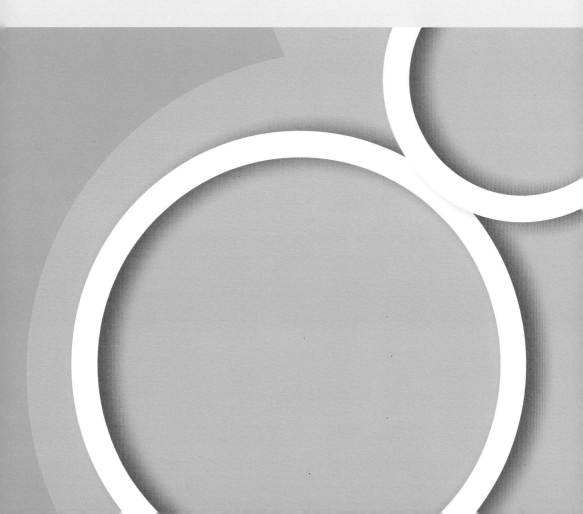

CHAPTER 1

The Pediatric Eye Examination

Children are not merely small adults, and most ophthalmic problems in children differ from those in adults. Each developmental level in children requires a different approach to the ophthalmologic examination. Proper preparation and attitude can make the ophthalmologic examination of pediatric patients both enjoyable and rewarding.

Preparation

If possible, a small room or corner of the waiting area should be designated for children. Both the parents and other adult patients will be grateful for this separation. A small table and chairs, some books, and some toys are sufficient.

A dedicated long pediatric examination lane with different types of distance fixation targets is optimal. Having several small toys readily available for near fixation is useful for the *1 toy, 1 look* rule (Fig 1-1). Light-colored plastic finger puppets become silent accommodative near targets that can also provide a corneal light reflex if placed over a muscle light or penlight.

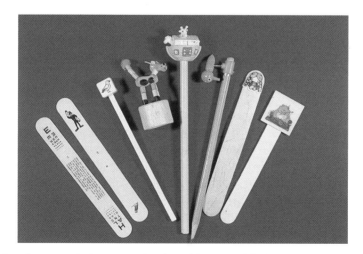

Figure 1-1 Small toys and pictures and reduced letter and E charts are used as near fixation targets. *(Reproduced with permission from Haldi BA, Mets MB. Nonsurgical treatment of strabismus.* Focal Points: Clinical Modules for Ophthalmologists. *San Francisco: American Academy of Ophthalmology; 1997, module 4. Photograph courtesy of Betty Anne Haldi, CO.)*

Because some children fear the white coat, many pediatric practitioners prefer not to wear one.

Examination: General Considerations and Strategies

When the patient is an infant, it is especially important to obtain information regarding the pregnancy and neonatal period, paying close attention to maternal health, gestational age at birth, birth weight, and neonatal history. The physician should also ask whether the child has reached applicable developmental milestones and whether there are any neurologic problems.

Past and present medications should be recorded, along with drug sensitivities and allergic responses. A family history regarding strabismus and other childhood eye disorders should be obtained. Previous ocular surgeries should be reviewed.

The examination begins with observation of the child as the practitioner enters the room. With practice, the practitioner may gather important information before the formal examination begins. Visual behavior, abnormal head position, dysmorphic features, ability to ambulate, familial disorders (note parents and siblings), and family social dynamics can be effectively observed at this time.

The practitioner should be seated at the child's eye level—some children are more comfortable sitting in a parent's lap. Introducing oneself to the child and the parent and establishing and maintaining eye contact with the child are important. Being relaxed, open, honest, and playfully engaging during the examination helps create a "safe" environment. Gaining the child's confidence makes for a faster and better examination, easier follow-up visits, and greater parental support.

It is helpful to begin by asking easy questions with simple answers. For example, children enjoy being regarded as "big" and correcting adults when they are wrong. The practitioner can tell them they look "so grown up"; grossly overestimate their age or grade level and then ask, "Is that right?" A simple joke can relax both child and parent.

To initiate physical contact with a child, the practitioner can say "give me five" or admire the patient's clothing or shoes. Pushing the "magic button" on the nose of a child as a video presentation or mechanical animals are surreptitiously activated with the foot pedal allows work to be done close to the child's face while he or she is distracted.

As there may be only a few moments of cooperation, the most important features should be checked at the beginning of the examination. If fusion is in doubt, it should be checked first before being disrupted with other tests, including those for vision. While checking vision, the practitioner can make children feel successful by initially giving them objects they can readily discern, then saying, "That's too easy—let's try this one."

A different vocabulary should be developed for working with children, such as "I want to show you something special" instead of "I want to examine you." Use "magic sunglasses" for the stereo glasses, "special flashlight" for the retinoscope, "funny hat" for the indirect ophthalmoscope, and "magnifying glass" for the indirect lens. Confrontation visual field testing can be performed as a counting-fingers game or Simon Says. Children might be talked into a slit-lamp examination if the practitioner says that they can "drive the motorcycle" by grabbing the handles of the slit lamp. Using the imagination to "play" with children as the examination proceeds can be beneficial. Children will be more cooperative if the practitioner is sharing an experience with them instead of doing something to them.

The most threatening or most unpleasant part of the examination should be reserved for the end. The least expensive test that can be ordered is a return office visit. Children who become totally uncooperative can return later to finish the examination.

For the follow-up examination of an infant who is fussy during the first visit, ask the parent to bring the child in hungry and then feed him or her during the examination.

When dealing with a vision-threatening or life-threatening problem, the practitioner must persist with the examination and even use sedation or anesthesia when necessary.

Examination: Specific Elements

Visual Acuity Assessment

Visual acuity assessment requires different approaches depending on the age and cooperativeness of the child. Ideally, measurements at distance with crowded Snellen or Sloan letter optotypes guide amblyopia diagnosis and management. Commonly, however, the child suspected of having amblyopia is preverbal, preliterate, or not fully cooperative. In such cases, clinical options include assessing fixation behavior and using preliterate eye charts. Table 1-1 lists the expected acuity for various tests at different ages. Copies of whatever optotypes are appropriate for the child (eg, Allen cards, LEA symbols) can be given to the parent for at-home rehearsal to help distinguish not seeing the test object from not understanding the test.

In infants and toddlers, fixation behavior is observed to qualitatively assess vision. Fixation and following (tracking) behavior is observed as the child's attention is directed to the examiner's face or a small toy in the examiner's hand. Fixation preference is determined by observing a child's response to covering 1 eye compared with covering the other. Children typically resist occlusion of the eye with better vision. It is also important to determine whether each eye can maintain fixation through smooth pursuit or a blink; strong fixation preference for 1 eye indicates decreased vision in the nonpreferred eye.

Fixation behavior may be characterized by the *CSM* (Central, Steady, and Maintained) method. *Central* refers to foveal fixation with a centrally located corneal light reflex, tested

Table 1-1 Normal Visual Acuity Using Various Tests in Children

Age (Years)	Vision Test	Normal
0–2	Visually evoked potential (VEP)	20/30 (age 1)
0–2	Preferential looking	20/30 (age 2)
0–2	Fixation behavior	CSM (see text)
2–5	LEA symbols	20/40–20/20
2–5	HOTV chart	20/40–20/20
5+	Snellen chart	20/30–20/20

monocularly. If the fixation target is viewed eccentrically, fixation is termed *uncentral (UC)*. *Steady* refers to the absence of nystagmus and other motor disruptions of fixation. The S assessment is also performed monocularly. *Maintained* refers to fixation that is held after the opposite eye is uncovered. An eye that does not maintain fixation under binocular conditions may be presumed to have lower visual acuity than the opposite eye. Maintained fixation is easier to identify in a strabismic patient. For children with small-angle strabismus or no strabismus, the *induced tropia test* may be performed. First, the examiner directs the child's attention to a target. Then a 10–15 prism diopter base-down prism is placed in front of 1 eye, and the eyes are observed. If the eyes move up, the child is using the eye under the prism, and vice versa. The test should be repeated a few times on each eye. If the child consistently chooses the eye with the prism or the eye without the prism regardless of which eye has the prism, or if fixation spontaneously alternates between the eyes while the prism is in place, no preference is present. If the child consistently fixates with the same eye, the opposite eye likely has decreased vision. The visual acuity of an eye that has eccentric fixation and nystagmoid movements when attempting fixation would be designated *uncentral, unsteady,* and *unmaintained (UC, US, UM)*.

Monocular recognition testing—which involves having the patient identify letters, numbers, or symbols, all generically referred to as optotypes—is the preferred method of assessing visual acuity. The optotypes may be presented on a wall chart, computer monitor, or handheld card. The acuity test should be calibrated for the test distance used. Because of the potential for variable or inaccurate viewing distances when testing at near, measurement at distance is preferred for managing amblyopia.

Various optotypes are available for testing preliterate children. LEA symbols and the HOTV test are reliable for preschool-aged children. Testability may be improved by having a shy child point and match rather than verbalize the optotypes. Other optotypes such as the Allen figures do not conform to accepted parameters of optotype design and therefore provide less accurate results. Most pediatric ophthalmologists consider letter (Sloan or Snellen) acuity optotypes the most accurate, followed in decreasing order of accuracy by HOTV and LEA symbols, the tumbling E, Allen figures, and fixation behavior. The examiner should use the most sophisticated test that the child can perform.

For patients with amblyopia, a line of optotypes (linear acuity) or single optotypes surrounded by *contour interaction bars* ("crowding bars"; Fig 1-2) should be used, because acuity is overestimated if vision is measured with isolated optotypes. The lines should

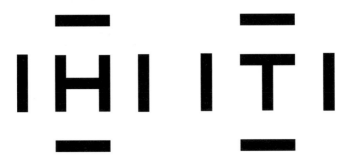

Figure 1-2 Crowded optotypes. *(Courtesy of the Good-Lite Company and Robert W. Hered, MD.)*

be spaced such that the distance between optotypes is no greater than the width of the optotypes on a given line. The Bailey-Lovie and ETDRS (Early Treatment of Diabetic Retinopathy Study) chart designs incorporate appropriate linear optotype spacing, a consistent number of optotypes on each line, and a logarithmic (logMAR) change in letter size between chart lines (Fig 1-3). See also BCSC Section 3, *Clinical Optics*.

By convention, visual acuity is determined first for the right eye and then for the left. A patch or other occluder is used in front of the left eye as the acuity of the right eye is checked, then vice versa. An adhesive patch is the most effective occluder because it reduces the possibility that the child will "peek" with the fellow eye. Computerized visual acuity test systems allow for more variety in optotype presentation, reducing errors due to memorization of letters. Patients with nystagmus may show better binocular visual acuity than monocular visual acuity with either eye occluded. To assess distance monocular visual acuity in this situation, the fellow eye should be fogged with a translucent occluder or a lens +5 diopters (D) greater than the refractive error in that eye. Patients with poor vision may need to move closer to the chart until they can see the 20/400 line. In such cases, visual acuity is recorded as the distance in feet (numerator) over the size of the letter (denominator); for example, if the patient is able to read 20/400 optotypes at 5 ft, the acuity is recorded as 5/400. See the visual acuity conversion chart on the inside front cover of the book, which provides conversions of visual acuity measurements for the various methods in use—the Snellen fraction, decimal notation (Visus), visual angle minute of arc, and base-10 logarithm of the minimum angle of resolution (logMAR).

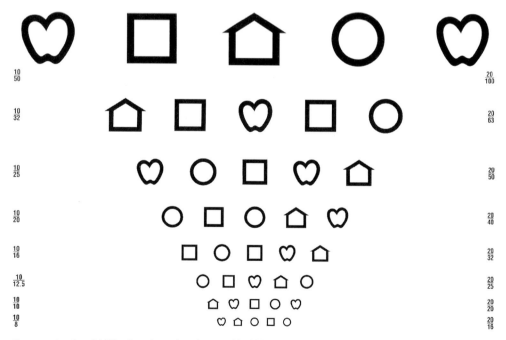

Figure 1-3 LogMAR visual acuity chart with LEA symbols. *(Courtesy of the Good-Lite Company and Robert W. Hered, MD.)*

The line with the smallest figures in which the majority of letters can be read accurately is recorded; if the patient misses a few of the figures on a line, a notation is made. In addition to recording the results, the clinician should identify the type of test used, including the optotype and whether crowding was used, to facilitate comparison with measurements taken at other times.

Uncorrected and corrected near visual acuity is determined, again using age-appropriate optotypes. Because of the potential for inaccuracy related to viewing distance, near visual acuities should not be compared with distance acuities in children. Measuring near visual acuity in children with reduced vision is helpful in determining how they will function at school.

Alternative Methods of Visual Acuity Assessment in Preverbal Children

Two major methods are used to quantitate visual acuity in preverbal infants and toddlers: *preferential looking (PL)* and *visually evoked potential (VEP)*.

Preferential looking tests

These tests assess visual acuity by observing the child's response to a visual stimulus. Teller Acuity Cards II (Stereo Optical Co, Chicago, IL) are a series of rectangular cards on which alternating black and white stripes are printed on a gray background. The stripes are printed on one side of the card only (Fig 1-4). Movement of the eyes toward the side with the stripes indicates that the child is able to see them. Stripe width decreases on successive cards. Seeing narrower stripes denotes better vision. The Cardiff Acuity Test, which is popular in Europe, uses vanishing optotypes.

Visually evoked potential

A special form of visually evoked potential (VEP), a sweep VEP, can also be used to assess visual acuity in preverbal patients. In this test, electrodes are placed over the occipital

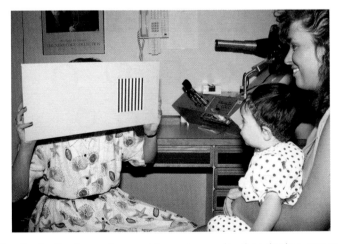

Figure 1-4 Teller Acuity Cards can be used to measure visual acuity in a preverbal child. *(Courtesy of John W. Simon, MD.)*

lobe. The child views a stimulus with a series of bar or grid patterns. If the stripes are large enough for the child to discriminate, a visual impulse is recorded by the electrodes. The stripe width narrows to the point that the stimulus appears uniformly gray, at which point no impulse is recorded. Visual acuity is estimated based on the smallest line width that produces a response.

Red Reflex Examination (Brückner Test)

The Brückner test is performed in a semidark room using a direct ophthalmoscope to assess the red reflex from both eyes simultaneously at a distance of approximately 1 m. Most infants and children will look toward the light from the direct ophthalmoscope. The clinician can quickly determine the clarity and symmetry of the red reflex and identify significant or asymmetric refractive errors and ocular misalignment. This is an essential technique for pediatricians and pediatric primary care providers.

Dynamic Retinoscopy

Dynamic retinoscopy is a useful measure of accommodation. The child is given a distance fixation target and then quickly switched to a near fixation target while the retinoscopic reflex is observed. A child with normal accommodation will neutralize the reflex at near focus. A poor accommodation reflex indicates a possible need for bifocal or reading glasses. Hypoaccommodation occurs more frequently in children with Down syndrome or cerebral palsy.

Visual Field Testing

Visual field information can be obtained in very young patients, once they have developed visual fixation (usually by 4 months of age), by presenting a peripheral target while the child fixates on an interesting central target. Movement of the eyes toward the peripheral target (an *evoked* saccade) confirms the field. Visual fields can be approximated by confrontation in children old enough to count or match fingers placed in each quadrant. School-aged children can often be evaluated with manual or automated perimetry testing.

Pupil Testing

The pupillary light reflex is not reliably present until approximately 30 weeks' gestational age. Newborns usually have a miotic pupil that gradually increases in size until the preteen years. Accurate pupil testing in young children is complicated by the smaller pupil and difficulty controlling accommodation with near focus response to a test light. Careful observation, remote or foot control of the room lights for continued observation during changes in room illumination, and use of appropriate distance fixation targets greatly facilitate pupil evaluation. Digital photography can be useful for accurate assessment and documentation.

Anterior Segment Examination

In children, a successful anterior segment examination is usually possible but often requires persistence and different techniques. Children old enough to sit by themselves can usually be enticed to hold the "motorcycle handles" of the slit lamp and place their chin on the "pillow" long enough for a brief examination of both eyes. Longer looks are possible if, while at the slit lamp, they watch a cartoon behind the examiner. Younger children may also be placed at the slit lamp while in a parent's lap or held with the chin positioned in the chin rest. Children unable or unwilling to cooperate with standard slit-lamp examination can be examined with a portable slit lamp, surgical loupes, or a 20 D or 28 D hand-held lens used with an indirect ophthalmoscope. Children with suspicious findings who cannot be adequately assessed with these techniques may require a restrained or sedated examination.

Intraocular Pressure Measurement

It is not easy or always possible to perform formal tonometry in children. Ocular palpation, though not quantitative, can allow a gross assessment of whether pressure is normal or abnormal. This requires practice involving correlation with formal tonometry performed on the same patient. Formal tonometry requires a noncrying, relaxed patient. With a non-threatening approach and practice, the practitioner may find that many young children permit accurate testing when handheld devices such as the Tono-Pen (Reichert Ophthalmic Instruments, Depew, NY) or Icare (Icare Finland Oy, Helsinki, Finland) are used. The Tono-Pen or the Perkins Tonometer (Haag-Streit USA, Mason, OH) may be used to test infants when they are sleeping or feeding in the supine position. Children at risk for glaucoma may require sedated examination if accurate readings cannot be obtained in the clinic.

Cycloplegic Refraction

Because of the relationship between accommodation and ocular convergence, one of the most important tests in the evaluation of any patient with issues relating to binocular vision and ocular motility is refraction with cycloplegic agents. *Cyclopentolate* (1.0%) is the preferred drug for routine use in children, especially when combined with phenylephrine, which has no cycloplegic effect. Use of 0.5% concentration is suggested in infants. The clinician should remember that adverse effects may occur in children receiving cyclopentolate. *Homatropine* (5.0%) and *scopolamine* (0.25%) are occasionally used instead of cyclopentolate, but neither is as rapid acting or as effective. *Tropicamide* (0.5% or 1.0%) is usually not strong enough for effective cycloplegia in children. Some ophthalmologists use a combination of cyclopentolate and tropicamide to achieve maximum dilatation. Some ophthalmologists use *atropine* (1.0%) drops or ointment, but this drug causes prolonged blurring and is more often associated with adverse effects (see the section "Adverse effects"). Nonetheless, 1.0% atropine drops are frequently used without problems in the treatment of amblyopia (see Chapter 4).

Table 1-2 shows the schedule of administration and duration of action for commonly used cycloplegics. The duration of action varies greatly, and the pupillary effect occurs earlier and lasts longer than the cycloplegic effect, so a dilated pupil does not necessarily indicate complete cycloplegia. For patients with accommodative esodeviations, frequent cycloplegic examinations are essential when control is precarious. Having the patient fixate at distance helps prevent false readings due to residual accommodative effort.

Table 1-2 Administration and Duration of Cycloplegics

Medication	Administration Schedule	Onset of Action	Duration of Cycloplegic Action
Tropicamide	1 drop every 5 min × 2; wait 30 min	20–40 min	4–6 hr
Cyclopentolate	1 drop every 5 min × 2; wait 30 min	30–60 min	6–24 hr
Scopolamine	1 drop every 5 min × 2; wait 1 hr	30–60 min	4–7 d
Homatropine	1 drop every 5 min × 2; wait 1 hr	30–60 min	1 d
Atropine	1–3 drops per day × 3–4 days; then 1 drop morning of appointment	45–120 min	1–2 wk

Eyedrops in children

Almost all children are apprehensive about eyedrops. There are many approaches to giving eyedrops. If possible, someone other than the examining physician should administer the drops. Some practitioners use a cycloplegic spray, some use a topical anesthetic drop first, and some simply use the cycloplegic drops. The drops can be described as being "like a splash of swimming pool water" that will "feel funny for about 30 seconds." Do not give children a long time to think about it. Dark irides are more difficult to dilate. In some cases, the parent can put the cycloplegic drops in at home. See also BCSC Section 2, *Fundamentals and Principles of Ophthalmology.*

Adverse effects

Adverse reactions to cycloplegic agents include allergic (or hypersensitivity) reaction with conjunctivitis, edematous eyelids, and dermatitis. These reactions are more frequent with atropine than with any of the other agents. Atropine drops may also cause systemic symptoms, including fever, dry mouth, flushing of the face, rapid pulse, nausea, dizziness, delirium, and erythema. Treatment is discontinuation of the medicine, with supportive measures as necessary. If the reaction is severe, physostigmine may be given. The ophthalmologist should remember that 1 drop of 1.0% atropine is 0.5 mg atropine. In addition, hypnotic effects can be seen with scopolamine and occasionally with cyclopentolate or homatropine.

Refraction technique

Refraction is generally performed after cycloplegia. The ophthalmologist's working distance and the child's visual axis are important considerations. Retinoscopy must be performed on axis in order to provide accurate refraction information. The 2 main methods for refraction are loose lenses for infants and younger children and the phoropter for those old enough to sit in an exam chair. A surprising number of 2-year-olds are interested in and willing to use the phoropter, especially if they can watch a cartoon during the refraction.

Fundus Examination

The fundus examination is frequently the final component of the pediatric eye examination. Although it can be challenging, particularly in young children, it is important to obtain an adequate view of the fundus regardless of the patient's age. After appropriate dilation, infants and small children can be examined with the indirect ophthalmoscope using decreased illumination and a 28 D or 20 D lens. This may require restraint in some infants, particularly those being screened for retinopathy of prematurity (in which a topical anesthetic, use of an eyelid speculum, and scleral depression are needed for a complete retinal evaluation). For children older than 2–3 years, the practitioner can obtain brief but sufficient views of the optic nerve, macula, and surrounding retina by using diversionary targets such as illuminated toys and cartoons. Abnormal findings or incomplete evaluation may require examination under anesthesia.

Examination of the Uncooperative Child

Most infants and children can be accurately examined in the clinic setting. Even difficult children usually respond to some combination of rest periods, persuasion, persistence, bribery, and, if indicated, a repeat visit. There are times when, despite best attempts, significant concerns are present and adequate information cannot be obtained. In infants and younger children, brief restraint may prevail. However, the practitioner must consider the physical and emotional consequences of restraining a child, for both the patient and the parents. Depending on the nature of the ocular problem, a sedated examination or an examination under anesthesia may be the best solution.

CHAPTER 2

Strabismus Terminology

The term *strabismus* is derived from the Greek word *strabismos*—"to squint, to look obliquely or askance"—and means ocular misalignment. This misalignment may be caused by abnormalities in binocular vision or by anomalies of neuromuscular control of ocular motility. Many terms are employed in discussions of strabismus, and unless these terms are used correctly, confusion and misunderstanding can occur. Unfortunately, some terms still in use are not correct physiologically.

Orthophoria is the ideal condition of perfect ocular alignment. In reality, orthophoria is seldom encountered, as a small heterophoria can be found in most people. Some ophthalmologists therefore prefer *orthotropia* to mean correct direction or position of the eyes under binocular conditions. Both terms are commonly used to describe eyes without manifest strabismus. *Heterophoria* is an ocular deviation kept latent by the fusional mechanism (latent strabismus). *Heterotropia* is a deviation that is manifest and not kept under control by the fusional mechanism (manifest strabismus). It is sometimes helpful to identify the deviating eye. This practice is particularly helpful when the clinician is measuring vertical deviations or restrictive or paretic strabismus, or when amblyopia is present in a preverbal child.

Prefixes and Suffixes

A detailed nomenclature has evolved to describe the various types of ocular deviations. This vocabulary uses many prefixes and suffixes based on the relative positions of the visual axes of both eyes to account for the multiple strabismic patterns encountered.

Prefixes

Eso- The eye is rotated so that the cornea is deviated nasally. Because the visual axes align at a point closer than the fixation target, this state is also known as *convergent strabismus,* one type of horizontal strabismus.

Exo- The eye is rotated so that the cornea is deviated temporally. Because the visual axes are diverging from the fixation target, this state is also known as *divergent strabismus,* another form of horizontal strabismus.

Hyper- The eye is rotated so that the cornea is deviated superiorly. This describes one type of *vertical strabismus.*

Hypo- The eye is rotated so that the cornea is deviated inferiorly. This describes another type of *vertical strabismus*.

In- The eye is rotated so that the superior pole of the vertical meridian is torted nasally. This state is known as *intorsional strabismus*.

Ex- The eye is rotated so that the superior pole of the vertical meridian is torted temporally. This state is known as *extorsional strabismus*.

Suffixes

-phoria A latent deviation (eg, esophoria, exophoria, right hyperphoria) that is controlled by the fusional mechanism so that the eyes remain aligned under binocular conditions.

-tropia A manifest deviation (eg, esotropia, exotropia, right hypertropia) that exceeds the control of the fusional mechanism so that the eyes are misaligned under binocular conditions. Tropias can be constant or intermittent.

Strabismus Classification Terms

No classification is perfect or all-inclusive, and several methods of classifying eye alignment and motility disorders are used. Following are terms used in these classifications.

Age of Onset

Infantile A deviation documented before age 6 months, presumably related to a defect present at birth. The term *congenital* is also sometimes used, although it may be less accurate because the deviation is usually not present at birth.

Acquired A deviation with onset after 6 months of age, after a period of presumably normal visual development.

Fixation

Alternating Spontaneous alternation of fixation from one eye to the other.

Monocular Definite preference for fixation with one eye.

Variation of the Deviation Size With Gaze Position or Fixating Eye

Comitant (concomitant) The size of the deviation does not vary by more than a few prism diopters in different positions of gaze or with either eye used for fixating.

Incomitant (noncomitant) The deviation varies in size in different positions of gaze or with the eye used for fixating. Most incomitant strabismus is paralytic or restrictive. *Primary deviation* is the deviation measured when the nonparetic or nonrestricted eye is fixating. *Secondary deviation* is the deviation measured when the paretic or restricted eye is fixating.

Miscellaneous Terms

Consecutive A strabismus that is in the direction opposite that of a previous strabismus. For example, a consecutive exotropia is an exotropia that follows a history of esotropia.

Dissociated strabismus complex (DSC) DSC consists of dissociated vertical deviation, dissociated horizontal deviation, and dissociated torsional deviation. The number of components present varies, with some patients having all 3 and others having only 1. Dissociated vertical deviation is the most prevalent of the 3 components. The complex can be bilateral or unilateral, and the degree of control of the deviation can vary between eyes.

Overelevation/overdepression in adduction These motility anomalies are also commonly called *inferior oblique overaction* and *superior oblique overaction*, respectively, but the terms *overelevation* and *overdepression in adduction* are preferred because the anomalies can be due to several etiologies, including muscle pulley heterotopy, overaction or underaction of the oblique muscles, orbital dystopia, and synkinesis of extraocular muscles.

Underelevation/underdepression in adduction These motility anomalies are also called *inferior oblique underaction* and *superior oblique underaction*, respectively, but the terms *underelevation* and *underdepression in adduction* are preferred for the reasons noted above.

Abbreviations for Types of Strabismus

The addition of a prime (′) to any of the following indicates that measurement of ocular alignment is made at near fixation (eg, E′ indicates esophoria at near).

0, EX = 0 Orthophoria (orthotropia).

E, X, RH, LH Esophoria, exophoria, right hyperphoria, left hyperphoria at distance fixation, respectively.

ET, XT, RHT, LHT Constant esotropia, exotropia, right hypertropia, left hypertropia at distance fixation, respectively.

E(T), X(T), RH(T), LH(T) Intermittent esotropia, exotropia, right hypertropia, left hypertropia at distance fixation, respectively. The addition of parentheses around the *T* indicates an intermittent tropia.

RHoT, LHoT Right hypotropia, left hypotropia at distance fixation, respectively.

IOOA, IOUA Inferior oblique overaction, inferior oblique underaction, respectively.

OEAd, ODAd Overelevation in adduction, overdepression in adduction, respectively.

SOOA, SOUA Superior oblique overaction, superior oblique underaction, respectively.

UEAd, UDAd Underelevation in adduction, underdepression in adduction, respectively.

DSC Dissociated strabismus complex.

DHD, DTD, DVD Dissociated horizontal deviation, dissociated torsional deviation, dissociated vertical deviation, respectively.

CHAPTER 3

Anatomy of the Extraocular Muscles

Origin, Course, Insertion, Innervation, and Action of the Extraocular Muscles

There are 7 extraocular muscles (EOMs) in the human eye: the 4 rectus muscles (lateral, medial, superior, and inferior), the 2 oblique muscles, and the levator palpebrae superioris muscle. Figure 3-1 shows an anterior view of the EOMs and their relationships to one another. Cranial nerve (CN) VI (abducens) innervates the lateral rectus muscle; CN IV (trochlear), the superior oblique muscle; and CN III (oculomotor), the levator palpebrae, superior rectus, medial rectus, inferior rectus, and inferior oblique muscles. CN III has an upper and a lower division: the upper division supplies the levator palpebrae and superior rectus muscles; the lower division supplies the medial rectus, inferior rectus, and inferior oblique muscles. The parasympathetic innervation of the sphincter pupillae and ciliary muscle travels with the branch of the lower division of CN III that supplies the inferior oblique muscle. BCSC Section 5, *Neuro-Ophthalmology,* discusses the ocular motor nerves in more detail, and Section 2, *Fundamentals and Principles of Ophthalmology,* extensively illustrates the anatomical structures mentioned in this chapter.

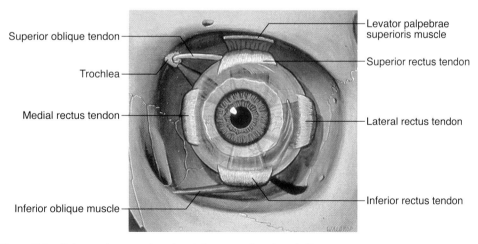

Figure 3-1 Extraocular muscles, frontal composite view, left eye. *(Reproduced with permission from Dutton JJ. Atlas of Clinical and Surgical Orbital Anatomy. Philadelphia: Saunders; 1994:23.)*

When the eye is directed straight ahead and the head is also straight, the eye is said to be in *primary position.* The *primary action* of a muscle is its major effect on the position of the eye when the muscle contracts while the eye is in primary position. The secondary and tertiary actions of a muscle are the additional effects on the position of the eye in primary position (see also Chapter 5 and Table 5-1). The globe usually can be moved approximately 50° in each direction from primary position. Under normal viewing circumstances, however, the eyes move only about 15°–20° from primary position before head movement occurs.

Table 3-1 summarizes the characteristics of the EOMs.

Horizontal Rectus Muscles

The horizontal rectus muscles are the medial and lateral rectus muscles. Both arise from the annulus of Zinn. The *medial rectus muscle* courses along the medial orbital wall. The proximity of the medial rectus muscle to the medial orbital wall means that the medial rectus can be injured during ethmoid sinus surgery. The *lateral rectus muscle* courses along the lateral orbital wall.

Vertical Rectus Muscles

The vertical rectus muscles are the superior and inferior rectus muscles. The *superior rectus muscle* originates from the annulus of Zinn and courses anteriorly, upward over the eyeball, and laterally, forming an angle of 23° with the visual axis or the midplane of the eye in primary position (Fig 3-2; see also Chapter 5, Fig 5-4). The *inferior rectus muscle* also arises from the annulus of Zinn, and it then courses anteriorly, downward, and laterally along the floor of the orbit, forming an angle of 23° with the visual axis or midplane of the eye in primary position (see Chapter 5, Fig 5-5).

Oblique Muscles

The *superior oblique muscle* originates from the orbital apex, above the annulus of Zinn, and passes anteriorly and upward along the superomedial wall of the orbit. The muscle becomes tendinous before passing through the trochlea, a cartilaginous saddle attached to the frontal bone in the superior nasal orbit. The combination of the trochlea and the superior oblique tendon is known as the *tendon–trochlea complex.* A bursalike cleft separates the trochlea from the loose fibrovascular sheath surrounding the tendon (Fig 3-3). The discrete fibers of the tendon telescope as they move through the trochlea, the central fibers moving farther than the peripheral ones. The function of the trochlea is to redirect the tendon inferiorly, posteriorly, and laterally, with the tendon forming an angle of 51° with the visual axis or midplane of the eye in primary position (see Chapter 5, Fig 5-6). The tendon penetrates the Tenon capsule 2 mm nasally and 5 mm posteriorly to the nasal insertion of the superior rectus muscle. Passing under the superior rectus muscle, the tendon inserts posterior to the equator in the superotemporal quadrant of the eyeball, almost or entirely laterally to the midvertical plane or center of rotation.

The *inferior oblique muscle* originates from the periosteum of the maxillary bone, just posterior to the orbital rim and lateral to the orifice of the lacrimal fossa. It courses laterally, superiorly, and posteriorly, going inferior to the inferior rectus muscle and inserting under

Table 3-1 Extraocular Muscles

Muscle	Approx. Length of Active Muscle (mm)	Origin	Anatomical Insertion and Distance From Limbus (mm)	Direction of Pull	Tendon Length (mm)	Arc of Contact (mm)	Innervation
Medial rectus (MR)	40	Annulus of Zinn	Up to 5.5 mm from medial limbus	90°	4.5	7	Lower CN III
Lateral rectus (LR)	40	Annulus of Zinn	Up to 6.9 mm from lateral limbus	90°	7	12	CN VI
Superior rectus (SR)	40	Annulus of Zinn	Up to 7.7 mm from superior limbus	23°	6	6.5	Upper CN III
Inferior rectus (IR)	40	Annulus of Zinn	Up to 6.5 mm from inferior limbus	23°	7	6.5	Lower CN III
Superior oblique (SO)	32	Orbital apex, above annulus of Zinn (functional origin at the trochlea)	Posterior to equator in superotemporal quadrant	51°	26	7–8	CN IV
Inferior oblique (IO)	37	Behind inferior orbital rim, lateral to lacrimal fossa	Lateral to area of macula	51°	1	15	Lower CN III
Levator palpebrae superioris (LPS)	40	Orbital apex, above annulus of Zinn	Septa of pretarsal orbicularis and anterior surface of tarsus	—	14–20	—	Upper CN III

CN = cranial nerve.
See also Figures 5-3 through 5-7 in Chapter 5.

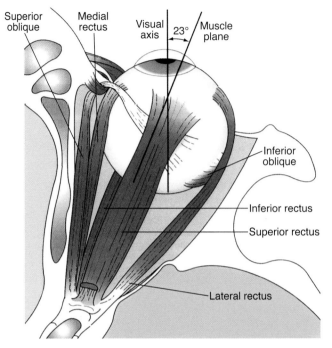

Figure 3-2 The extrinsic muscles of the right eyeball in primary position, seen from above. Note that only the origin and insertion of the inferior oblique muscle are visible in this view. *(Modified with permission from Yanoff M, Duker J, eds.* Ophthalmology. *2nd ed. London: Mosby; 2004:549.)*

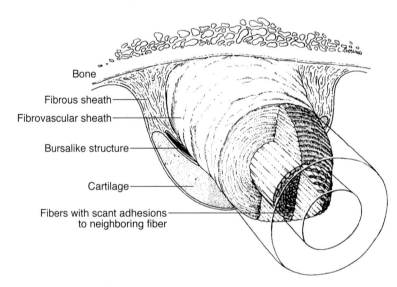

Figure 3-3 Components of the trochlea. *(Modified with permission from Helveston EM, Merriam WW, Ellis FD, et al. The trochlea: a study of the anatomy and physiology.* Ophthalmology. *1982;89:124–133.)*

the lateral rectus muscle in the posterolateral portion of the globe, in the area of the macula. The inferior oblique muscle forms an angle of 51° with the visual axis or midplane of the eye in primary position (see Chapter 5, Fig 5-7). A stiff neurofibrovascular bundle (NFVB) containing the nerve to the inferior oblique runs anteriorly, along the lateral border of the inferior rectus muscle, to the myoneural junction. Most inferior oblique muscles have a single belly, but approximately 10% have 2 bellies; in rare cases, there are 3.

DeAngelis DD, Kraft SP. The double-bellied inferior oblique muscle: clinical correlates. *J AAPOS.* 2001;5(2):76–81.

Stager DR. Costenbader lecture. Anatomy and surgery of the inferior oblique muscle: recent findings. *J AAPOS.* 2001;5(4):203–208.

Levator Palpebrae Superioris Muscle

The levator palpebrae superioris muscle arises at the orbital apex from the lesser wing of the sphenoid bone just superior to the annulus of Zinn. At its origin, the muscle blends with the superior rectus muscle inferiorly and with the superior oblique muscle medially. The levator palpebrae superioris passes anteriorly, lying just above the superior rectus muscle; the fascial sheaths of these 2 muscles are connected. The levator palpebrae superioris muscle becomes an aponeurosis in the region of the superior fornix. This muscle has both a cutaneous and a tarsal insertion. BCSC Section 7, *Orbit, Eyelids, and Lacrimal System,* discusses this muscle in detail.

Relationship of the Rectus Muscle Insertions

Starting at the medial rectus and proceeding to the inferior rectus, lateral rectus, and superior rectus muscles, the rectus muscle tendons insert progressively farther from the limbus. Drawing a continuous curve through these insertions yields a spiral, known as the *spiral of Tillaux* (Fig 3-4). The temporal side of each vertical rectus muscle insertion is farther from the limbus (ie, more posterior) than is the nasal side.

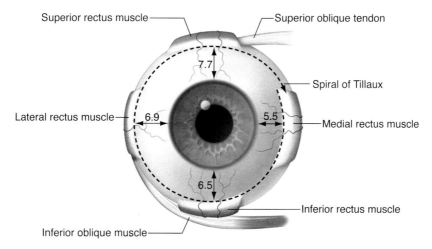

Figure 3-4 Spiral of Tillaux, right eye. *Note:* The insertion distances, given in millimeters, are maximum values. Insertion distances vary in individuals. *(Illustration by Christine Gralapp.)*

Blood Supply of the Extraocular Muscles

Arterial System

The muscular branches of the ophthalmic artery provide the most important blood supply to the EOMs. The *lateral muscular branch* supplies the lateral rectus, superior rectus, superior oblique, and levator palpebrae superioris muscles; the *medial muscular branch,* the larger of the 2, supplies the inferior rectus, medial rectus, and inferior oblique muscles.

The lateral rectus muscle is partially supplied by the *lacrimal artery;* the *infraorbital artery* partially supplies the inferior oblique and inferior rectus muscles. The muscular branches give rise to the *anterior ciliary arteries* accompanying the rectus muscles; each rectus muscle has 1–4 anterior ciliary arteries. These pass to the episclera of the globe and then supply blood to the anterior segment. The commonly held notion that the lateral rectus has fewer ciliary vessels than the other rectus muscles has been challenged by recent anatomical work, which shows that the number of ciliary vessels is similar for the lateral rectus and the other rectus muscles and that these vessels may, in fact, contribute substantially to the blood supply of the anterior segment.

Johnson MS, Christiansen SP, Rath PP, et al. Anterior ciliary circulation from the horizontal rectus muscles. *Strabismus.* 2009;17(1):45–48.

Venous System

The venous system parallels the arterial system, emptying into the *superior* and *inferior orbital veins.* Generally, 4 or more *vortex veins* are located posterior to the equator; these are often found near the nasal and temporal margins of the superior rectus and inferior rectus muscles. Although their number and positions can vary, the location of 2 vortex veins in the orbit is consistent: the inferotemporal quadrant just posterior to the inferior oblique muscle and the superotemporal quadrant just posterior to the superior oblique tendon.

Structure of the Extraocular Muscles

The important functional characteristics of muscle fibers are contraction speed and fatigue resistance. The eye muscles participate in motor acts that are among the fastest (saccadic eye movements) in the human body and among the most sustained (gaze fixation and vergence movements). Like skeletal muscle, EOM is voluntary striated muscle. However, EOM differs from typical skeletal muscle developmentally, biochemically, structurally, and functionally. The EOMs are innervated at a ratio of nerve fiber to muscle fiber up to 10 times that of skeletal muscle. This difference may allow for more accurate eye movements controlled by an array of systems ranging from the primitive vestibulo-ocular reflex to highly evolved vergence movements.

The EOMs exhibit a distinct 2-layer organization: an outer *orbital layer,* which acts only on connective tissue pulleys (see the section Pulley System), and an inner *global layer,* whose tendon inserts on the sclera to move the globe. The muscle fibers comprising the orbital and global layers can be either singly or multiply innervated.

Singly innervated fibers are fast-twitch generating and resistant to fatigue. Eighty percent of the fibers comprising the orbital layer muscle are singly innervated. Ninety percent of the fibers making up the global layer muscle are singly innervated, and they can be subdivided into 3 groups (red, intermediate, and white), based on mitochondrial content, with the red fibers being the most fatigue resistant and the white fibers, the least. The orbital singly innervated fibers are considered the major contributor to sustained EOM force in primary and deviated positions. Of all muscle fiber types, this type is the most affected by denervation from damage to the motor nerves or the end plates, as occurs after botulinum toxin injection.

The function of the multiply innervated fibers of the orbital and global layers is not clear. These fibers are not seen in the levator palpebrae superioris, and it is thought that they are involved in the finer control of fixation and in smooth and finely graded eye movements, particularly vergence control.

These novel properties of eye muscles lead to differential responses to local anesthetics and pharmaceuticals such as botulinum toxin and calcium channel blockers, as well as to disease processes such as myasthenia gravis and muscular dystrophy.

Finally, there is recent evidence for compartmentalization of rectus muscle innervation. For example, studies in primates and humans have shown distinct superior and inferior zones within the horizontal rectus muscles. The clinical significance of these observations is currently being investigated.

da Silva Costa RM, Kung J, Poukens V, Yoo L, Tychsen L, Demer JL. Intramuscular innervation of primate extraocular muscles: unique compartmentalization in horizontal recti. *Inv Ophthalmol Vis Sci.* 2011;52(5):2830–2836.

Orbital and Fascial Relationships

Within the orbit, a complex musculofibroelastic structure suspends the globe, supports the EOMs, and compartmentalizes the fat pads (Fig 3-5). In recent years, the interconnectedness of the orbital tissues, as well as its extent and complexity, has come to light. The intense fibrous connections throughout the orbit can be illustrated clinically by the consequences of tissue entrapment in blowout fractures and of post–retrobulbar hemorrhage fibrosis of delicate fibrous septa. This topic remains under investigation.

Adipose Tissue

The eye is supported and cushioned within the orbit by a large amount of fatty tissue. External to the muscle cone, fatty tissue comes forward with the rectus muscles, stopping about 10 mm from the limbus. Fatty tissue is also present inside the muscle cone, kept away from the sclera by the Tenon capsule (see Fig 3-5).

Muscle Cone

The muscle cone lies posterior to the equator. It consists of the EOMs, their sheaths, and the intermuscular septum. High-resolution magnetic resonance imaging (MRI) has

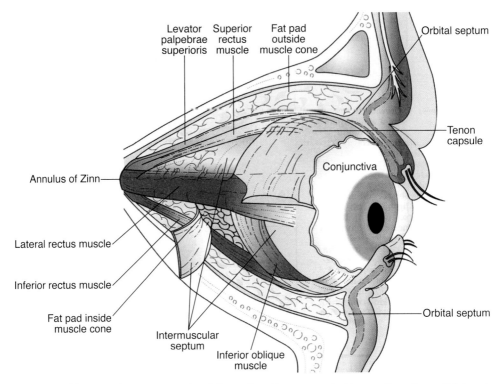

Figure 3-5 The muscle cone contains 1 fat pad and is surrounded by another; these 2 fat pads are separated by the rectus muscles and intermuscular septum. Note that the intermuscular septum does not extend all the way back to the apex of the orbit. *(Modified with permission from Yanoff M, Duker J, eds. Ophthalmology. 2nd ed. London: Mosby; 2004:553.)*

shown that the muscle cone does not extend back to the orbital apex; rather, it ends in the area of the globe–optic nerve junction.

Muscle Capsule

Each rectus muscle has a surrounding fascial capsule that extends with the muscle from its origin to its insertion. These capsules are thin posteriorly, but near the equator they thicken as they pass through the sleeve of the Tenon capsule, continuing anteriorly with the muscles to their insertions. Anterior to the equator, between the undersurface of the muscle and the sclera, there is almost no fascia, only connective tissue footplates that connect the muscle to the globe. The smooth, avascular surface of the muscle capsule allows the muscles to slide easily over the globe.

The Tenon Capsule

The Tenon capsule (*fascia bulbi*) is the principal orbital fascia and forms the envelope within which the eyeball moves (Fig 3-6). The Tenon capsule fuses posteriorly with the

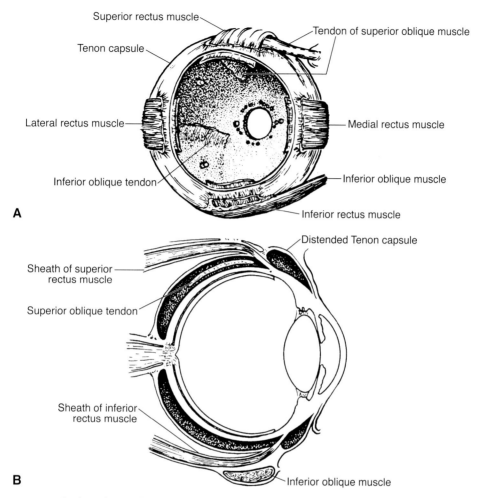

Superior rectus muscle

Tendon of superior oblique muscle

Tenon capsule

Lateral rectus muscle

Medial rectus muscle

Inferior oblique tendon

Inferior oblique muscle

Inferior rectus muscle

A

Distended Tenon capsule

Sheath of superior rectus muscle

Superior oblique tendon

Sheath of inferior rectus muscle

Inferior oblique muscle

B

Figure 3-6 A, Anterior and posterior orifices of the Tenon capsule shown after enucleation of the globe. **B,** The Tenon space shown by injection with India ink. *(Modified with permission from von Noorden GK, Campos EC. Binocular Vision and Ocular Motility: Theory and Management of Strabismus. 6th ed. St Louis: Mosby; 2002:45.)*

optic nerve sheath and anteriorly with the intermuscular septum at a position 3 mm from the limbus. The posterior portion of the Tenon capsule is thin and flexible, allowing for free movement of the optic nerve, ciliary nerves, and ciliary vessels as the globe rotates, while separating the orbital fat inside the muscle cone from the sclera. At and just posterior to the equator, the Tenon capsule is thick and tough, suspending the globe like a trampoline by means of connections to the periorbital tissues. The global layer of the 4 rectus muscles penetrates this thick fibroelastic tissue approximately 10 mm posterior to their insertions. The oblique muscles penetrate the Tenon capsule anterior to the equator. The Tenon capsule continues forward over these 6 EOMs and separates them from the orbital fat and structures lying outside the muscle cone.

Pulley System

The 4 rectus muscles are surrounded by fibroelastic pulleys that maintain the position of all of the EOMs relative to the orbit. The pulleys consist of collagen, elastin, and smooth muscle, allowing them to contract and relax. Dynamic MRI studies show that, in some cases, the pulleys act mechanically as the rectus muscle origins. The pulleys may also serve to stabilize the muscle path, preventing sideslipping or movement perpendicular to the muscle axis (Fig 3-7). Anteriorly, the pulleys merge with the *intermuscular septum,* which fuses with the conjunctiva 3 mm posterior to the limbus. The posterior section of the intermuscular septum separates the intraconal fat pads from the extraconal fat pads. Numerous extensions from all of the EOM sheaths attach to the orbit and help support the globe.

The inferior oblique muscle originates inferonasally on the maxillary bone near the orbital rim, adjacent to the anterior lacrimal crest, and it continues laterally, entering its connective tissue pulley inferior to the inferior rectus muscle, at the site where the inferior oblique muscle also penetrates the Tenon capsule. The inferior oblique pulley and inferior rectus pulley join to form the Lockwood ligament (Fig 3-8). Attached to the conjoined

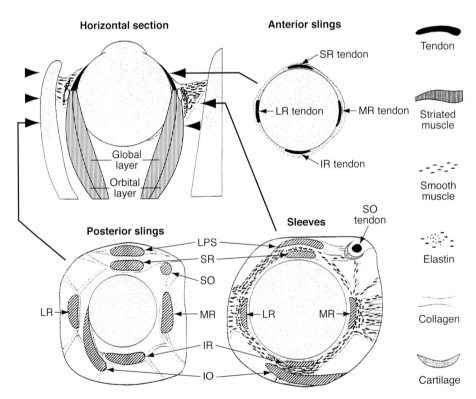

Figure 3-7 Structure of orbital connective tissues. *IO,* inferior oblique; *IR,* inferior rectus; *LPS,* levator palpebrae superioris; *LR,* lateral rectus; *MR,* medial rectus; *SO,* superior oblique; *SR,* superior rectus. The 3 coronal views are represented at the levels indicated by arrows in horizontal section. *(Modified with permission from Demer JL, Miller JM, Poukens V. Surgical implications of the rectus extraocular muscle pulleys. J Pediatr Ophthalmol Strabismus. 1996;33(4):208–218.)*

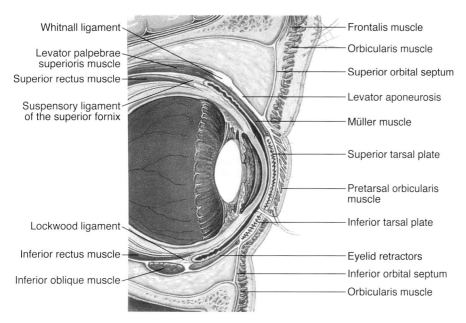

Whitnall ligament

Levator palpebrae superioris muscle

Superior rectus muscle

Suspensory ligament of the superior fornix

Lockwood ligament

Inferior rectus muscle

Inferior oblique muscle

Frontalis muscle

Orbicularis muscle

Superior orbital septum

Levator aponeurosis

Müller muscle

Superior tarsal plate

Pretarsal orbicularis muscle

Inferior tarsal plate

Eyelid retractors

Inferior orbital septum

Orbicularis muscle

Figure 3-8 Attachments of the upper and lower eyelids to the vertical rectus muscles. *(Modified with permission from Buckley EG, Freedman S, Shields MB, eds.* Atlas of Ophthalmic Surgery, Vol III: Strabismus and Glaucoma. *St Louis: Mosby-Year Book; 1995:15.)*

inferior oblique and inferior rectus pulley complex is the dense NFVB containing the inferior oblique motor nerve.

The *active pulley hypothesis* proposes that the pulley positions are shifted by the contraction of the orbital layer against the elasticity of the pulley suspension. This concept remains controversial: whether there is actual innervational control of the pulleys is still debated. However, high-resolution MRI scans have shown that the pulleys are located only a short distance from the globe center; therefore, small shifts in pulley location would confer large shifts in EOM pulling direction. Normal pulleys shift only slightly in the coronal plane, even during large ductions. *Heterotopy (malpositioning)* of the rectus pulleys may cause some cases of incomitant strabismus and A or V patterns, and these anomalies can mimic oblique muscle dysfunction by misdirecting the forces of the rectus muscles (see Chapters 10 and 11). Bony abnormalities such as those seen with craniosynostosis can also alter the direction of pull of rectus muscles by causing malpositioning of the pulleys. Posterior fixation sutures (*fadenoperation;* posterior fixation of an EOM to the underlying sclera) were designed to reduce an EOM's effect in its field of action by decreasing the arc of contact and rotational lever arm. However, MR imaging suggests that the actual effect of the fadenoperation is to hinder the posterior shift of the contracting EOM pulley, mechanically restricting EOM action.

The pulley model and its implications have been challenged by other high-resolution MRI studies, which show that, during eye movements into eccentric fields, the posterior portions of rectus muscles shift. These findings are consistent with the more traditional model of eye muscle function, which is the "restrained shortest-path model."

Demer JL. Mechanics of the orbita. *Dev Ophthalmol.* 2007;40:132–157.

Anatomical Considerations During Surgery

The nerves to the rectus muscles and the superior oblique muscle enter the muscles approximately one-third of the distance from the origin to the insertion (or trochlea, in the case of the superior oblique muscle). Damaging these nerves during anterior surgery is unlikely but not impossible. An instrument thrust more than 26 mm posterior to a rectus muscle's insertion may cause injury to the nerve.

Cranial nerve IV is outside the muscle cone and is not affected by a retrobulbar block. However, any EOM could be reached by a retrobulbar needle and injured by injection of local anesthetic.

The nerve supplying the inferior oblique muscle enters the lateral portion of the muscle, where it crosses the inferior rectus muscle; the nerve can be damaged by surgery in this area. Because parasympathetic fibers to the sphincter pupillae (for pupil constriction) and the ciliary muscle (for accommodation) accompany the nerve to the inferior oblique muscle, with a synapse in the ciliary ganglion, surgery in this area may also result in an enlarged pupil. These nerves and the inferior oblique muscle can be injured by an inferotemporal retrobulbar block as well.

Surgery on the inferior oblique muscle requires careful inspection of the inferolateral quadrant to ensure that all bellies are identified. If, during a weakening or strengthening procedure, a second or third belly is not identified, the action of the muscle may not be sufficiently altered and additional surgery may be required as a result.

The NFVB along the lateral border of the inferior rectus muscle can become an ancillary insertion site for the inferior oblique muscle when the muscle is anteriorly or medially transposed. Anterior transposition of the inferior oblique creates an anti-elevation effect.

Maintaining the integrity of the muscle capsules during surgery decreases intraoperative bleeding and provides a smooth muscle surface with less risk of adhesion formation. If only the muscle capsule is sutured to the globe, the muscle can retract backward, causing a slipped muscle.

The intermuscular septum between rectus muscles and especially between the rectus and oblique muscles can help locate a lost muscle during surgery. Extensive dissections of the intermuscular septum are not necessary for rectus muscle recession surgery. However, during resection surgery, these connections should be severed to prevent, for example, the inferior oblique muscle from being advanced with the lateral rectus muscle. Often, there are 2 frenula: one that connects the lateral rectus muscle to the underlying inferior oblique at its insertion and another that connects the superior rectus to the underlying superior oblique tendon. Usually, these have to be disconnected during recessions and resections of either of these 2 rectus muscles.

The medial rectus muscle is the only rectus muscle that does not have an oblique muscle running tangential to it. This makes surgery on the medial rectus less complicated but means that there is neither a point of reference if the surgeon becomes disoriented nor a point of attachment if the muscle is lost.

The inferior rectus muscle is distinctly bound to the lower eyelid by the fascial extension from its sheath. *Recession,* or weakening, of the inferior rectus muscle tends to widen the palpebral fissure and result in lower eyelid retraction. *Resection,* or strengthening, of the inferior rectus muscle tends to narrow the fissure by elevating the lower eyelid. There-fore, any alteration of the inferior rectus muscle may be associated with a change in the palpebral fissure (see Fig 3-8).

The superior rectus muscle is loosely bound to the levator palpebrae superioris mus-cle. The eyelid may be pulled downward following resection of the superior rectus muscle, thus narrowing the palpebral fissure. In contrast, the eyelid is not usually retracted up-ward with small or moderate recessions. In hypotropia, a pseudoptosis may be present because the upper eyelid tends to follow the superior rectus muscle (see Fig 3-8).

The blood supply to the EOMs provides almost all of the temporal half of the anterior segment circulation and the majority of the nasal half of the anterior segment circulation, which also receives some blood from the long posterior ciliary artery. Therefore, simul-taneous surgery on 3 rectus muscles may induce anterior segment ischemia, particularly in older patients.

Whenever muscle surgery is performed, special care must be taken to avoid pen-etration of the Tenon capsule 10 mm or more posterior to the limbus. If the integrity of the Tenon capsule is violated posterior to this point, fatty tissue may prolapse through the capsule and form a restrictive adhesion to sclera, muscle, intermuscular septum, or con-junctiva, limiting ocular motility.

When surgery is performed near the vortex veins, accidental severing of a vein is pos-sible. The procedures that present the greatest risk of damaging a vortex vein are recession or resection of the inferior rectus or superior rectus muscle, weakening of the inferior oblique muscle, and exposure of the superior oblique muscle tendon. Hemostasis can be achieved with cautery or with an absorbable hemostatic sponge.

The sclera is thinnest just posterior to the 4 rectus muscle insertions. As this area is the site of most eye muscle surgery, especially recession procedures, scleral perforation is always a risk during eye muscle surgery. The surgeon can minimize this risk by

- using spatulated needles with swaged sutures
- working with a clean, dry, and blood-free surgical field
- using loupe magnification or the operating microscope

Chapter 14 discusses these procedures and complications in greater detail.

CHAPTER 4

Amblyopia

Amblyopia is a unilateral or, less commonly, bilateral reduction of best-corrected visual acuity (also referred to as *corrected distance visual acuity*) that cannot be attributed directly to the effect of any structural abnormality of the eye or visual pathways. Amblyopia signifies a failure of normal neural development in the immature visual system (see Chapter 6) and is caused by abnormal visual experience early in life resulting from one of the following:

- strabismus
- refractive error: anisometropia or high bilateral refractive errors (isoametropia)
- visual deprivation

Epidemiology

Amblyopia is responsible for more cases of childhood-onset unilateral decreased vision than all other causes combined, with a prevalence of 2%–4% in the North American population. In addition, this condition is the most common cause of unilateral visual impairment in adults younger than 60 years. The prevalence of amblyopia is increased in children with a family history of amblyopia, children born prematurely, and those with developmental delay.

Detection and Screening

Amblyopic vision loss is preventable or reversible with timely detection and intervention. Thus, it is important that children with or at risk for amblyopia be identified at a young age, when the prognosis for successful treatment is best. Risk factors for amblyopia include strabismus, ocular media opacities, anisometropia, and isoametropia. Regular screening throughout childhood, whether performed in primary care offices or as part of community-based programs, allows for timely detection of vision problems, including amblyopia. Screening techniques for amblyopia vary based on the age of the child and include direct measurement of visual acuity and testing for risk factors. The latter includes corneal light reflex tests and cover testing for detection of strabismus and the Brückner test (see Chapter 7) for detection of ocular media opacities, strabismus, anisometropia, and isoametropia. Instrument-based pediatric vision screening is effective in preschool-aged and younger children. It includes the use of portable autorefraction devices to detect refractive errors and photoscreening devices, which use optical images of the eye to detect strabismus, refractive errors, and abnormalities of the red reflex.

Miller JM, Lessin HR; American Academy of Pediatrics Section on Ophthalmology; Committee on Practice and Ambulatory Medicine; American Academy of Ophthalmology; American Association for Pediatric Ophthalmology and Strabismus; American Association of Certified Orthoptists. Instrument-based pediatric vision screening policy statement. *Pediatrics*. 2012;130(5):983–986. Epub 2012 Oct 29.

Pathophysiology

Amblyopia is primarily a defect of central vision; the peripheral visual field is usually normal. In early postnatal development, there are critical periods of cortical development during which neural circuits display a heightened sensitivity to environmental stimuli and are dependent on natural sensory experience for proper formation. (See Chapter 6 for additional discussion of the neural basis of amblyopia.) During these periods, the child's developing visual system is vulnerable to abnormal input due to visual deprivation, strabismus, or significant uncorrected refractive errors. Also during these periods, the visual system's plasticity allows the greatest opportunity for reversal of amblyopia. In general, the critical period for development of visual deprivation amblyopia is earlier than that of strabismic or anisometropic amblyopia (see the Classification section). Furthermore, amblyopia due to visual deprivation develops more rapidly and is deeper than that due to strabismus or anisometropia.

Abnormal early visual experience can also result in profound disturbances of neuron function within the visual system, resulting in the vision loss of amblyopia. Cells of the primary visual cortex can lose their innate ability to respond to stimulation of 1 or both eyes, and cells that remain responsive can show significant functional deficiencies. Abnormalities also occur in neurons within the lateral geniculate body. However, very little change has been found in the retinas of subjects with amblyopia.

The receptive fields of neurons in the amblyopic visual system are abnormally large. This may account for the *crowding phenomenon* (also known as *contour interaction*), a characteristic of amblyopia in which optotypes of a given size are easier to recognize when presented singly than when closely surrounded by similar forms, such as a full line of letters (see Chapter 1).

Classification

Amblyopia can be categorized by the disorders responsible for its occurrence.

Strabismic Amblyopia

One of the most common forms of amblyopia, strabismic amblyopia develops in the deviating eye of a child with strabismus. Constant, nonalternating heterotropias are the type most likely to cause significant amblyopia. Strabismic amblyopia is thought to result from competitive or inhibitory interaction between neurons carrying nonfusible input from the 2 eyes. This interaction leads to domination of cortical vision centers by input from the fixating eye and also results in reduced responsiveness to input from the nonfixating eye. In young children with strabismus, suppression develops rapidly. This visual adaptation occurs to avoid diplopia and visual confusion (see Chapter 6). Amblyopia does not always prevent diplopia, however. For example, older patients with long-standing strabismus have a small risk of developing diplopia after strabismus surgery, despite the presence of significant amblyopia.

Several features that are typical of strabismic amblyopia are less common in other forms of amblyopia. In strabismic amblyopia, *grating acuity,* the ability to detect patterns composed of uniformly spaced stripes, is often reduced considerably less than recognition acuity measured with optotype charts. This discrepancy must be considered when the results of tests based on grating detection, such as Teller Acuity Cards II (Stereo Optical Co, Inc, Chicago, IL) and the LEA Grating Acuity Test (Good-Lite Co, Elgin, IL), are interpreted.

When visual acuity is measured through a neutral density filter, the acuity of an eye with strabismic amblyopia tends to decline less sharply than that of an eye with organic disease. This phenomenon is called the *neutral density filter effect.*

Eccentric fixation is the consistent use of a nonfoveal region of the retina for monocular viewing. Minor degrees of eccentric fixation, detectable only with special tests such as visuscopy, are present in many patients with strabismic amblyopia and relatively mild vision loss. Clinically evident eccentric fixation can be detected by observing a decentered position of the corneal light reflex from the fixating amblyopic eye while the dominant eye is covered. It implies visual acuity of 20/200 or worse and a poorer prognosis for visual recovery with treatment.

Refractive Amblyopia

Refractive amblyopia is another common form of amblyopia, the etiology of which is consistent defocus of the retinal image in 1 or both eyes. There are 2 types: anisometropic and isoametropic.

Anisometropic amblyopia

In anisometropic amblyopia, dissimilar refractive errors in the 2 eyes cause the image on 1 retina to be chronically defocused. Considered more prevalent than strabismic amblyopia in some recent studies, this condition is thought to result partly from the direct effect of image blur and partly from interocular competition or inhibition similar (but not identical) to that responsible for strabismic amblyopia. Levels of anisometropia that can lead to amblyopia are greater than 1.50 D of anisohyperopia, 2.00 D of anisoastigmatism, and 3.00 D of anisomyopia. Higher levels are associated with greater risk. The eyes of a child with anisometropic amblyopia usually appear normal to the family and primary care physician, which may cause a delay in detection and treatment.

Isoametropic amblyopia

Isoametropic amblyopia (bilateral ametropic amblyopia) is a bilateral decrease in visual acuity that results from large, approximately equal, uncorrected refractive errors in the

2 eyes of a young child. The mechanism of this form of amblyopia involves the deleterious effect of blurred retinal images on the immature visual system. Hyperopia exceeding 4.00–5.00 D and myopia exceeding 5.00–6.00 D carry a risk of inducing isoametropic amblyopia. Uncorrected bilateral astigmatism in early childhood may result in loss of resolving ability limited to the chronically blurred meridians (meridional amblyopia). The degree of cylindrical isoametropia that produces meridional amblyopia is not known, but most ophthalmologists recommend correction when there is more than 2.00–3.00 D of cylinder.

Visual Deprivation Amblyopia

The least common but most severe and difficult to treat of the forms of amblyopia, visual deprivation amblyopia occurs because of an eye abnormality that obstructs the visual axis or otherwise interferes with central vision. The most common cause of visual deprivation amblyopia (also known as *stimulus deprivation amblyopia, deprivation amblyopia, visual stimulus deprivation amblyopia,* and *form-vision deprivation amblyopia*) is a congenital or early-acquired cataract, but blepharoptosis, periocular lesions that obstruct the visual axis, corneal opacities, and vitreous hemorrhage may also be causal. Because amblyopia is responsible for permanent vision loss in many ocular abnormalities of early childhood, there is greater urgency in their management compared to similar conditions in adults. Unilateral visual deprivation amblyopia tends to be worse than amblyopia produced by bilateral deprivation of similar degree, because interocular competition adds to the direct developmental impact of severe image degradation (see Chapter 6). Even in bilateral cases, however, visual acuity can be 20/200 or worse.

In children younger than 6 years, dense cataracts occupying the central 3 mm or more of the lens are capable of causing severe visual deprivation amblyopia. Similar lens opacities acquired after age 6 years are generally less harmful. Small anterior polar cataracts, around which retinoscopy can be readily performed, and lamellar cataracts, through which a reasonably good view of the fundus can be obtained, may cause mild to moderate amblyopia or may have no effect on visual development. Unilateral anterior polar cataracts, however, are associated with anisometropia and subtle optical distortion of the surrounding clear portion of the lens, which may cause anisometropic and/or mild visual deprivation amblyopia.

Reverse amblyopia is a form of visual deprivation amblyopia that develops in the fellow eye as a result of patching (occlusion amblyopia) or penalization.

Evaluation

Amblyopia is diagnosed when a patient has a condition known to cause amblyopia and has decreased visual acuity that cannot be fully explained by physical abnormalities of the eye. Characteristics of vision alone cannot reliably differentiate amblyopia from other forms of vision loss. The crowding phenomenon, for example, is typical of amblyopia but not pathognomonic or uniformly demonstrable. Subtle afferent pupillary defects occur rarely and only in severe cases of amblyopia. Amblyopia sometimes coexists with vision loss directly caused by an uncorrectable structural abnormality of the eye such as optic nerve hypoplasia or coloboma. When the clinician encounters a doubtful or borderline case of this type and the patient is a young child, it is appropriate to undertake a trial of amblyopia treatment. Improvement in vision confirms that amblyopia was indeed present.

Multiple assessments of visual acuity are sometimes required in order to determine the presence and severity of amblyopia. (Assessment of visual acuity is discussed in Chapter 1.) In some circumstances, it is appropriate to assume that amblyopia is present and to begin treatment even before decreased vision has been conclusively determined. Examples include initiating occlusion therapy with the presence of a high degree of anisometropia or shortly after surgery for a unilateral cataract.

When determining the severity of amblyopia in a young patient, the clinician should keep certain considerations in mind. Assessment of fixation preference is sensitive for detecting amblyopia, but false-positive results can occur. For example, a child with small-angle strabismus may show a strong fixation preference despite visual acuity in the 2 eyes being equal or nearly so. In addition, the young child's brief attention span frequently results in measurements that fall short of the true limits of acuity; these measurements can mimic those of bilateral amblyopia or obscure or falsely suggest a significant interocular difference.

Treatment

Treatment of amblyopia involves the following steps:

1. Eliminate (if needed) any obstruction of the visual axis, such as a cataract.
2. Correct any significant refractive error.
3. Force use of the amblyopic eye by limiting use of the better eye.

Cataract Removal

Cataracts capable of producing amblyopia require timely surgery. Removal of unilateral visually significant congenital lens opacities during the first 4–6 weeks of life is necessary for optimal recovery of vision. Significant cataracts with uncertain time of onset also deserve prompt and aggressive treatment if recent development is at least a possibility. See Chapter 23 for further discussion of childhood cataract.

Refractive Correction

In general, optical prescription for amblyopic eyes should be based on the refractive error as determined with cycloplegia. Because an amblyopic eye's ability to control accommodation tends to be impaired, this eye cannot be relied on to compensate for uncorrected hyperopia as would a normal child's eye. Sometimes, however, symmetric reductions in plus lens power may be required in order to foster acceptance of spectacle wear. Refractive correction for aphakia following cataract surgery in childhood must be provided promptly to avoid prolonging the visual deprivation that occurs because of a severe uncorrected refractive error. Anisometropic, isoametropic, and even strabismic amblyopia may improve or resolve with only refractive correction. Given this, many ophthalmologists initiate treatment with refractive correction alone, adding occlusion or penalization later if needed (see the next section). The role of refractive surgery in patients who fail conventional treatment with spectacles and/or contact lenses is under investigation.

Paysse EA, Coats DK, Hussein MA, Hamill MB, Koch DD. Long-term outcomes of photo-refractive keratectomy for anisometropic amblyopia in children. *Ophthalmology*. 2006;113(2): 169–176.

Writing Committee for the Pediatric Eye Disease Investigator Group; Cotter SA, Foster NC, Holmes JM, et al. Optical treatment of strabismic and combined strabismic-anisometropic amblyopia. *Ophthalmology*. 2012;119(1):150–158. Epub 2011 Sep 29.

Occlusion and Penalization

Occlusion therapy (patching) is commonly employed to treat unilateral amblyopia. The sound eye is covered, obligating the child to use the amblyopic eye. Adhesive patches are usually used for occlusion therapy, but spectacle-mounted occluders or opaque contact lenses can be utilized instead if skin irritation or inadequate adhesion is a problem. With spectacle-mounted occluders, close supervision is necessary to ensure that the patient does not peek around the occluder.

Part-time occlusion, defined as occlusion for 2–6 hours per day, has been shown to achieve results similar to those of prescribed full-time occlusion. The relative duration of patch-on and patch-off intervals should reflect the degree of amblyopia. For severe deficits (visual acuity of 20/100–20/400), 6 hours per day is preferred. Maintenance patching of 1–2 hours per day is often prescribed to prevent recurrence of amblyopia after successful patching.

Full-time occlusion of the sound eye is defined as occlusion during all waking hours. In rare cases, with aggressive patching, strabismus may occur because of lack of binocular viewing and tenuous fusion. Therefore, the child whose eyes are consistently or intermittently straight may benefit from being given some opportunity to see binocularly. Part-time occlusion reduces the likelihood of occlusion amblyopia or induced strabismus.

The timing of follow-up should be related to the intensity of treatment and the age of the child. An examination is typically scheduled within 2–3 months after initiation of treatment. Subsequent visits can be scheduled at longer intervals based on early response. Part-time occlusion and penalization methods allow for less frequent observation.

The desired endpoint of therapy for unilateral amblyopia is free alternation of fixation, linear recognition acuity that differs by no more than 1 line between the 2 eyes, or both. The time required for completion of treatment depends on several factors, including the severity of amblyopia, choice and intensity of therapeutic approach, adherence to treatment, and age of the patient.

More severe amblyopia and older age correlate with a need for more intensive or longer treatment. Consistent occlusion during infancy may reverse substantial strabismic amblyopia in less than 1 month. In contrast, an older child who wears a patch only after school and on weekends may require several months to overcome a moderate deficit.

Adherence to occlusion therapy for amblyopia declines with increasing age. However, studies in older children and teenagers with strabismic or anisometropic amblyopia have shown that treatment can still be beneficial beyond the first decade of life. This is especially true in children who have not previously undergone treatment. The effectiveness of part-time patching regimens in older children is being investigated.

Other methods of amblyopia treatment involve pharmacologic and/or optical degradation of the better eye's vision such that it becomes temporarily inferior to the amblyopic eye's vision, an approach referred to as *penalization*. Use of the amblyopic eye is thus promoted without complete occlusion of the fellow eye. An advantage of penalization over occlusion therapy in patients with orthotropia or small-angle strabismus is that penalization allows a degree of binocularity, which is particularly beneficial in children with latent nystagmus.

Studies have demonstrated that pharmacologic penalization can successfully treat moderate degrees of amblyopia. A cycloplegic agent (usually atropine 1% solution) is administered to the better-seeing eye so that it is unable to accommodate. As a result, the better eye experiences blur with near viewing and also, if hyperopia is undercorrected, with distance viewing. This form of treatment has been demonstrated to be as effective as patching for mild to moderate amblyopia (visual acuity of 20/100 or better). Atropine may be administered daily, but weekend administration is as effective for milder amblyopia. Depending on the depth of amblyopia and the response to prior treatment, hyperopic correction of the dominant eye can be reduced to enhance the effect. Regular follow-up of patients whose amblyopia is being treated with cycloplegia is important in order to monitor for reverse amblyopia (see Complications of Therapy). Pharmacologic penalization offers the advantage of being difficult for the child to thwart. It does not work well for myopic patients, however, because clear near vision persists in the penalized eye despite cycloplegia.

Optical penalization involves the prescription of excessive plus lenses (fogging) or diffusing filters for the sound eye. This form of treatment avoids potential pharmacologic adverse effects and may be capable of inducing greater blur. If the child wears glasses, application of a translucent filter, such as Scotch Magic Tape (3M, St Paul, MN) or a Bangerter foil (Ryser Optik AG, St Gallen, Switzerland), to the spectacle lens can be tried. Optical penalization may be more acceptable than occlusion therapy to many children and their parents, but patients must be closely monitored to ensure proper utilization (no peeking) of spectacle-borne devices.

Complications of Therapy

With occlusion therapy and penalization, there is a risk of overtreatment, which can result in reverse amblyopia in the sound eye. Development of strabismus is also a risk. Full-time occlusion carries the greatest risk of reverse amblyopia and of strabismus and thus requires close monitoring. Consequently, most ophthalmologists do not use full-time occlusion in younger children. The parents of a strabismic child should be instructed to watch for a switch in fixation preference and to report its occurrence promptly. Iatrogenic reverse amblyopia can usually be treated successfully with judicious patching of the formerly better-seeing eye or by alternating occlusion. Sometimes, simply stopping treatment leads to equalization of vision.

Adherence issues

Lack of adherence to the therapeutic regimen is a common problem that can prolong the treatment period or lead to outright failure. If difficulties derive from a particular treatment method, the clinician should seek a suitable alternative. Families who appear to lack sufficient motivation should be counseled concerning the importance of the therapy and the need for consistency in carrying it out. They can be reassured that once an appropriate routine is established, the daily effort required is likely to diminish, especially if the amblyopia improves.

Methods to improve a resistant child's adherence to treatment vary according to age. In infants and toddlers, physical methods such as wearing arm splints or mittens or making the patch more adhesive with tincture of benzoin may be useful. For children older than 3 years, creating goals and offering rewards tend to work well, as does linking patching to play activities (eg, decorating the patch or patching while the child plays a video game). Authoritative words directed specifically at the child by the clinician may also help.

In some patients, skin irritation due to the adhesive may develop. Switching to a different brand of patch or preparing the skin with tincture of benzoin or ostomy adhesive can eliminate most skin-related problems.

Unresponsiveness

In some cases, even conscientious application of an appropriate therapeutic program fails to improve vision at all or beyond a certain level. Complete or partial unresponsiveness to treatment occasionally affects younger children but more often occurs in patients older than 5 years. A repeat comprehensive eye examination to look for potential subtle optic nerve or retinal anomalies is indicated when there is a significant deviation from expected response to amblyopia treatment in the face of good adherence to the program. Neuroimaging might be considered in cases that inexplicably fail to respond to treatment.

The decision whether to initiate or continue treatment in a prognostically unfavorable situation should take into account the wishes of the patient and family. Primary therapy should generally be terminated if there is a lack of demonstrable progress over 3–6 months despite good treatment adherence. Amblyopia is not always fully correctable, even at younger ages of treatment.

Recurrence

When amblyopia treatment is discontinued after complete or partial improvement of vision, approximately one-third of patients show some degree of recurrence. Reducing the occlusion regimen to 1–2 hours per day or the frequency of pharmacologic penalization for a few months before cessation decreases the incidence of recurrence. If recurrence occurs, visual acuity can usually be improved again with resumption of therapy. If the need for maintenance therapy is established, treatment must be continued until stability of vision is demonstrated with no treatment other than regular spectacles. This may require periodic monitoring until age 8–10 years. As long as vision remains stable, intervals of up to 12 months between follow-up visits are acceptable. The improvement in vision that is obtained in most children treated between 7 and 12 years of age is sustained following cessation of treatment.

CHAPTER 5

Motor Physiology

Basic Principles and Terms

Axes of Fick and Ocular Rotations

Ocular rotations have commonly been described as involving movements about the 3 *axes of Fick,* designated as *x* (transverse), *y* (sagittal), and *z* (vertical) (Fig 5-1). However, current thinking more conveniently describes ocular rotations as *horizontal rotations* about a vertical axis, corresponding to medial and lateral gaze; *vertical rotations* about a horizontal axis, corresponding to upward and downward gaze; and *torsional rotations* about the line of sight. The final orientation of the eye after a change in gaze position depends on the sequence of the rotations; this order, therefore, is not commutative. The most common sequence of rotations is the *Fick sequence:* horizontal rotation, followed by a vertical rotation, and then rotation about the line of sight. Another order is the *Helmholtz sequence,* which is helpful in the analysis of horizontal vergences: vertical rotation, then horizontal, and finally torsional. Small and moderate eye rotations can be reasonably approximated using the

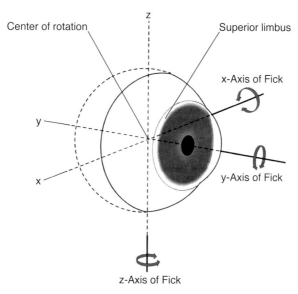

Figure 5-1 Axes of Fick. *(Adapted with permission from Yanoff M, Duker J, eds.* Ophthalmology. *2nd ed. London: Mosby; 2004:557.)*

independent horizontal and vertical components as if they did not interact. This approximation is not applicable if large horizontal and vertical rotations occur simultaneously.

Historically, *Listing's equatorial plane* was used as a reference plane for describing multiplanar eye movements. However, current thinking utilizes the concept of rotational sequencing.

Positions of Gaze

- *Primary position* is the position of the eyes when they are fixating straight ahead.
- *Secondary diagnostic positions* are straight up, straight down, right gaze, left gaze.
- *Tertiary diagnostic positions* are the 4 oblique positions of gaze: up and right, up and left, down and right, down and left, as well as the right and left head-tilt positions.
- *Cardinal positions* are up and right, up and left, right, left, down and right, down and left (Fig 5-2).

See Chapter 7 for additional discussion of positions of gaze.

Extraocular Muscle Action

The 4 rectus muscles are traditionally thought of as fixed straight strings running directly from the orbital apex to the muscle insertions. The oblique muscles were historically thought to simply attach obliquely to the globe. In light of ongoing discoveries that lend support to the active pulley hypothesis (discussed in Chapter 3), some of these older concepts, as well as descriptions of extraocular muscles (EOMs) and their actions, have undergone revision.

Arc of contact

The point of effective, or physiologic, insertion is the tangential point where the muscle first contacts the globe. The action of the eye muscle may be considered a vector of force that acts at this tangential point to rotate the eye. The length of muscle actually in contact with the globe constitutes the arc of contact.

The traditional concepts of arc of contact and muscle plane are based on straight-line, 2-dimensional models of orbital anatomy and do not take into account muscle pulleys and their effect on the linearity of muscle paths. Magnetic resonance imaging scans have

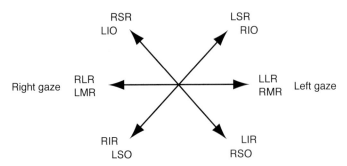

Figure 5-2 Cardinal positions and yoke muscles. *RSR,* right superior rectus; *LIO,* left inferior oblique; *LSR,* left superior rectus; *RIO,* right inferior oblique; *RLR,* right lateral rectus; *LMR,* left medial rectus; *LLR,* left lateral rectus; *RMR,* right medial rectus; *RIR,* right inferior rectus; *LSO,* left superior oblique; *LIR,* left inferior rectus; *RSO,* right superior oblique.

shown that the rectus muscles may not follow the shortest or straightest paths from the orbital apex to the scleral insertions. In the active pulley model, the direction of pull of a muscle is partially determined by the relationship between the muscle's pulley and its scleral insertion. This view has been challenged by some authors, who have shown magnetic resonance evidence that the traditional shortest-path model may still have validity. See Chapter 3 for further discussion of these models.

Eye Movements

Motor Units

An individual motor nerve fiber and its several muscle fibers constitute a motor unit. The electrical activity of motor units can be recorded by *electromyography.* An electromyogram (EMG) is a useful research tool in the investigation of normal and abnormal innervation of eye muscles. A portable EMG device connected to an insulated needle is often used during injection of botulinum toxin into eye muscles, helping the surgeon localize the appropriate muscle within the orbit, especially when the muscle has been operated on previously.

Recruitment during fixation or following movement

As the eye moves farther into abduction, more and more lateral rectus motor units are activated and brought into play by the brain to help pull the eye. This process is called *recruitment.* In addition, as the eye fixates farther into abduction, the frequency of activity of each motor unit increases until it reaches a peak number of contractions per second (several hundred, for some motor units).

Monocular Eye Movements

Ductions

Ductions are monocular rotations of the eye. *Adduction* is movement of the eye nasally; *abduction* is movement of the eye temporally. *Elevation* (*supraduction* or *sursumduction*) is an upward rotation of the eye; *depression* (*infraduction* or *deorsumduction*) is a downward rotation of the eye. *Intorsion (incycloduction)* is defined as a nasal rotation of the superior portion of the vertical corneal meridian. *Extorsion (excycloduction)* is a temporal rotation of the superior portion of the vertical corneal meridian.

The following are important terms relating to the muscles used in monocular eye movements:

- *agonist:* the primary muscle moving the eye in a given direction
- *synergist:* the muscle in the same eye as the agonist that acts with the agonist to produce a given movement (eg, the inferior oblique muscle is a synergist with the agonist superior rectus muscle for elevation of the eye)
- *antagonist:* the muscle in the same eye as the agonist that acts in the direction opposite to that of the agonist (eg, the medial rectus and lateral rectus muscles are antagonists)

Sherrington's law of reciprocal innervation states that increased innervation and contraction force of a given EOM are accompanied by a reciprocal decrease in innervation and contraction force of its antagonist. For example, as the right eye abducts, innervation of the right lateral rectus muscle is increased, generating increased force; simultaneously, innervation of the right medial rectus is reduced, creating a matching reduction in this muscle's force.

Field of action

The term *field of action* refers to the gaze position (one of the cardinal positions) in which the effect of the muscle is most readily observed. For the lateral rectus muscle, the direction of rotation and the position of gaze are both abduction; for the medial rectus, they are both adduction. However, the direction of rotation and the gaze position are not the same for the vertical muscles. For example, the inferior oblique muscle, acting alone, is an abductor and elevator, pulling the eye up and out—but its elevation action is best observed in adduction. Similarly, the superior oblique muscle, acting alone, is an abductor and depressor, pulling the eye down and out—but its depression action is best observed in adduction.

The clinical significance of fields of action is that a deviation (strabismus) which increases with gaze in some directions may result from weakness of the muscle normally pulling the eye in that direction, from restriction of its action by its antagonist muscle, or from a combination of these 2 factors.

Primary, secondary, and tertiary action

With the eye in primary position, the horizontal rectus muscles are purely horizontal movers around the vertical axis and therefore have a primary horizontal action. Recent anatomical studies have shown compartmentalization of the innervation to the horizontal rectus muscles in some patients; this may explain the finding of small vertical actions of these muscles in these cases (see Chapter 3). The vertical rectus muscles have a direction of pull that is mostly vertical as their primary action, but the angle of pull from origin to insertion is inclined 23° to the visual axis (or midplane of the eye), giving rise also to *torsion,* which is defined as any rotation of the vertical corneal meridians. Intorsion is the secondary action of the superior rectus; extorsion is the secondary action of the inferior rectus; and adduction is the tertiary action of both muscles. Because the oblique muscles are inclined 51° to the visual axis (or midplane of the eye), torsion is their primary action. Vertical rotation (depression/elevation) is their secondary action, and abduction is their tertiary action). The levator palpebrae superioris is also an EOM, and its sole action is elevation of the upper eyelid. See Table 5-1 for a summary of the EOM actions.

Changing muscle action with different gaze positions

The gaze position determines the effect of EOM contractions on the rotation of the eye. There are 7 gaze positions: primary position and the 6 cardinal positions (see Fig 5-2). In each of the cardinal positions, each of the 6 oculorotatory EOMs has different effects on the eye's rotation based on the relationship between the *visual axis* of the eye and the orientation of the muscle plane to the visual axis. In each cardinal position, the angle between the visual axis and the direction of pull of the muscle being tested is minimized, thus maximizing the horizontal effect of the medial or lateral rectus or the vertical effect

Table 5-1 Action of the Extraocular Muscles Referenced to Primary Position

Muscle*	Primary	Secondary	Tertiary
Medial rectus	Adduction	—	—
Lateral rectus	Abduction	—	—
Inferior rectus	Depression	Extorsion	Adduction
Superior rectus	Elevation	Intorsion	Adduction
Inferior oblique	Extorsion	Elevation	Abduction
Superior oblique	Intorsion	Depression	Abduction
Levator palpebrae superioris	Elevation of upper eyelid	—	—

*The superior muscles are intortors; the inferior muscles, extortors. The vertical rectus muscles are adductors; the oblique muscles, abductors.

of the superior rectus, inferior rectus, superior oblique, or inferior oblique. By having the patient move the eyes to the 6 cardinal positions, the clinician can isolate and evaluate the ability of each of the 6 oculorotatory EOMs to move the eye. See also Binocular Eye Movements later in this chapter.

With the eye in primary position, the horizontal rectus muscles share a common horizontal plane that contains the visual axis (Fig 5-3). The clinician can assess the relative strength of the horizontal rectus muscles by observing the horizontal excursion of the eye as it moves medially from primary position to test the medial rectus and laterally to test the lateral rectus.

The muscle actions of the vertical rectus muscles and the oblique muscles are more complex because, in primary position, the muscle axes are not parallel with the visual axis (see Figs 5-4 through 5-7).

In primary position, the superior and inferior rectus muscle planes form an angle of 23° with the visual axis (y-axis) and insert slightly anterior to the z-axis (Figs 5-4, 5-5). Therefore, from primary position, the contraction of the superior rectus has 3 effects: primary elevation around the x-axis, secondary intorsion around the y-axis, and adduction around the z-axis. In this position, the main pulling power of the superior rectus is medial to the center of rotation, which accounts for the adduction action of the muscle. The relative vertical strength of the superior rectus muscle can be most readily observed by aligning the visual axis parallel to the muscle plane axis—that is, when the eye is rotated 23° into abduction. In this position, the superior rectus becomes a pure elevator and its elevating action is maximal. To minimize the elevation action of the superior rectus, the visual axis should be perpendicular to the muscle axis at a position of 67° of adduction. In this position, the superior rectus would become a pure intortor. Because the globe cannot be adducted this far, the superior rectus maintains significant elevating action in maximal voluntary adduction.

The actions of the inferior rectus muscle mirror the vertical and torsional actions of the superior rectus. Because the inferior rectus is attached to the globe inferiorly, its action from primary position is primarily depression and secondarily extorsion. However, as with the superior rectus, its tertiary action is adduction (see Fig 5-5). Its action as a depressor is maximally demonstrated in 23° of abduction and reduced, though not absent, in adduction.

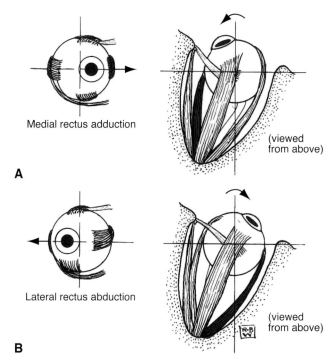

Medial rectus adduction

(viewed from above)

A

Lateral rectus abduction

(viewed from above)

B

Figure 5-3 The right horizontal rectus muscles. **A,** Right medial rectus muscle. **B,** Right lateral rectus muscle. *(Modified with permission from von Noorden GK. Atlas of Strabismus. 4th ed. St Louis: Mosby; 1983:3.)*

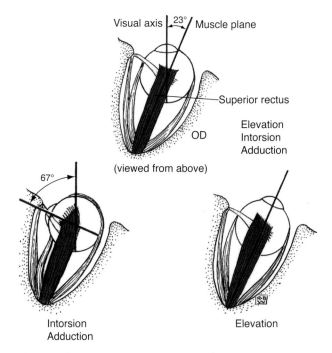

Visual axis 23° Muscle plane

Superior rectus

Elevation
Intorsion
Adduction

OD

(viewed from above)

67°

Intorsion
Adduction

Elevation

Figure 5-4 The right superior rectus muscle, viewed from above. *(Modified with permission from von Noorden GK. Atlas of Strabismus. 4th ed. St Louis: Mosby; 1983:3.)*

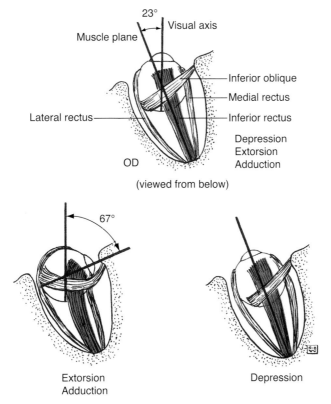

Figure 5-5 The right inferior rectus muscle, viewed from below. *(Modified with permission from von Noorden GK. Atlas of Strabismus. 4th ed. St Louis: Mosby; 1983:5.)*

The direction in which the 2 oblique muscles lie is from the anteromedial aspect of the globe to the posterolateral area, forming an angle of approximately 51° with the visual axis (Figs 5-6, 5-7). Because of the large angle formed in primary position, the primary action of the superior oblique is intorsion, with its secondary action being depression and its tertiary action, abduction. Because the muscle plane is aligned with the visual axis in extreme adduction, the superior oblique muscle action can be seen as mainly depression. When the eye abducts about 40° from primary position, the visual axis becomes perpendicular to the muscle plane, and the muscle action is one of mainly intorsion. A clinical application of this principle is the fact that in a complete third nerve palsy, the eye develops a large-angle exotropia. With the eye in this exotropic position, the superior oblique is a pure intortor. This intorsion can be observed by asking the patient to attempt to gaze downward and inward with the involved eye: the eye will intort even though it cannot be voluntarily moved into that field of gaze.

The vertical and torsional actions of the inferior oblique mirror those of the superior oblique (see Fig 5-7). In primary position, the primary action is extorsion, and the secondary action is elevation. However, as with the superior oblique, the tertiary action is abduction. The inferior oblique's action as an elevator is best seen in adduction and, as an extortor, in abduction.

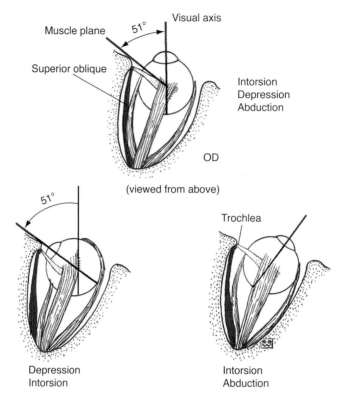

Figure 5-6 The right superior oblique muscle, viewed from above. *(Modified with permission from von Noorden GK.* Atlas of Strabismus. *4th ed. St Louis: Mosby; 1983:7)*

Binocular Eye Movements

When binocular eye movements are conjugate and the eyes move in the same direction, such movements are called *versions*. When the eye movements are disconjugate and the eyes move in opposite directions, such movements are known as *vergences* (eg, convergence, divergence, vertical vergence, and cyclovergence).

Versions

Right gaze *(dextroversion)* is movement of both eyes to the patient's right. Left gaze *(levoversion)* is movement of both eyes to the patient's left. *Elevation,* or *upgaze (sursumversion),* is an upward rotation of both eyes. *Depression,* or *downgaze (deorsumversion),* is a downward rotation of both eyes. In *dextrocycloversion,* both eyes rotate so that the superior portion of the vertical corneal meridian moves to the patient's right. Similarly, *levocycloversion* is movement of both eyes so that the superior portion of the vertical corneal meridian rotates to the patient's left.

The term *yoke muscles* is used to describe 2 muscles (1 in each eye) that are the prime movers of their respective eyes into a given position of gaze. For example, when the eyes move or attempt to move into right gaze, the right lateral rectus muscle and the left medial rectus muscle are simultaneously innervated and contracted. These muscles are said to be "yoked" together.

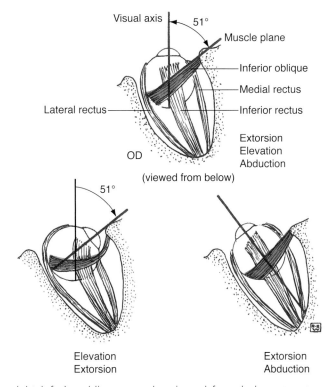

Figure 5-7 The right inferior oblique muscle, viewed from below. *(Modified with permission from von Noorden GK. Atlas of Strabismus. 4th ed. St Louis: Mosby; 1983:9.)*

Each EOM in one eye has a yoke muscle in the other eye. Because the effect of a muscle is usually best seen in a given direction of gaze, the concept of yoke muscles is used to evaluate the contribution of each EOM to eye movement. See Figure 5-2, which shows the 6 cardinal positions of gaze and the yoke muscles whose primary actions are in that field of gaze.

Hering's law of motor correspondence states that when the eyes move into a gaze direction, simultaneous innervation leads to yoke pairs of muscles having equal force. The most useful application of this law is in evaluation of binocular eye movements and, in particular, the yoke muscles involved.

Hering's law has important clinical implications, especially when the practitioner is dealing with a paralytic or restrictive strabismus. Because the amount of innervation to both eyes is always determined by the fixating eye, the angle of deviation varies according to which eye is fixating. When the unaffected eye is fixating, the amount of misalignment is called the *primary deviation.* When the paretic or restrictive eye is fixating, the amount of misalignment is called the *secondary deviation.* The secondary deviation is larger than the primary deviation because of the increased innervation necessary to move the paretic or restrictive eye to the position of fixation. This extra innervation is transmitted to the yoke muscle(s) in the fellow eye, which causes excessive action of this muscle and thus a larger angle of deviation. In cases where Hering's law does not appear to hold, the diagnosis may be a dissociated vertical deviation (see Chapter 11) or a dissociated horizontal deviation (DHD) (see Chapter 9).

Application of Hering's law is also useful in the explanation of muscle sequelae of a right superior oblique muscle palsy (see Chapter 11). If a patient uses the right eye to fixate on an object that is located up and to the left, the innervation of the right inferior oblique muscle required to move the eye into this gaze position is reduced because the right inferior oblique does not have to overcome the normal antagonistic effect of the right superior oblique muscle (Sherrington's law). According to Hering's law, less innervation is also received by the yoke muscle of the right inferior oblique muscle, the left superior rectus muscle. This decreased innervation could lead to the incorrect impression that the left superior rectus muscle is paretic, or what is referred to as an *inhibitional palsy of the contralateral antagonist* (Fig 5-8).

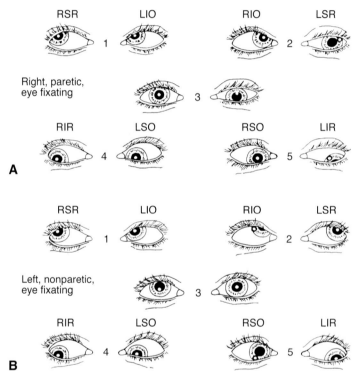

Figure 5-8 Palsy of right superior oblique muscle. **A,** With the palsied right eye fixating, little or no vertical difference appears between the 2 eyes in the right (uninvolved) field of gaze (*1* and *4*). In primary position *(3)*, a left hypotropia may be present because the right elevators require less innervation to stabilize the eye in primary position, and thus the left elevators will receive less than normal innervation. When gaze is up and left *(2)*, the RIO needs less than normal innervation to elevate the right eye because its antagonist, the RSO, is palsied. Consequently, its yoke, the LSR, will be apparently underacting, and pseudoptosis with pseudopalsy of the LSR will be present. When gaze is toward the field of action of the palsied RSO muscle *(5)*, maximum innervation is required to move the right eye down during adduction, and thus the yoke LIR will be overacting. **B,** With unaffected left eye fixating, no vertical difference appears in the right field of gaze (*1* and *4*). In primary position *(3)*, the right eye is elevated because of unopposed elevators. When gaze is up and left *(2)*, the RIO shows marked overaction because its antagonist is palsied. The action of the LSR is normal. When gaze is down and left *(5)*, normal innervation required by the fixating normal eye does not suffice to fully move the palsied eye into that field of gaze. (See also Chapter 7, Fig 7-10.) *(Reproduced with permission from von Noorden GK. Atlas of Strabismus. 4th ed. St Louis: Mosby; 1983:24–25.)*

Vergences

Convergence is movement of both eyes nasally relative to a given starting position; *divergence* is movement of both eyes temporally relative to a given starting position. The medial rectus muscles are yoked muscles for convergence; the lateral rectus muscles are yoked for divergence. *Incyclovergence* is a rotation of both eyes such that the superior portion of each vertical corneal meridian rotates nasally; *excyclovergence* is a rotation of both eyes such that the superior pole of each vertical corneal meridian rotates temporally. *Vertical vergence* movement, though less frequently encountered, can also occur: 1 eye moves upward and the other downward. (See also Chapter 6.) See Table 5-2 for a classification of the vergence system. The roles of its various components are described below.

Accommodative convergence of the visual axes Part of the synkinetic near reflex. A fairly consistent increment of accommodative convergence (AC) occurs for each diopter of accommodation (A), giving the *accommodative convergence/accommodation (AC/A) ratio.*

   Abnormalities of this ratio are common, and they are an important cause of strabismus (see Chapter 8). With an abnormally high AC/A ratio, the excess convergence tends to produce esotropia during accommodation on near targets. An abnormally low AC/A ratio tends to make the eyes less esotropic, or even exotropic, when the patient looks at near targets. For techniques of measuring this ratio, see the discussion of the AC/A ratio under Convergence in Chapter 7.

Fusional convergence A movement to converge and position the eyes so that similar retinal images project on corresponding retinal areas. Fusional convergence is accomplished without changing the refractive state of the eyes and is activated when a target in the midline is seen with bitemporal retinal image disparity. See also Chapter 6.

Proximal (instrument) convergence An induced convergence movement caused by a psychological awareness of near; this movement is particularly apparent when a person looks through an instrument such as a binocular microscope.

Tonic convergence The constant innervational tone to the EOMs when a person is awake and alert. Because of the anatomical shape of the bony orbits and the position of the rectus muscle origins, the alignment of the eyes under complete muscle paralysis is divergent. Therefore, convergence tone is necessary in the awake state to maintain straight eyes even in the absence of strabismus. A practical application of this can be seen in esotropic

Table 5-2 Classification of the Vergence System

Convergence	Divergence	Vertical Vergence	Cyclovergence
Accommodative convergence of the visual axes	Fusional divergence	Fusional vertical vergence	Excyclovergence
Fusional convergence	Nonfusional divergence		Incyclovergence
Proximal (instrument) convergence			
Tonic convergence			
Voluntary convergence			

patients under general anesthesia, who may show less esotropia or even exotropia with suspension of tonic convergence, which may lead to the incorrect assumption that a lesser amount of surgery should be done.

Voluntary convergence A conscious application of the near synkinesis.

Fusional divergence An optomotor reflex to diverge and align the eyes so that similar retinal images project on corresponding retinal areas. Fusional divergence is accomplished without changing the refractive state of the eyes and is activated when a target in the midline is seen with binasal retinal image disparity. See also Chapter 6.

Nonfusional divergence An optomotor reflex to diverge the eyes when vision in 1 eye is blurred and fusion is disrupted on a long-term basis, as seen in cases of sensory exotropia or in spontaneous consecutive exotropia with amblyopia.

Vertical vergence An optomotor reflex to reduce vertical disparity and realign the eyes when fusion is disrupted, so that similar retinal images project on corresponding retinal areas.

Cyclovergence An optomotor reflex to reduce the cyclotorsional disparity of the eyes so that similar retinal images project on corresponding retinal areas. Cyclovergence includes 2 components: incyclovergence and excyclovergence. In addition to a motor reflex, each of these subsystems has a sensory component to compensate for cyclotorsional disparity, and for most targets the sensory component is the more important of the two.

Supranuclear Control Systems for Eye Movement

There are several supranuclear eye movement systems. The *saccadic system* generates all fast (up to 400°–500°/sec) eye movements, such as eye movements of refixation. This system functions to place the image of an object of interest on the fovea or to move the eyes from one object to another. Saccadic movements require a sudden strong pulse of force from the EOMs to move the eye rapidly against the viscosity produced by the fatty tissue and the fascia in which the globe lies. The study of saccadic velocity is used in some centers to quantitate muscle paresis and abnormal innervation. However, a careful examiner can confirm the presence of a paretic muscle without sophisticated instrumentation by clinically detecting a "floating saccade."

The *smooth pursuit system* generates all following, or pursuit, eye movements. Pursuit latency is shorter than for saccades, but the maximum peak velocity of these slow pursuit movements is limited to 30°–60°/sec. The involuntary *optokinetic system* utilizes smooth pursuit to track a moving object and then introduces a compensatory saccade to refixate. Tests of this system, performed with an optokinetic stimulus, are often used to detect visual responses in an infant or child with apparent vision loss, such as with ocular motor apraxia (see Chapter 12). The *vergence system* controls disconjugate eye movement, as in convergence or divergence. Supranuclear control of vergence eye movements is not yet fully understood. There are also systems that integrate eye movements with body movements. The most clinically important of these systems is the *labyrinthine (vestibulo-ocular) reflex system*, which involves the semicircular canals of the inner ears. Other systems involve the utricle and saccule of the inner ears. The cervical, or neck, receptors provide input for this reflex control. See BCSC Section 5, *Neuro-Ophthalmology,* for in-depth discussion of these systems.

CHAPTER **6**

Sensory Physiology and Pathology

Physiology of Normal Binocular Vision

If an area of the retina is stimulated by any means—externally by light or internally by mechanical pressure or electrical processes—the resulting sensation is always one of light, and the light is subjectively localized as coming from a specific visual direction in space. The imaginary line connecting the fixation point and the fovea is termed the *visual axis,* and normally, with central fixation, it is subjectively localized straight ahead.

Retinal Correspondence

If retinal locations in each eye share a common subjective visual direction—that is, if stimulation of these 2 points results in the subjective sensation that the stimulating target or targets lie in the same direction—these retinal locations are said to be *corresponding.* When the image of an object in space falls on corresponding points, it is perceived as a single object. On the other hand, stimulation of *noncorresponding* or *disparate* retinal points results in the sensation of 2 visual directions for the same target, or diplopia.

With *normal retinal correspondence,* the foveae of the 2 eyes are corresponding points. Retinal areas in each eye that are essentially equidistant to the right or left and above or below the fovea are also corresponding points. The locus of points in space that stimulate corresponding points in each retina is known as the *horopter.* With symmetric convergence, the geometric relationship between corresponding points—for example, a point 1° nasal to the fovea in 1 eye would correspond to a point 1° temporal to the fovea in the other eye—gives a circle that passes through the optical center of each eye and the point of fixation. This theoretical horopter is known as the *Vieth-Müller circle.* When the horopter is determined experimentally, the locus of points that are seen singly falls not on a circle but on a curve called the *empirical horopter* (Fig 6-1).

The horopter exists in both the horizontal and vertical planes. Although it might seem that the horopter would be a surface in space, the horizontal separation of the eyes causes points in the oblique quadrants to be vertically disparate. For symmetric convergence, the 3-dimensional horopter of points that have both horizontal and vertical correspondence consists of a curved horizontal line and a sloped vertical line that intersect at the fixation point. Each fixation point has a unique horopter centered on that point.

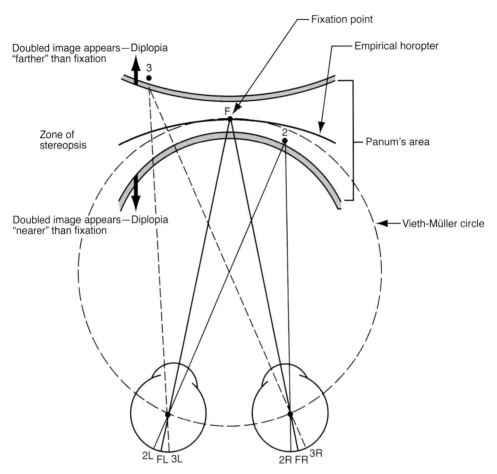

Figure 6-1 Empirical horopter. *F* = fixation point; *FL* and *FR* = left and right foveae, respectively. Point 2, falling within Panum's area, is seen singly and stereoscopically. Point 3 falls outside Panum's area and is therefore seen doubly.

If the horopter includes all points in space that stimulate corresponding retinal points, double vision would be expected when the target does not lie on the horopter. However, the visual system can combine slightly disparate points within a limited area surrounding the horopter, called *Panum's area of single binocular vision* (see Fig 6-1). Objects in this space fall on disparate retinal points but are physiologically seen singly. Objects outside Panum's area fall on widely disparate retinal points and are seen as lying in 2 visual directions, resulting in physiologic diplopia.

Fusion

Fusion is the cortical unification of visual objects from the 2 eyes into a single percept. For retinal images to be fused, they must be similar in size and shape. Fusion in areas near the fovea (central fusion) tolerates very little dissimilarity between the images in each eye before diplopia is elicited, because of the small receptive fields in this region. More dissimilarity is tolerated in the periphery (peripheral fusion), where the receptive fields are larger. Fusion has been artificially subdivided into sensory fusion, motor fusion, and stereopsis.

Sensory fusion

Sensory fusion is based on the innate, orderly topographic relationship between the retinas and the visual cortex, whereby images falling on corresponding (or nearly corresponding) retinal points in each eye are combined to form a single visual percept.

Motor fusion

Motor fusion is a vergence movement that causes similar retinal images to be maintained on corresponding retinal areas despite the tendency of natural (eg, heterophorias) or artificial causes to induce disparities. For example, if a progressive base-out prism is introduced before both eyes while a target is viewed, the retinal images move temporally over both retinas if the eyes remain in fixed position. However, fusional convergence movements maintain similar retinal images on corresponding retinal areas, and the eyes are observed to converge. This response is called *fusional convergence.* Measurement of fusional vergence amplitudes is discussed in Chapter 7.

Stereopsis

Stereopsis occurs when horizontal retinal disparity between the 2 eyes produces a subjective ordering of visual objects in depth, or 3 dimensions. It is the highest form of binocular cooperation and adds a unique quality to vision. The region of points with binocular disparities that result in stereopsis is slightly wider than Panum's area, so stereopsis is not simply a by-product of combining the disparate images from a point into a single object. The brain interprets nasal disparity between 2 similar retinal images of an object in the midline as indicating that the object is farther away from the fixation point, and temporal disparity as indicating that the object is nearer. Binasal or bitemporal images are not a requirement for stereopsis; objects not in the midline in front of or behind the horopter also elicit stereopsis, even though their images fall on the nasal retina in 1 eye and the temporal retina in the other.

Stereopsis and depth perception *(bathopsis)* are not synonymous. Monocular cues also contribute to depth perception. These cues include object overlap, relative object size, highlights and shadows, motion parallax, and perspective. Stereopsis is a *binocular* sensation of relative depth caused by horizontal disparity of retinal images. Although stereopsis operates at distances over 2000 ft, depth perception relies increasingly on monocular cues beyond 10–20 ft.

Selected Aspects of the Neurophysiology of Vision

The decussation of the optic nerves at the chiasm is essential for the development of binocular vision and stereopsis. With decussation, visual information from corresponding retinal areas in each eye runs through the lateral geniculate body (LGB) and optic tracts to the visual cortex, where the information from both eyes is commingled and modified by the integration of various inputs.

The *magnocellular (M), parvocellular (P),* and *koniocellular (K) systems* are parallel systems for processing visual information in the retinogeniculocortical pathway. The M system is represented predominantly in the peripheral retina and is especially sensitive to moving stimuli but not sensitive to stationary images. The M system is also relatively insensitive to color. The P system is represented predominantly in the fovea and gives a slow tonic response to visual stimulation, carries high-resolution information about object borders and color contrast, and is important for shape perception and the ability to see objects in detail. The K system is less well understood but is thought to be concerned with aspects of color vision, especially the color blue.

This monocular separation of the pathways is maintained through the lateral geniculate laminae into the *striate cortex* (also called the *primary visual cortex,* or *V1*), where the geniculate axon terminals from the right and left eyes are segregated into a system of alternating parallel stripes called *ocular dominance columns.* From there, the paired right and left monocular cells converge on the first binocular cells in layers 2, 3, and 4B of V1. Binocular vision and binocular motor fusion are made possible by horizontal connections that enable information from these monocular columns to be shared. There is also a projection from the visual cortex back to the LGB; this feedback pathway is thought to play a modulatory role.

Visual Development

In the human retina, most of the ganglion cells are generated between 8 and 15 weeks' gestation, reaching a plateau of 2.2–2.5 million by week 18. After week 30, the ganglion cell population decreases dramatically during a period of rapid cell death that lasts 6–8 weeks. Thereafter, cell death continues at a low rate into the first few postnatal months. The retinal ganglion cell population is reduced to a final count of approximately 1.0–1.5 million. The loss of about 1 million optic axons may serve to refine the topography and specificity of the retinogeniculate projection by eliminating inappropriate connections.

The continued development of visual function after birth is accompanied by major anatomical changes occurring simultaneously at all levels of the central visual pathways. The fovea is still covered by multiple cell layers and is sparsely packed with cones, which may account for the estimated visual acuity of 20/400 at birth. During the first years of life, the photoreceptors redistribute within the retina and foveal cone density increases fivefold to achieve the configuration found in the adult retina, improving visual acuity to 20/20. In newborns, the white matter of the visual pathways is not fully myelinated. Myelin sheaths enlarge rapidly for the first 2 years after birth and then more slowly through the first decade of life. At birth, the neurons of the LGB are only 60% of their average adult size. Their volume gradually increases until age 2 years. Refinement of synaptic connections in the striate cortex continues for many years after birth. The density of synapses declines by 40% over several years, attaining final adult levels at about age 10 years.

Effects of Abnormal Visual Experience on the Retinogeniculocortical Pathway

Abnormal visual experience resulting from visual deprivation, anisometropia, or strabismus can powerfully affect retinogeniculocortical development. Single-eyelid suturing in baby macaque monkeys usually produces axial myopia but no other significant anatomical changes in the eye. The lateral geniculate laminae that receive input from the deprived eye experience minor shrinkage, but these cells respond rapidly to visual stimulation, implying that a defect in the LGB is not likely to account for amblyopia. In the striate cortex, monocular visual deprivation causes the regions of the visual cortex driven predominantly by the closed eye (ocular dominance columns) to radically narrow (Fig 6-2). This happens because the 2 eyes compete for synaptic contacts in the cortex. As a result, the deprived eye loses many of the connections already formed at birth with postsynaptic cortical targets. The open eye profits by the sprouting of terminal arbors beyond their usual boundaries to occupy territory relinquished by the deprived eye (Fig 6-3). However, the benefit derived from invading the cortical territory of the deprived eye is unclear because visual acuity does not improve beyond normal. Positron emission tomography (PET) has shown that cortical blood flow and glucose metabolism are lower during stimulation of the amblyopic eye compared with the normal eye, suggesting the visual cortex as the primary site of amblyopia. Monocular deprivation also devastates binocularity because few cells can be driven by both eyes.

There is a critical period in which visual development of the macaque eye is vulnerable to the effects of eyelid suturing. This critical period corresponds to that in which the wiring of the striate cortex is still vulnerable to the effects of visual deprivation. During the critical period, the deleterious effects of suturing the right eyelid, for example, are correctable by reversal—that is, opening the sutured right eye and closing the left eye. After this reversal, the ocular dominance columns of the initially closed right eye appear practically normal, indicating that anatomical recovery of the initially shrunken columns was

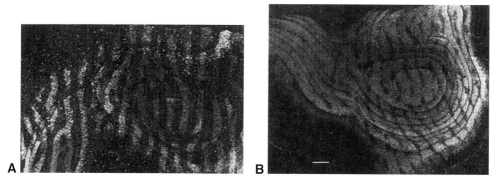

Figure 6-2 Change of ocular dominance columns in macaque visual cortex after monocular deprivation. Radioactive proline was injected into the normal eye and transported to the visual cortex to reveal the projections of that eye. In these sections, cut parallel to the cortical surface, white areas show labeled terminals in layer 4. **A,** Normal monkey. The stripes representing the injected eye (bright) and noninjected eye (dark) have roughly equal spacing. **B,** Monkey that had 1 eye sutured closed from birth for 18 months. The bright stripes (open, injected eye) are widened and the dark ones (closed eye) are greatly narrowed, showing the devastating physical effect of deprivation amblyopia. (Scale bar = 1 mm.) *(Reproduced with permission from Kaufman PL, Alm A. Adler's Physiology of the Eye. 10th ed. St Louis: Mosby; 2002:699. Originally from Hubel DH, Wiesel TN, LeVay S. Plasticity of ocular dominance columns in monkey striate cortex. Philos Trans R Soc Lond B Biol Sci. 1977;278(961):377–409.)*

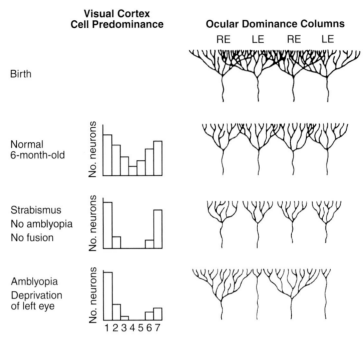

Figure 6-3 Anatomical and physiologic maturation of ocular dominance columns of the primary visual cortex in normal and deprived monkeys. *Birth:* Broad overlap of afferents from the lateral geniculate nucleus, hence little dominance by right eye *(RE)* versus left eye *(LE). Normal 6-month-old:* Regression of overlapping afferents from both eyes with distinct areas of monocular dominance. The bar graph shows the classic U-shaped distribution obtained by single-cell recordings from the visual cortex. About half the cells are driven predominantly by the right eye and the other half by the left eye. A small number are driven equally by the 2 eyes. *1* = driven only by right eye; *7* = driven only by left eye; *2–6* = driven binocularly. *Strabismus:* Effect of artificial eye misalignment in the neonatal period on ocular dominance. The monkey alternated fixation (no amblyopia) and lacked fusion. Lack of binocularity is evident as exaggerated segregation into dominance columns. The bar graph shows the results of single-cell recordings obtained from this animal after age 1 year. Almost all neurons are driven exclusively by the right or left eye, with little binocular activity. *Amblyopia:* Effect of suturing the left eyelid shut shortly after birth. Dominance columns of the normal right eye are much wider than those of the deprivationally amblyopic left eye. The bar graph shows markedly skewed ocular dominance and little binocular activity. *(Modified with permission from Tychsen L. Binocular vision. In: Hart WM, ed. Adler's Physiology of the Eye: Clinical Application. 9th ed. St Louis: Mosby; 1992:810.)*

induced by opening the right eye and closing the left eye. However, when the right eye is sewn closed beyond the critical period, the columns of the right eye do not re-expand if the right eye is opened and the left eye closed.

Eyelid suturing in the baby macaque is a good model for visual deprivation amblyopia. In children, this condition can be caused by any dense opacity of the ocular media or occlusion by the eyelid. Visual deprivation can rapidly cause profound amblyopia.

Amblyopia in children also has other causes. Optical defocus resulting from anisometropia causes the cortical neurons driven by the defocused eye to be less sensitive (particularly to higher spatial frequencies because they are most affected by blur) and to send out a weaker signal. This results in reduced binocular activity. Anisometropic amblyopia has a later-onset critical period than strabismic amblyopia and requires a prolonged period of unilateral blur. Meridional (astigmatic) amblyopia does not develop during the first year of life and may not develop until age 3.

Strabismus can be artificially created in monkeys by the sectioning of an extraocular muscle. Alternating fixation develops in some monkeys after this procedure; they maintain normal acuity in each eye. Examination of the striate cortex reveals cells with normal receptive fields and an equal number of cells responsive to stimulation of either eye. However, the cortex is bereft of binocular cells (see Fig 6-3). After 1 extraocular muscle is cut, some monkeys do not alternately fixate but constantly fixate with the same eye, and amblyopia develops in the deviating eye. An important factor in the development of strabismic amblyopia is interocular suppression due to uncorrelated images in the 2 eyes. Strabismus causes abnormal input to the striate cortex by preventing the synchronous firing of correlated images from the 2 foveae. Another factor is the optical defocus of the deviated eye. The dominant eye is focused on the object of regard, while the deviated eye is pointed in a different direction; for the deviated eye, the object may be too near or too far to be in focus. Either mechanism can cause asynchrony or inhibition of 1 set of signals in the striate cortex. The critical period for development of strabismic amblyopia begins at approximately 4 months of age, during the time of ocular dominance segregation and sensitivity to binocular correlation.

Abnormal sensory input alone is sufficient to alter the normal anatomy of the visual cortex. Other areas of the cerebral cortex may also depend on sensory stimulation to form the proper anatomical circuits necessary for normal adult visual function. This notion underscores the importance of providing children with a stimulating sensory environment.

Abnormalities of Binocular Vision

When a manifest deviation of the eyes occurs, the corresponding retinal elements of the eyes are no longer directed at the same object. This places the patient at risk for 2 distinct visual phenomena: visual confusion and diplopia.

Visual Confusion

Visual confusion is the simultaneous perception of 2 different objects projected onto corresponding retinal areas. The 2 foveal areas are physiologically incapable of simultaneous perception of dissimilar objects. The closest foveal equivalent is *retinal rivalry,* wherein the 2 perceived images rapidly alternate (Fig 6-4). Confusion may be a phenomenon of extrafoveal retinal areas only. Clinically significant visual confusion is rare.

Diplopia

Double vision, or *diplopia,* usually results from an acquired misalignment of the visual axes that causes an image to fall simultaneously on the fovea of 1 eye and on a nonfoveal point in the other eye. The object that falls on these noncorresponding points must be outside Panum's area to appear double. The same object is seen as having 2 locations in subjective space, and the foveal image is always clearer than the nonfoveal image of the

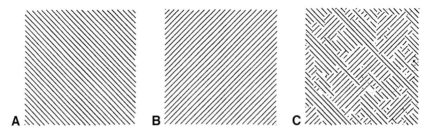

Figure 6-4 Rivalry pattern. **A,** Pattern seen by the left eye. **B,** Pattern seen by the right eye. **C,** Pattern seen with binocular vision. *(Reproduced with permission from von Noorden GK, Campos EC. Binocular Vision and Ocular Motility: Theory and Management of Strabismus. 6th ed. St Louis: Mosby; 2002:12.)*

nonfixating eye. The perception of diplopia depends on the age at onset, its duration, and the patient's subjective awareness of it. The younger the child, the greater the ability to suppress, or inhibit, the nonfoveal image.

Central fusion disruption is intractable diplopia, the features of which are absence of suppression and absence of fusional amplitudes. These findings, when accompanied by active motor avoidance of bifocal stimulation, are referred to as *horror fusionis.* The angle of strabismus may be small or may vary. Central fusion disruption can occur in a number of clinical settings: after disruption of fusion for a prolonged period; after head trauma; and, in rare cases, in long-standing strabismus. Management can be challenging.

Sensory Adaptations in Strabismus

To avoid visual confusion and diplopia, the visual system can use the mechanisms of suppression and anomalous retinal correspondence (Fig 6-5). It is important to realize that pathologic suppression and anomalous retinal correspondence develop only in the immature visual system.

Suppression

Suppression is the alteration of visual sensation that occurs when the images from 1 eye are inhibited or prevented from reaching consciousness during binocular visual activity. Physiologic suppression is the mechanism that prevents physiologic diplopia (diplopia elicited by objects outside Panum's area) from reaching consciousness. Pathologic suppression may result from strabismic misalignment of the visual axes or other conditions that result in discordant images in each eye, such as cataract or anisometropia. Such suppression can be seen as an adaptation of a visually immature brain to avoid diplopia. If a patient with strabismus and normal retinal correspondence (NRC) does not have diplopia, suppression is present, provided the sensory pathways are intact. In less obvious situations, several simple tests are available for clinical diagnosis of suppression (see Chapter 7).

The following classification of suppression may be useful for the clinician:

- *Central versus peripheral. Central suppression* is the mechanism that keeps the foveal image of the deviating eye from reaching consciousness, thereby preventing visual confusion. *Peripheral suppression* is the mechanism that eliminates diplopia

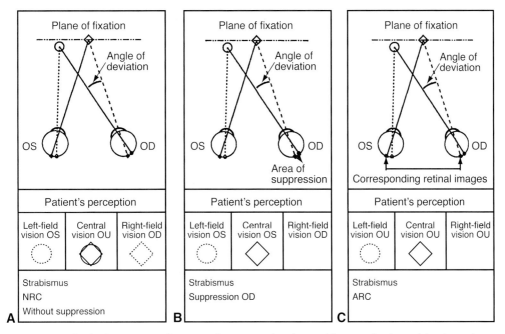

Figure 6-5 Retinal correspondence and suppression in strabismus. **A,** A strabismic patient with normal retinal correspondence (NRC) and without suppression would have diplopia and visual confusion, which is the perception of a common visual direction for 2 separate objects (represented by the superimposition of the images of the fixated diamond and the circle, which is imaged on the fovea of the deviating eye). **B,** The elimination of diplopia and confusion by suppression of the retinal image of the deviating right eye. **C,** The elimination of diplopia and confusion by anomalous retinal correspondence (ARC), an adaptation of visual directions in the deviated right eye. *(Adapted with permission from Kaufman PL, Alm A. Adler's Physiology of the Eye. 10th ed. St Louis: Mosby; 2003:490.)*

by preventing awareness of the image that falls on the peripheral retina in the deviating eye that corresponds to the image falling on the fovea of the fixating eye. This form of suppression is clearly pathologic, developing as a cortical adaptation only within an immature visual system. Adults may be unable to develop peripheral suppression and therefore may be unable to eliminate the peripheral second image without closing or occluding the deviating eye.

- *Nonalternating versus alternating.* If suppression always causes the image from the dominant eye to predominate over the image from the deviating eye, the suppression is *nonalternating.* This may lead to amblyopia. If the process switches between the 2 eyes, the suppression is described as *alternating.*
- *Facultative versus constant.* Suppression may be considered *facultative* if present only when the eyes are in the deviated state and absent in all other states. Patients with intermittent exotropia, for instance, often experience suppression when the eyes are divergent but may experience high-grade stereopsis when the eyes are straight. In contrast, *constant suppression* is always present, whether the eyes are deviated or aligned. The suppression scotoma in the deviating eye may be either *relative* (permitting some visual sensation) or *absolute* (permitting no perception of light).

Management of suppression

Therapy for suppression often includes the following:

- proper refractive correction
- occlusion or pharmacologic penalization, to treat amblyopia
- alignment of the visual axes, to permit simultaneous stimulation of corresponding retinal elements by the same object

Orthoptic exercises may be attempted to overcome the tendency of the image from 1 eye to suppress the image from the other eye when both eyes are open. These exercises are designed to first make the patient aware of diplopia, then have the patient attempt to fuse the images—both on an instrument and in free space. However, suppression is a useful adaptation to avoid diplopia in patients who are unable to fuse, so eliminating it is problematic in a patient for whom subsequent fusion training is unsuccessful. The role of orthoptics in the treatment of suppression is therefore controversial.

Anomalous Retinal Correspondence

Anomalous retinal correspondence (ARC) is a condition wherein the fovea of the fixating eye has acquired an anomalous common visual direction with a peripheral retinal element in the deviated eye; that is, the 2 foveae have different visual directions. ARC is an adaptation that restores some degree of binocular cooperation despite manifest strabismus. Anomalous binocular vision is a functional state that is superior to total suppression. In the development of ARC, normal sensory development is replaced only gradually and not completely. The more long-standing the deviation, the more deeply rooted the ARC may become. The period during which ARC may develop probably extends through the first decade of life.

Paradoxical diplopia can occur when ARC persists after surgery. When esotropic patients whose eyes have been set straight or nearly straight report a crossed diplopic localization of foveal or parafoveal stimuli, they are experiencing paradoxical diplopia (Fig 6-6). Paradoxical diplopia is typically a fleeting postoperative phenomenon, seldom lasting longer than a few days to weeks, but in rare cases it can persist much longer.

Testing for ARC

Testing for ARC is performed to determine how patients use their eyes in normal life and to seek out any vestiges of normal correspondence. As discussed earlier, ARC is a sensory adaptation to abnormal ocular alignment. Because the depth of the sensory rearrangement can vary widely, an individual can test positive for both NRC and ARC. Tests that closely simulate everyday use of the eyes are more likely to give evidence of ARC. The more dissociative the test, the more likely the test will produce an NRC response, unless the ARC is deeply rooted. Some of the more common tests (discussed at length in Chapter 7), in order of most to least dissociating, are the afterimage test, the Worth 4-dot test, the red-glass test (dissociation increases with the density of the red filter), amblyoscope testing, and testing with Bagolini striated glasses. If an anomalous localization response occurs in the more dissociative tests, the depth of ARC is greater.

Note that ARC is a binocular phenomenon, tested for and documented in both eyes simultaneously. It is not necessarily related to eccentric fixation (see Chapter 4), which

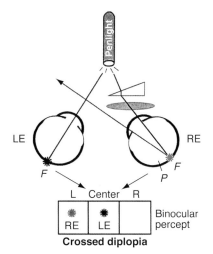

Crossed diplopia

Figure 6-6 Paradoxical diplopia. Diagram of esotropia and ARC, wherein the deviation is being neutralized with a base-out prism. A red glass and base-out prism are placed over the right eye. The prism neutralizes the deviation by moving the retinal image of the penlight temporally, off the pseudofovea *(P)* to the true fovea *(F)*. Because the pseudofovea is the center of orientation, the image is perceived to fall on the temporal retina and is projected to the opposite field, thus resulting in crossed diplopia. *(Modified with permission from Wright KW, Spiegel PH.* Pediatric Ophthalmology and Strabismus. *St Louis: Mosby; 1999:219.)*

is a monocular phenomenon found on testing 1 eye alone. Because some tests for ARC depend on separate stimulation of each fovea, the presence of eccentric fixation can significantly affect the test results (see also Chapter 7).

Monofixation Syndrome

The term *monofixation syndrome* is used to describe a particular presentation of a sensory state in strabismus. The essential feature of this syndrome is the presence of peripheral fusion with the absence of bifoveal fusion due to a central scotoma. *Microtropia* is a term that was separately introduced to describe small-angle strabismus with a constellation of findings that largely overlap those of monofixation syndrome.

A patient with monofixation syndrome may have no manifest deviation but usually has a small (<8Δ) heterotropia; the heterotropia is most commonly an esotropia but is sometimes an exotropia or hypertropia. Stereoacuity is present but reduced. Amblyopia is a common finding.

Monofixation syndrome is a favorable outcome of infantile strabismus surgery and is present in a substantial minority of patients with intermittent exotropia. It can also be a primary condition that causes unilaterally decreased vision when no obvious strabismus is present. Monofixation syndrome can result from anisometropia or macular lesions as well. If associated amblyopia is clinically significant, occlusion therapy is indicated.

Diagnosis

To diagnose monofixation syndrome, the clinician must demonstrate the absence of bimacular fusion, by documenting a macular scotoma in the nonfixating eye under binocular conditions, and the presence of peripheral binocular vision (peripheral fusion).

Vectographic projections of Snellen letters can be used to document the facultative scotoma of monofixation syndrome. Snellen letters are viewed through polarized analyzers or goggles equipped with liquid-crystal shutters so that some letters are seen with only the right eye, some with only the left eye, and some with both eyes. Patients with monofixation syndrome omit letters that are imaged only in the nonfixating eye. There are a variety of other tests for central suppression that are more commonly used (see Chapter 7).

Testing stereoacuity is an important part of the monofixation syndrome evaluation. Any amount of gross stereopsis confirms the presence of peripheral fusion. Most patients with monofixation syndrome demonstrate stereopsis of 200–3000 seconds of arc. However, because some patients with this syndrome have no demonstrable stereopsis, other tests for peripheral fusion, such as the Worth 4-dot test and testing with Bagolini glasses, must be used in conjunction with stereoacuity measurement. Fine stereopsis (better than 67 seconds of arc) is present only in patients with bifoveal fixation.

Kushner BJ. The occurrence of monofixational exotropia after exotropia surgery. *Am J Ophthalmol.* 2009;147(6):1082–1085.

Lang J. Microtropia. *Arch Ophthalmol.* 1969;81(6):758–762.

Parks MM. The monofixation syndrome. *Trans Am Ophthalmol Soc.* 1969;67:609–657.

Diagnostic Evaluation of Strabismus and Torticollis

History and Presenting Features of Strabismus

When obtaining the history from a patient with strabismus, the clinician should document, if possible, the age of onset of a deviation or symptom. Old photographs may be useful for this purpose. In addition, the clinician should seek to answer the following questions about the deviation or symptom:

- Did its onset coincide with trauma or illness?
- Is the deviation constant or intermittent?
- Is it present for distance or near vision or both?
- Is it unilateral or alternating?
- Is it present only when the patient is inattentive or fatigued?
- Does the child close 1 eye (squint)?
- Is the deviation associated with double vision or eyestrain?

Previous treatment should be reviewed, including amblyopia therapy, spectacle correction, and eye muscle surgery. While obtaining the history, the clinician should observe the patient, noting such factors as head positioning, head movement, attentiveness, and motor control. See Chapter 1 for discussion of general considerations and strategies for examination of the pediatric patient.

Assessment of Ocular Alignment

Positions of Gaze

The *primary position of gaze* is the position of the eyes when fixating straight ahead on an object at infinity. For practical purposes, infinity is considered to be 6 m (20 ft), and for this position the head should be straight.

The *cardinal positions* are the 6 positions of gaze in which the prime mover is 1 muscle of each eye, together called *yoke muscles* (see Chapter 5). The *midline positions* are straight up and straight down from primary position. These latter 2 gaze positions help the clinician determine the elevating and depressing capabilities of the eye, but they do not isolate any 1 muscle because 2 elevator and 2 depressor muscles affect midline gaze positions.

The *diagnostic positions of gaze* consist of these 9 gaze positions: the 6 cardinal positions, straight up and straight down, and primary position. For patients with vertical strabismus, the diagnostic positions of gaze also include forced head tilt to the right and left (see the section 3-Step Test, later in the chapter). Near fixation and reading position (depending on the patient's symptoms) complete the list of clinically important alignment measurements. Several formats are available for documenting findings of these tests (Fig 7-1).

Tests for measuring ocular alignment can be grouped into 3 basic types: cover tests, corneal light reflex tests, and subjective tests.

Cover Tests

Foveal fixation in each eye, attention, cooperation, and the ability to make eye movements are all necessary for cover testing. If a patient is unable to maintain constant fixation on an accommodative target, cover tests should not be used. There are 3 main types of cover tests: the cover-uncover test, the alternate cover test, and the simultaneous prism and cover test. All can be performed at distance or near fixation.

The monocular *cover-uncover test* is the most important test for detecting manifest strabismus and for differentiating a heterophoria from a heterotropia (Fig 7-2). As each eye is covered, the examiner watches for any movement in the opposite, *noncovered* eye; such movement indicates a heterotropia. If there is no movement of the noncovered eye, movement of the *covered* eye as the cover is applied and movement in the opposite direction (a fusional movement) as the cover is removed indicates a heterophoria. If the patient has a heterophoria, the eyes will be straight before and after the cover-uncover test; the deviation appears during the test as a result of interruption of binocular vision. A patient with a heterotropia, however, starts with a deviated eye and, after testing, ends with the same eye or—in the case of an *alternating heterotropia*—the opposite eye deviated. In some patients with heterophoria, the eyes are straight before testing, but they dissociate into a manifest deviation (heterotropia) after the occlusion interrupts binocular vision.

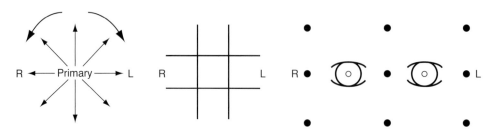

Figure 7-1 Three examples of methods for recording the results of ocular alignment testing.

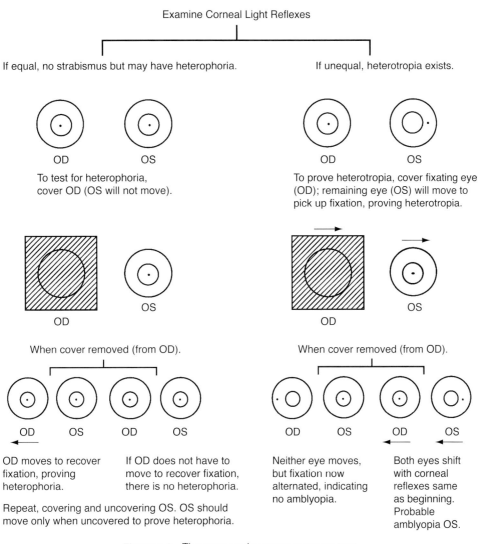

Figure 7-2 The monocular cover-uncover test.

The *alternate cover test* (Fig 7-3A) detects both latent and manifest deviations. Testing should be performed at both distance and near fixation. The deviation is quantified by using prisms to eliminate the eye movement as the occluder is switched from eye to eye (*prism alternate cover test;* Fig 7-3B). It may be necessary to use both horizontally and vertically placed prisms. This measures the total deviation; it does not distinguish between latent (heterophoria) and manifest (heterotropia) components of the deviation.

Two horizontal or 2 vertical prisms should not be stacked because doing so can induce significant measurement errors. A more accurate method for measuring deviations larger than those a single prism can correct is to place prisms in front of each eye, although this is not perfectly additive either. However, it is acceptable to stack a horizontal

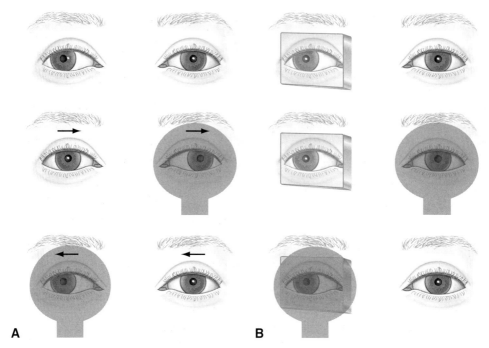

Figure 7-3 **A,** The alternate cover test. *Top:* Exotropia, left eye fixating. *Middle and bottom:* Both eyes move each time the cover alternates from 1 eye to the other. **B,** The prism alternate cover test. *Top:* The exotropia is neutralized with a prism of the correct power. *Middle and bottom:* The eyes do not move as the cover alternates from 1 eye to the other. *(Illustration developed by Steven Archer, MD; original illustration by Mark Miller.)*

and a vertical prism over the same eye, if necessary. For the most accurate results, plastic prisms should be held with the back surface (the surface closest to the patient) in the patient's frontal plane, regardless of the size of the deviation. If the patient's head is tilted, the prisms must be tilted accordingly. With incomitant (paretic or restrictive) strabismus, the clinician can measure the primary and secondary deviations by holding the prism over the paretic or restricted eye and the sound eye, respectively.

The *simultaneous prism and cover test* is used to determine the manifest deviation without occlusion (only the heterotropia). The test is performed by placing a prism in front of the deviating eye and covering the fixating eye at the same time. The test is repeated using increasing prism powers until the deviated eye no longer shifts. This test has special application in monofixation syndrome. Under binocular conditions, patients with this condition often use peripheral fusion to exert some control over their deviation. The heterotropia alone is smaller than the total deviation (heterotropia plus heterophoria) measured by the prism alternate cover test. The simultaneous prism and cover test provides the best indication of the size of the deviation under real-life conditions.

Thompson JT, Guyton DL. Ophthalmic prisms. Measurement errors and how to minimize them. *Ophthalmology.* 1983;90(3):204–210.

Corneal Light Reflex Tests

Corneal light reflex tests rely on the location of the first Purkinje image of a fixation light to assess the alignment of the eyes. The Hirschberg and Krimsky tests are the main tests of this type. Although they are not as accurate as cover tests, they are a useful alternative for uncooperative patients and those with poor or eccentric fixation, in whom cover testing is not possible.

The *Hirschberg test* is based on the correlation between the decentration of the corneal light reflection and the ocular deviation. The ratio is about 22Δ/mm but can vary by as much as 20% from one individual to the next. With an uncooperative child, it is not always possible to accurately measure the light reflex displacement, so gross estimates of the deviation are often used: 30Δ if the reflex is at the pupil margin, 60Δ if the reflex is in the middle of the iris, and 90Δ if the reflex is at the limbus (Fig 7-4).

The *Krimsky test* uses prisms to quantify the decentration of the corneal reflections and is best suited for near fixation measurement. This is done by holding a prism over either eye. By adjusting the prism power to center the corneal reflection symmetrically in each eye, it is possible to approximate the near deviation (Fig 7-5).

The angle kappa (Fig 7-6) can affect corneal light reflex measurements. *Angle kappa* is the angle between the visual axis and the anatomical pupillary axis of the eye. If the fovea is slightly temporal to the pupillary axis (as is usually the case), the corneal light reflection will be slightly nasal to the center of the cornea. This is termed *positive angle kappa*. A large positive angle kappa can simulate exotropia. If the position of the fovea is nasal to the pupillary axis, the corneal light reflection will be temporal to the center of the cornea. This is termed *negative angle kappa;* it simulates esotropia. The angle kappa does not affect any of the cover tests.

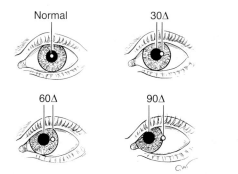

Figure 7-4 Hirschberg test. The extent to which the corneal light reflex is displaced from the center of the pupil provides an approximation of the angular size of the deviation (in this example, a left esotropia). *(Modified with permission from Simon JW, Calhoun JH. A Child's Eyes: A Guide to Pediatric Primary Care. Gainesville, FL: Triad Publishing Company; 1997:72.)*

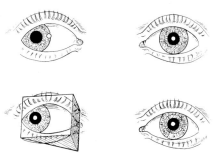

Figure 7-5 Krimsky test. The right exotropia is measured by the size of the prism required to center the pupillary reflexes, as shown at bottom. *(Reprinted with permission from Simon JW, Calhoun JH. A Child's Eyes: A Guide to Pediatric Primary Care. Gainesville, FL: Triad Publishing Company; 1997:72.)*

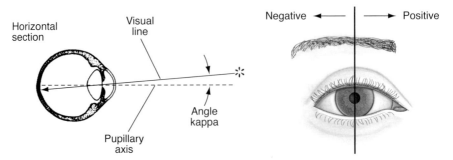

Figure 7-6 Angle kappa. A positive angle (in which the corneal light reflex is medial to the vertical line) simulates exotropia, whereas a negative angle (in which the light reflex is lateral to the vertical line) simulates esotropia. *(Reprinted with permission from Parks MM. Ocular Motility and Strabismus. Hagerstown, MD: Harper & Row; 1975.)*

The *Brückner test* uses the red reflex to test for bifoveal fixation. The direct ophthalmoscope is used to obtain a red reflex simultaneously in both eyes. Foveation of the ophthalmoscope filament dims the red reflex. If strabismus is present, the deviated eye will have a lighter and brighter reflex than the fixating eye. The Brückner test is used mainly by primary care practitioners to screen for strabismus; observation of the red reflex in this setting can also identify opacities in the visual axis and refractive errors. See also Chapter 1.

Subjective Tests

The *Maddox rod test* uses a device consisting of a series of parallel cylinders that converts a point source of light into a line image. The optical properties of the cylinders cause the streak of light to be situated 90° to the orientation of the parallel cylinders. Because fusion is precluded by the Maddox rod, heterophorias and heterotropias cannot be differentiated. The Maddox rod can be used to test for horizontal and vertical deviations and, when used in conjunction with another Maddox rod, for cyclodeviations.

To test for horizontal deviations, the clinician places the Maddox rod in front of 1 eye (for this example, the right eye) with the cylinders positioned horizontally. The patient fixates on a point source of light; he or she sees a vertical line with the right eye and the point source of white light with the left eye. If the light superimposes on the line, orthophoria is present. If the light is to the left of the line, an esodeviation is present; if the light is to the right of the line, an exodeviation is present. To measure the amount of deviation, the examiner finds the prism that superimposes the point source on the line. The Maddox rod test cannot be used satisfactorily to quantitate horizontal deviations, however, because accommodative convergence cannot be controlled. A similar procedure, with the cylinders aligned vertically, is used to test for vertical deviations.

The *double Maddox rod test* (Fig 7-7) is used to measure cyclotropia. Maddox rods are placed in a trial frame or phoropter and positioned in front of each eye, with the rods aligned vertically so that the patient sees 2 horizontal lines. The patient or examiner

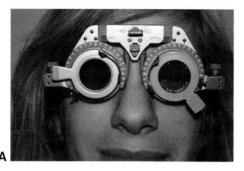 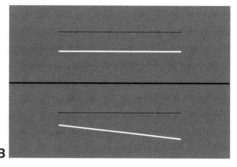

A **B**

Figure 7-7 Double Maddox rod test. **A,** The cylinders are aligned vertically to produce 2 horizontal lines. **B,** *Top:* View of a patient with a small left hypertropia and no torsion. *Bottom:* View of a patient with a small left hypertropia and extorsion. *(Part A courtesy of Scott Olitsky, MD; part B courtesy of Steven Archer, MD.)*

rotates the axes of the rods until the lines are perceived to be parallel. To facilitate the patient's recognition of the 2 lines, it is often helpful to dissociate the lines by placing a small prism base-up or base-down in front of 1 eye. The angle of rotation that causes the line images to appear parallel determines the magnitude and direction (intorsion or extorsion) of cyclotropia. Traditionally, a red Maddox rod is placed before the right eye and a white Maddox rod before the left, but evidence suggests that the different colors can cause fixation artifacts; these artifacts do not occur if the same color is used bilaterally. In congenital conditions such as congenital superior oblique palsy, the patient often does not subjectively appreciate the torsion and will not indicate any torsion with the double Maddox rod test. In these cases, observation of the fundus with an indirect ophthalmoscope for torsion can aid diagnosis.

The *Lancaster red-green test* (and variations such as the Hess, Harms, and Lee screening tests) uses red-green goggles that can be reversed, a red-slit projector, a green-slit projector, and a screen ruled into squares. The patient's head is held steady; by convention, the test is begun with the red filter in front of the right eye. The examiner projects a red slit onto the screen, and the patient is asked to place the green slit so that it appears to coincide with the red slit. The relative positions of the 2 streaks are then recorded. The test is repeated for the diagnostic positions of gaze, and the goggles are then reversed so that the deviation that occurs with the fellow eye fixating can be recorded. The Lancaster red-green test is used primarily for patients with complicated incomitant strabismus and requires that the patient have normal retinal correspondence (see Chapter 6).

The *major amblyoscope* (Fig 7-8A) is a versatile instrument that can be used to measure ocular alignment subjectively or with cover testing. For subjective measurements, dissimilar targets are presented to each eye, and the patient is asked to superimpose them. If the patient has normal retinal correspondence, the horizontal, vertical, and torsional deviations can be read directly from the calibrated scale of the amblyoscope (Fig 7-8B). Also see the section Amblyoscope Testing, later in this chapter.

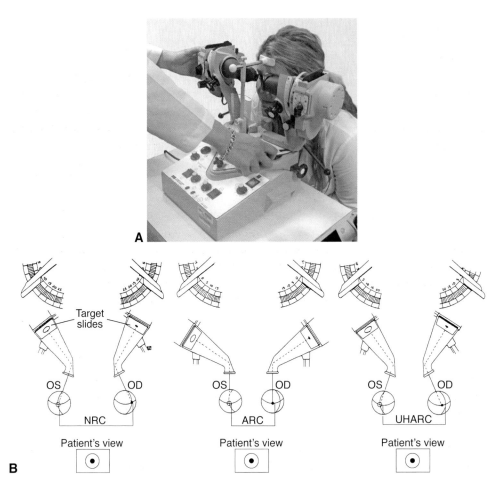

Figure 7-8 A, The major amblyoscope. Targets can be placed in each arm of the device to be presented separately to each eye. The arms can then be moved to compensate for ocular misalignment. **B,** Testing with a major amblyoscope for retinal correspondence in a patient with 20Δ of esotropia. *NRC* = (harmonious) normal retinal correspondence; *ARC* = anomalous retinal correspondence; *UHARC* = unharmonious anomalous retinal correspondence. *(Part A courtesy of Steven Archer, MD; part B modified with permission from von Noorden GK, Campos EC. Binocular Vision and Ocular Motility: Theory and Management of Strabismus. 6th ed. St Louis: Mosby; 2002:229.)*

Assessment of Eye Movements

Ocular Rotations

Generally, when eye movements are assessed, versions are tested first. The examiner should pay particular attention to the movements of both eyes into the 9 diagnostic positions of gaze. Limitations in movement into these positions and asymmetric excursion of the 2 eyes (such as "overaction") should be noted. Spinning the child, or provoking the doll's head maneuver, may be helpful in eliciting vestibular-stimulated eye movements. If versions are not full, duction movements should be tested for each eye separately. BCSC Section 5, *Neuro-Ophthalmology,* also discusses testing of the ocular motility system.

Convergence

Alignment at near fixation is usually measured at 33 cm directly in front of the patient in the horizontal plane. Comparing the alignment in primary position at both distance and near fixation helps the examiner assess the accommodative convergence (synkinetic near) reflex. The *near point of convergence* is determined by placing a fixation object at 40 cm in the midsagittal plane of the patient's head. As the patient fixates on the object, it is moved toward the patient until 1 eye loses fixation and turns out. The point at which this occurs is the near point of convergence. The eye that maintains fixation is considered the dominant eye. The normal near point of convergence is 8–10 cm or less. This determination does not distinguish between fusional convergence and accommodative convergence.

Accommodative convergence/accommodation ratio

The *accommodative convergence/accommodation (AC/A) ratio* is defined as the amount of convergence (in prism diopters) per unit change in accommodation (in diopters). There are 2 methods of clinical measurement (see also BCSC Section 3, *Clinical Optics*): the gradient method and the heterophoria method.

1. The *gradient method* arrives at the AC/A ratio by dividing the change in deviation in prism diopters by the change in lens power. An accommodative target must be used, and the working distance (typically .33 m or 6 m) is held constant. Plus or minus lenses (eg, +1.00, +2.00, +3.00, −1.00, −2.00, −3.00) are used to vary the accommodative requirement. This method measures the *stimulus AC/A ratio,* which is not necessarily identical to the *response AC/A ratio.* The latter can be determined only with the use of an optometer that records the change in accommodation actually produced.
2. In the *heterophoria method,* the distance and near deviations are used, along with the interpupillary distance, to calculate the AC/A ratio. A rough clinical estimate can be made by comparing distance and near fixation alignment. If the patient is more exotropic or less esotropic at near fixation, too little convergence, or a low AC/A ratio, is present; if the patient is more esotropic or less exotropic at near, a high AC/A ratio is present. In accommodative esotropia, a difference in esotropia of 10Δ or more between distance and near fixation is considered to represent a high AC/A ratio.

Fusional Vergence

Vergences are movements of the 2 eyes in opposite directions; they are also discussed in Chapter 5. Fusional vergences are motor responses that serve to eliminate horizontal, vertical, or, to a limited degree, torsional image disparity. They can be grouped by the following functions:

- *Fusional convergence* eliminates bitemporal retinal disparity and controls an exophoria.
- *Fusional divergence* eliminates binasal retinal disparity and controls an esophoria.
- *Vertical fusional vergence* controls a hyperphoria or hypophoria.
- *Torsional fusional vergence* controls an incyclophoria or excyclophoria.

Table 7-1 Average Normal Fusional Vergence Amplitudes in Prism Diopters (Δ)

Testing Distance	Convergence	Divergence	Vertical
6 m	14	6	2.5
25 cm	38	16	2.6

Fusional vergence can be measured by using a major amblyoscope, a rotary prism, or a bar prism and gradually increasing the prism power until diplopia occurs. Accommodation must be controlled during fusional vergence testing. Normal fusional vergence amplitudes are listed in Table 7-1. Fusional vergence can be altered by the following:

- *Compensatory mechanisms:* As a tendency to deviate evolves, a larger-than-normal fusional vergence develops for that deviation. Very large fusional vergences are common in compensated, long-standing vertical deviations and in exodeviations.
- *Change in visual acuity:* An improvement in acuity may improve the fusional vergence mechanism and change a symptomatic intermittent deviation to an asymptomatic heterophoria.
- *State of awareness:* Fatigue, illness, or drug or alcohol ingestion may decrease the fusional vergence mechanism, converting a heterophoria to a heterotropia.
- *Orthoptics:* Orthoptic exercises may increase the magnitude of the fusional vergence mechanism (mainly fusional convergence). This treatment works best for near fusional convergence, particularly convergence insufficiency.
- *Optical stimulation of fusional vergence:* In controlled accommodative esotropia, reducing the strength of the hyperopic or bifocal correction induces an esophoria that stimulates fusional divergence. In other cases, the power of prisms used to control diplopia may be gradually reduced to stimulate compensatory fusional vergence.

Special Tests

Motor Tests

Special motor tests include the forced-duction test, active force generation, and saccadic velocity measurement. See also BCSC Section 5, *Neuro-Ophthalmology.*

- In the *forced-duction test,* forceps are used to move the eye into various positions and thereby determine resistance to passive movement. This test is usually performed at the time of surgery but can sometimes be performed in the clinic with topical anesthesia in cooperative patients.
- *Active force generation* assesses the relative strength of a muscle. The patient is asked to move the eye in a given direction while the observer grasps the eye with an instrument. If the muscle tested is paretic, the examiner feels less-than-normal tension.
- *Saccadic velocity measurement* can be performed using a special instrument that graphically records the speed and direction of eye movement. This test is useful for

distinguishing paralysis from restriction. If the muscle is paralyzed, the saccadic velocity remains low throughout the movement of the involved eye, whereas if the muscle is restricted, the velocity is initially normal but rapidly decelerates when the eye reaches the limit of its movement. Clinical observation can allow qualitative assessment of saccadic velocity; with this method, *floating saccades* indicate muscle paresis.

Assessment of the Field of Single Binocular Vision

The field of single binocular vision may be tested on a Goldmann perimeter. This is useful for following the recovery of a paretic muscle or for measuring the outcome of surgery to alleviate diplopia. A small white test object is followed by both eyes in the cardinal positions throughout the visual field. When the patient indicates that the test object is seen double, the point is plotted. The field of binocular vision normally measures about 45°–50° from the fixation point except where it is blocked by the nose (Fig 7-9). Weighted templates that reflect the greater importance of single binocular vision in primary and reading positions can be used to quantify the diplopia field.

> Sullivan TJ, Kraft SP, Burack C, O'Reilly C. A functional scoring method for the field of binocular single vision. *Ophthalmology.* 1992;99(4):575–581.

3-Step Test

There are 8 cyclovertical muscles (4 in each eye): the 2 *depressors* of each eye are the *inferior rectus (IR)* and *superior oblique (SO) muscles;* the 2 *elevators* of each eye are the *superior rectus (SR)* and *inferior oblique (IO) muscles.* Weakness of the cyclovertical muscles, especially the superior oblique muscles, is often responsible for hyperdeviations. The *3-step test* is an algorithm that can be used to help identify the weak cyclovertical muscle. As helpful as the test is, however, it is not always diagnostic and can be misleading, especially in patients in whom more than 1 muscle is paralyzed, in patients who have undergone strabismus surgery, in the presence of a skew deviation, and in the presence of restrictions or dissociated vertical deviation (see Chapter 11). The 3-step test is performed as outlined in the following subsections (Fig 7-10; also see Chapter 11, Fig 11-4).

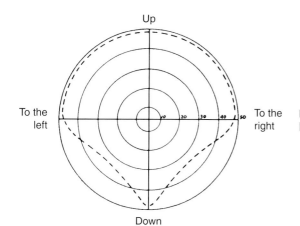

Figure 7-9 The normal field of single binocular vision.

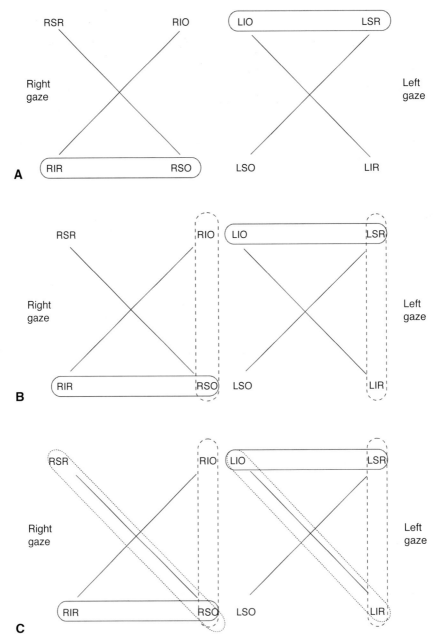

Figure 7-10 The 3-step test. **A,** Step 1: A right hypertropia suggests weakness in 1 of the 2 depressors of the right eye (RIR or RSO) or in 1 of the 2 elevators of the left eye (LIO or LSR). **B,** Step 2: Worsening of the right hypertropia on left gaze implicates either the RSO or the LSR. Note that at the end of step 2, 1 depressor and 1 elevator of opposite eyes will be identified as the possible weak muscle. **C,** Step 3: The right head tilt causes intorsion of the right eye. Because this rotation depends on activation of both the RSO (a depressor) and the RSR (an elevator), weakness of the RSO will cause the right hypertropia to increase.

Step 1

Determine which eye is hypertropic (see Fig 7-2). Step 1 narrows the number of possible underacting muscles from 8 to 4. In the example shown in Figure 7-10, the right eye has been found to be hypertropic. This means that the paralysis will be found in either the depressors of the right eye (RIR, RSO) or the elevators of the left eye (LIO, LSR). Draw an oval around these 2 muscle groups (see Fig 7-10A).

Step 2

Determine whether the vertical deviation is greater in right gaze or in left gaze. In the example, the deviation is larger in left gaze. This implicates 1 of the 4 vertically acting muscles used in left gaze. Draw an oval around the 4 vertically acting muscles that are used in left gaze (see Fig 7-10B). At the end of step 2, the 2 remaining possible muscles (1 in each eye) are either both intortors or both extortors and are either both superior or both inferior muscles (1 rectus and 1 oblique). Note that in Figure 7-10B, the increased left-gaze deviation eliminates 2 inferior muscles and implicates 2 superior muscles.

Step 3

Known as the *Bielschowsky head-tilt test,* the final step involves tilting the head to the right and left during distance fixation. Head tilt to the right stimulates intorsion of the right eye (RSR, RSO) and extorsion of the left eye (LIR, LIO). Head tilt to the left stimulates extorsion of the right eye (RIR, RIO) and intorsion of the left eye (LSR, LSO). Normally, the 2 intortors and the 2 extortors of each eye have *opposite* vertical actions that cancel each other. If 1 intortor or 1 extortor is weak, the vertical action of the other ipsilateral torting muscle becomes manifest.

To continue the example, Figure 7-10C shows that when the head is tilted to the right, the right eye moves upward as it attempts to intort to maintain fixation, increasing the vertical deviation. This suggests that the vertical action of the right superior rectus muscle is unopposed, indicating that the right superior oblique muscle is weak and is the palsied muscle. (See also Chapter 11, Fig 11-3.)

Prism Adaptation Test

In the prism adaptation test, the patient is fitted with prisms to align the visual axes, which can help predict whether fusion may be restored following surgery.

Torticollis: Differential Diagnosis and Evaluation

Torticollis is an abnormal head position (AHP) due to rotation of the head around any of the 3 axes (head turn, chin-up or chin-down, or tilt), alone or in combination. Patients with torticollis are often referred to ophthalmologists as part of a comprehensive evaluation because torticollis can be associated with a variety of eye movement disorders, including strabismus. Early diagnosis and correction of ocular causes of torticollis is particularly important in children, because prolonged AHP may result in permanent facial asymmetry or secondary musculoskeletal changes. Common causes of both ocular and nonocular torticollis appear in Table 7-2.

Ocular Torticollis

Although the association between an AHP and ocular abnormality can be simply a shared underlying cause (eg, ocular tilt reaction), more often the AHP is a compensatory response to the ocular condition that results in improved binocularity, visual acuity, or centration of a limited visual field.

A patient with incomitant strabismus can often improve binocular alignment by adopting an AHP. Conditions that commonly cause an AHP include superior oblique palsy, Duane retraction syndrome, Brown syndrome, blowout fractures, and thyroid eye disease. Patients with unilateral ptosis may use a chin-up head posture to maintain binocularity.

Congenital nystagmus that damps at a null point is the most common condition in which better visual acuity is the motivation for an AHP. An AHP can also develop in jerk

Table 7-2 Differential Diagnosis of Torticollis (Abnormal Head Position)

Ocular torticollis	Nonocular torticollis
Nystagmus	Congenital muscular torticollis
Congenital nystagmus (null point)	Skeletal abnormalities
Manifest latent nystagmus (damp in	Congenital abnormalities (eg, Klippel-Feil
adduction)	syndrome)
Periodic alternating nystagmus	Traumatic abnormalities
Spasmus nutans	Neurologic conditions
Acquired adult jerk nystagmus	Syringomyelia
Paretic strabismus	Dystonia
Superior oblique palsy	Posterior fossa lesions
Duane retraction syndrome	Deafness in one ear
Sixth nerve palsy	Sandifer syndrome
Third nerve palsy	Psychogenic disease
Inferior oblique palsy	
Restrictive strabismus	
Brown syndrome	
Thyroid eye disease	
Orbital fracture	
Congenital fibrosis of extraocular muscles	
Supranuclear disorders	
Monocular elevation deficiency	
Dorsal midbrain syndrome	
Gaze palsy	
A- or V-pattern esotropia or exotropia	
Dissociated vertical deviation	
Ocular tilt reaction	
Monocular blindness (due to associated	
manifest latent nystagmus or for	
centration of remaining field)	
Homonymous hemianopia	
Ptosis	
Refractive errors	

nystagmus that damps with gaze in the direction of the slow phase (eg, manifest latent nystagmus [fusion maldevelopment nystagmus syndrome]). Other conditions in which a need for better visual acuity drives the AHP include bilateral ptosis and refractive errors. With bilateral duction deficits (eg, congenital fibrosis of extraocular muscles), an AHP may be needed for foveation.

Patients with homonymous hemianopia and monocular patients may turn their head toward their blind side to center their visual field relative to their body. In rare cases, patients with superior oblique palsy have a paradoxical head tilt to the wrong side, which increases the separation between diplopic images, possibly to reduce the conflict between the 2 images when fusion is not possible.

Diagnostic evaluation of ocular torticollis

Ophthalmologic evaluation of the patient with torticollis focuses on determining whether there is an ocular cause for the AHP. The duration of the torticollis can be a diagnostic clue, but the history is sometimes misleading. Parents may not recognize chronic AHP; examining old photographs can be helpful in this situation. Cycloplegic retinoscopy is performed to look for uncorrected refractive errors. Motility testing should be done with particular attention to gaze positions opposite those favored by the AHP. Nystagmus is usually obvious, but subtle nystagmus may be visible only during slit-lamp or fundus examination. Fundus examination may reveal extorsion suggestive of superior oblique palsy or conjugate torsion (extorsion in 1 eye and intorsion in the other), as seen in the ocular tilt reaction. If placing the patient in the supine position eliminates the head tilt, a musculoskeletal etiology is unlikely. If the diagnosis is uncertain, a period of monocular occlusion may be tried; elimination of the AHP during this period can establish that the purpose of the torticollis is to maintain binocular vision.

The axis of the AHP can be an important diagnostic consideration. Some conditions are uniquely associated with one type of AHP. For example, a head turn is associated with sixth nerve palsy, a chin-up posture with ptosis, and a chin-down posture with V-pattern esotropia or A-pattern exotropia. Other conditions most commonly produce an AHP in a particular axis but can sometimes produce an AHP in other axes. For example, patients with left superior oblique palsy usually assume a right head tilt to minimize the left hypertropia; however, the deviation is smaller in left gaze, leading some patients to employ a right head turn, either alone or in combination with a right head tilt. Patients with congenital nystagmus usually adopt a head turn to take advantage of a horizontal null point, but sometimes, a vertical or torsional component of the null point results in an AHP that includes components of chin-up posture, chin-down posture, or a head tilt.

Tests of Sensory Adaptation and Binocular Cooperation

Assessment of the vergence system indicates the extent to which the 2 eyes can be directed at the same object. Sensory binocularity involves the use of both eyes together to form a unified perception. In general, normal sensory binocularity depends on normal fusional vergence. Ideally, testing should therefore be performed before binocularity is disrupted by occlusion of either eye. When the vergence system fails and manifest strabismus occurs, the sensory response is diplopia, suppression, or anomalous retinal correspondence (ARC) (see Chapter 6). While a variety of sensory tests have historically provided a framework for understanding sensory adaptations in strabismus, only the Worth 4-dot test and stereopsis testing are used routinely in clinical practice. A shortcoming of all tests is the inability of the testing conditions to reproduce the patient's condition of normal seeing. The more dissociative the test, the less the test simulates everyday use of the eyes. The examiner should always perform these tests in conjunction with a cover test to determine whether a fusion response is due to orthophoria or ARC.

Red-Glass Test

In a patient with strabismus, the red-glass (diplopia) test involves stimulation of both the fovea of the fixating eye and an extrafoveal area of the other eye. First, the patient's deviation is measured objectively. Then a red glass is placed before the nondeviating eye while the patient fixates on a white light, such as the light from a Finhoff transilluminator. This test can be performed at both distance and near fixation. If the patient sees only 1 light (either red or white), suppression is present (Fig 7-11A). A 5Δ or 10Δ prism base-up in front of the deviated eye can be used to move the image out of the suppression scotoma, causing the patient to experience diplopia. With normal retinal correspondence (NRC), the white image will be localized correctly: the white image is seen below and to the side of the left image (Fig 7-11B). With ARC, the white image will be localized incorrectly: it is seen directly below the image (Fig 7-11C).

In the absence of suppression, the following responses are possible with the red-glass test:

- If the patient has esotropia, the images appear uncrossed (eg, if the red glass is over the left eye, the red light is to the left of the white light). This response is known as *homonymous,* or *uncrossed, diplopia.* This can easily be remembered because the esotropic patient sees the red light on the same side as the red glass (Fig 7-11D). If the patient has exotropia, the images appear crossed (eg, if the red glass is over the left eye, the red light is to the right of the white light). This response is known as *heteronymous,* or *crossed, diplopia* (Fig 7-11E). If the separation between the 2 images equals the previously determined deviation, the patient has NRC.
- If the patient sees the 2 lights superimposed so that they appear pinkish despite a measurable esotropia or exotropia, the localization of retinal points is abnormal. This condition is known as *harmonious anomalous retinal correspondence.*
- If the patient sees 2 lights (with uncrossed diplopia in esotropia and with crossed diplopia in exotropia) but the separation between the 2 images is less than the previously determined deviation, the patient has *unharmonious anomalous retinal correspondence.* Some investigators consider unharmonious ARC to be an artifact of testing.

Bagolini Lenses

Bagolini striated lenses have many narrow striations running parallel in 1 meridian that function like Maddox cylinders and cause the fixation light to appear as an elongated streak. The lenses are usually placed at 135° in front of the right eye and at 45° in front of the left eye. The advantages of the Bagolini glasses are that they afford the most natural

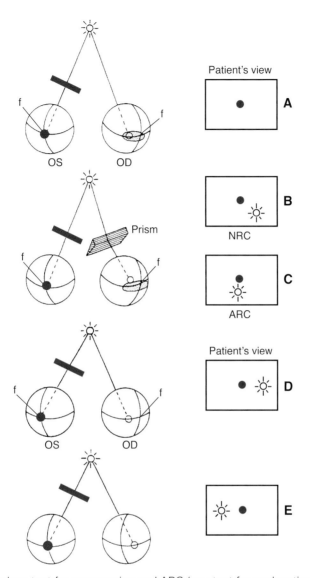

Figure 7-11   Red-glass test for suppression and ARC (see text for explanation; see also Chapter 6, Fig 6-5). *(Modified with permission from von Noorden GK, Campos EC.* Binocular Vision and Ocular Motility: Theory and Management of Strabismus. *6th ed. St Louis: Mosby; 2002:223.)*

testing conditions and permit the examiner to perform cover testing during the examination. Figure 7-12 summarizes some of the possible subjective results of this test. In monofixation syndrome, the central scotoma is perceived as a gap in one of the lines surrounding the fixation light.

4Δ Base-Out Prism Test

The 4Δ base-out prism test is a diagnostic maneuver performed primarily to document the presence of a small facultative scotoma in a patient with monofixation syndrome and

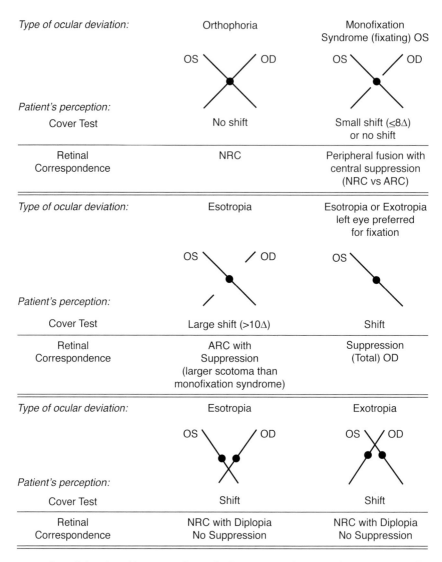

Figure 7-12 Bagolini striated lens test for retinal correspondence and suppression. For these figures, the Bagolini lenses are oriented at 135° in front of the right eye and at 45° in front of the left eye. The perception of the oblique lines seen by each eye under binocular conditions is shown. Examples of the types of strabismus in which these responses are commonly found are given.

no manifest deviation (see Chapter 6). In this test, a 4Δ base-out prism is quickly placed before 1 eye and then the other during binocular viewing, and motor responses are observed (Fig 7-13). Patients with bifixation usually show a version (bilateral) movement away from the eye covered by the prism followed by a unilateral fusional convergence movement of the eye not behind the prism. A similar response occurs regardless of which eye the prism is placed over. Often in monofixation syndrome, no movement is seen when the prism is placed before the nonfixating eye. A refixation version movement is seen

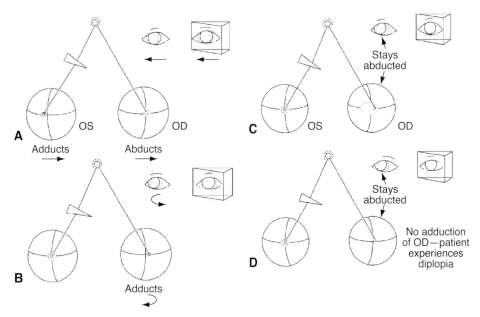

Figure 7-13 The 4Δ base-out prism test. **A,** When a prism is placed over the left eye, dextroversion occurs during refixation of that eye, indicating absence of foveal suppression in the left eye. If a suppression scotoma is present in the left eye, neither eye will move when the prism is placed before the left eye. **B,** Slow fusional adduction movement of the right eye is then observed, indicating absence of foveal suppression in the right eye. **C,** In a second patient, the right eye stays abducted, and the absence of adduction movement, as shown in part **B,** indicates foveal suppression in the right eye. **D,** Weak fusion is another cause of absence of adduction movement; such patients experience diplopia until refusion occurs spontaneously. *(Modified with permission from von Noorden GK, Campos EC.* Binocular Vision and Ocular Motility: Theory and Management of Strabismus. *6th ed. St Louis: Mosby; 2002:220.)*

when the prism is placed before the fixating eye, but the expected subsequent fusional convergence does not occur.

The 4Δ base-out prism test is the least reliable method of documenting the presence of a macular scotoma. Occasionally, a patient with bifixation recognizes diplopia when the prism is placed before an eye but makes no convergence movement to correct for it. Patients with monofixation syndrome may switch fixation each time the prism is placed and show no movement, regardless of which eye is tested.

Afterimage Test

This test involves the stimulation, or labeling, of the macula of each eye with a different linear afterimage, 1 horizontal and 1 vertical. Because suppression scotomata extend along the horizontal retinal meridian and may obscure most of a horizontal afterimage, the vertical afterimage is placed on the macula of the deviating eye and the horizontal afterimage on the macula of the fixating eye by having each eye fixate on a linear light filament separately. The test can also be performed by covering a camera flash with black paper and exposing only a narrow slit; the center of the slit is covered with black tape to serve as a fixation point, as well as to protect the fovea from exposure. In the presence of eccentric fixation (see Chapter 4), there is no assurance that the afterimage will be aligned with the fovea; thus, the test cannot be interpreted. The patient is then asked to draw the relative positions of the perceived afterimages. Possible perceptions are shown in Figure 7-14.

Amblyoscope Testing

Although its use has declined, the major amblyoscope (discussed earlier; see Fig 7-8A) was a mainstay in the assessment and treatment of strabismus for decades. The amblyoscope can measure horizontal, vertical, and torsional deviations. Because it can neutralize torsion, it is still useful for distinguishing between central fusion disruption (see Chapter 6) and inability to fuse because of a large cyclodeviation. It can also assess suppression, retinal correspondence, fusional amplitudes, and stereopsis and may be used for exercises designed to overcome suppression and increase fusional amplitudes.

Worth 4-Dot Test

The Worth 4-dot test (Fig 7-15) is often considered a test of sensory fusion; however, it does not test sensory fusion directly as there is no fusible feature in the test. Its best use is to test for a suppression scotoma. The test uses red-green glasses—traditionally, the red lens is placed in front of the right eye and the green lens in front of the left—and a target consisting of 4 dots: 1 red, 2 green, and 1 white. The red lens blocks the green light, and the green lens blocks the red light, so the red and green dots are each seen by only 1 eye. The white dot is the only feature seen by both eyes, but it is seen in color rivalry in a patient with fusion ability. The polarized Worth 4-dot test uses polarized glasses rather than red and green ones. The stimulus dots can be presented in a wall-mounted display or by a handheld flashlight. The test should be administered in good ambient light so that

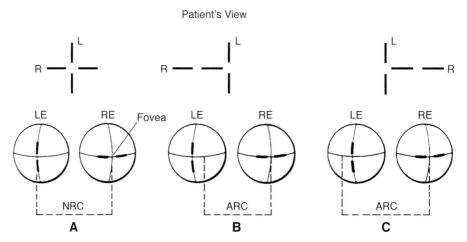

Figure 7-14 Afterimage test. **A,** Normal retinal correspondence. **B,** Crossed ARC in a case of esotropia. **C,** Uncrossed ARC in a case of exotropia. *(Modified with permission from von Noorden GK, Campos EC. Binocular Vision and Ocular Motility: Theory and Management of Strabismus. 6th ed. St Louis: Mosby; 2002:227.)*

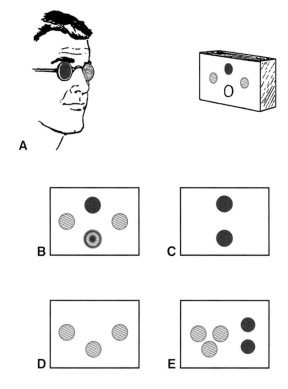

Figure 7-15 Worth 4-dot test. **A,** Looking through a pair of red-green glasses, the patient views a box with 4 lights (1 red, 2 green, 1 white) at 6 m and at 33 cm (with the 4 lights mounted on a flashlight). The possible responses are given in parts B to E. **B,** Patient sees all 4 lights: Peripheral fusion with orthophoria or strabismus with ARC. The light in the 6 o'clock position is seen in color rivalry or, depending on ocular dominance, as predominantly red or predominantly green. **C,** Patient sees 2 red lights: Suppression in left eye. **D,** Patient sees 3 green lights: Suppression in right eye. **E,** Patient sees 5 lights: Uncrossed diplopia with esotropia if the red lights appear to the right of the green lights, as in this figure; crossed diplopia with exotropia if the red lights appear to the left. *(Modified with permission from von Noorden GK, Campos EC. Binocular Vision and Ocular Motility: Theory and Management of Strabismus. 6th ed. St Louis: Mosby; 2002:221.)*

peripheral features in the room can stimulate motor fusion. The patient then reports the number of dots seen:

- Seeing 2 dots indicates a suppression scotoma in the left eye.
- Seeing 3 dots indicates a suppression scotoma in the right eye.
- Seeing 4 dots indicates that there is some degree of sensory fusion and that the patient has NRC (if there is no manifest strabismus) or harmonious ARC (if there is manifest strabismus). If there is a scotoma, the perception of 4 dots indicates that the scotoma must be smaller than the test target.
- Seeing 5 dots is a diplopia response. The patient has manifest strabismus without suppression or ARC.

In *monofixation syndrome* (see Chapter 6), the Worth 4-dot test can be used to demonstrate both the presence of peripheral fusion and the absence of bifixation. The standard Worth 4-dot flashlight projects onto a central retinal area of 1° or less when viewed at 3 m (10 ft), well within the 1°–4° scotoma characteristic of monofixation syndrome. Therefore, patients with monofixation syndrome will report seeing 2 or 3 lights, depending on their ocular fixation preference. As the Worth 4-dot flashlight is brought closer to the patient, the dots project onto more peripheral retina outside the central monofixation scotoma and a fusion response (4 lights) is obtained. This usually occurs between 0.67 m and 1 m (2–3 ft).

Stereoacuity Testing

Stereopsis occurs when the 2 retinal images—which have small disparities due to the horizontal separation of the eyes—are cortically integrated. There are 2 types of stereopsis tests: *contour* and *random dot. Contour stereopsis tests* involve horizontal separation of physical contours presented to each eye (with polarized or red-green glasses). At larger disparities, monocular cues are present in this type of test. *Random-dot stereopsis tests* avoid the problem of monocular cue artifacts by embedding the stereoscopic figures in a background of random dots.

In the *Stereo Fly test* (a contour stereopsis test), a card with superimposed images of a fly is shown to the patient. Ability to detect the elevation of the fly's wings above the plane of the card indicates stereopsis. Because the separation of the superimposed images is 3000 seconds of arc, this test is one of gross stereopsis. In other figures on the card, there is less separation between the superimposed images. Thus, quantitation of finer stereoacuity is possible in cooperative patients.

Several types of random-dot stereopsis tests are clinically useful. The *Randot test,* in which polarized glasses are worn, can measure stereoacuity down to 20 seconds of arc. The *Random-Dot E test* employs a preferential looking strategy to test stereopsis and is used in pediatric vision screening programs. In the *TNO test,* red-green glasses are used to separate the images seen by each eye. The *Lang stereopsis tests* do not require glasses to produce a random-dot stereoscopic effect and therefore may be useful in young children who object to wearing glasses.

Stereopsis can also be measured at distance using a chart projector with a vectographic slide, the Smart System PC-Plus (M&S Technologies, Niles, IL) or the Frisby Davis Distance Stereotest (Stereotest Ltd, Sheffield, United Kingdom). Distance stereoacuity tests may be helpful in monitoring control of intermittent exotropia.

Related Videos

The following videos contain additional information on topics covered in this chapter and are available at www.aao.org/bcscvideo. Mobile-device users can scan the QR code below to access the videos.

- Versions and Ductions (1 min, 50 sec)
- Cover Test (55 sec)
- Alternate Prism Cover Test (54 sec)
- Simultaneous Prism Cover Test (13 sec)

CHAPTER 8

Esodeviations

An *esodeviation* is a latent or manifest convergent misalignment of the visual axes. Esodeviations are the most common type of strabismus, accounting for more than 50% of ocular deviations in the pediatric population.

Epidemiology

Esodeviations occur in equal frequency in males and females, and they are more common in Caucasian and African American ethnic groups than in Asian ethnic groups in the United States. Risk factors for the development of esotropia include anisometropia and hyperopia, neurodevelopmental impairment, prematurity, low birth weight, craniofacial or chromosomal anomalies, maternal smoking during pregnancy, and family history of strabismus. The prevalence of esotropia increases with age (higher prevalence at 48–72 months compared with 6–11 months), moderate anisometropia, and moderate amounts of hyperopia. In some families, a mendelian inheritance pattern has been observed. Amblyopia develops in approximately 50% of children who have esotropia.

Esodeviations can result from innervational, anatomical, mechanical, refractive, or accommodative factors. There are several major types of esodeviations, and they can be classified as comitant or incomitant (Table 8-1).

Cotter SA, Varma R, Tarczy-Hornoch K, et al; Joint Writing Committee for the Multi-Ethnic Pediatric Eye Disease Study and the Baltimore Pediatric Eye Disease Study Groups. Risk factors associated with childhood strabismus. *Ophthalmology.* 2011;118(11):2251–2261.

Pseudoesotropia

Pseudoesotropia refers to the false appearance of esotropia when the visual axes are actually aligned. The appearance may be caused by a flat, broad nasal bridge; prominent epicanthal folds, a narrow interpupillary distance, or a negative angle kappa (see Chapter 7). The observer sees less sclera nasally than would be expected, which creates the impression that the eye is turned in toward the nose. This is especially noticeable when the child gazes to either side. Because no real deviation exists, results of both corneal light reflex testing and cover testing are normal.

Table 8-1 Major Types of Esodeviation

Comitant Esotropia

Infantile (congenital) esotropia
  Ciancia syndrome
Accommodative esotropia
  Refractive (normal AC/A ratio)
  Nonrefractive (high AC/A ratio)
  Partially accommodative
Acquired nonaccommodative esotropia
  Basic
  Cyclic
  Sensory (deprivation)
  Divergence insufficiency and divergence paralysis
    Primary
    Secondary
  Spasm of the near reflex
  Consecutive
    Spontaneous
    Postsurgical
Nystagmus and esotropia
  Fusion maldevelopment nystagmus syndrome
  Nystagmus blockage syndrome

Incomitant Esotropia

Sixth nerve palsy
Medial rectus muscle restriction following excessive resection
Thyroid eye disease
Medial orbital wall fracture
Congenital fibrosis of the extraocular muscles
Esotropia associated with high myopia
Duane retraction syndrome
Möbius syndrome

AC/A = accommodative convergence/accommodation.

Infantile (Congenital) Esotropia

Infantile esotropia is defined as an esotropia that is present by 6 months of age. Some ophthalmologists refer to this disorder as *congenital esotropia*. However, because the onset is usually not at birth, the term *infantile esotropia* is more accurate and will be used in this volume.

Variable, transient, intermittent strabismus is commonly observed in the first 2–3 months of life. Also, it is common to see both intermittent esotropia and exotropia in the same infant (termed *ocular instability of infancy*). This condition should resolve by 3 months of age but can sometimes persist, especially in premature infants. If an esotropia is present after age 2 months, is constant, and measures 30 prism diopters (Δ) or more, it is unlikely to resolve and will probably require surgical intervention.

Patients with infantile esotropia often have a family history of esotropia or strabismus, but well-defined genetic patterns are unusual. Infantile esotropia occurs in up to 30% of children with neurologic and developmental problems, including cerebral palsy, hydrocephalus, and prematurity. Infantile esotropia has been associated with an increased risk of development of mental illness by early adulthood (2.6 times higher compared with controls).

> Olson JH, Louwagie CR, Diehl NN, Mohney BG. Congenital esotropia and the risk of mental illness by early adulthood. *Ophthalmology.* 2012;119(1):145–149.

Pathogenesis

The cause of infantile esotropia remains unknown. The debate regarding its etiology has focused on the implications of 2 conflicting theories. The Worth "sensory" concept proposes that infantile esotropia results from a congenital deficit in a "fusion center" in the brain. According to this theory, the goal of restoring binocularity is futile. In contrast, the Chavasse theory proposes that the primary problem in infantile esotropia is one of motor development, which is potentially curable if ocular alignment is achieved in infancy. Several authors have reported favorable sensory results in infants operated on between 6 months and 2 years of age, and these encouraging results have become the basis for the practice of early surgery for infantile esotropia.

Evaluation

Visual behavior or visual acuity of the 2 eyes can be equal, in which case alternating fixation will be present. Amblyopia is commonly associated, however. If amblyopia is present, a fixation preference can be observed. Cross-fixation, in which a large-angle esotropia is associated with the use of the adducted eye for fixation of objects in the contralateral temporal field, is also frequent (Fig 8-1).

Versions and ductions are often normal initially. The deviation is comitant and characteristically larger than 30Δ. Overelevation in adduction and dissociated strabismus complex develop in more than 50% of patients, usually after 1–2 years of age. There may be an apparent abduction deficit because of cross-fixation; children with equal vision in both eyes have no need to abduct either eye on side gaze. If amblyopia is present, the better-seeing eye will fixate in all fields of gaze, making the amblyopic eye appear to have an abduction deficit. The infant's ability to abduct each eye can be demonstrated with the doll's head maneuver or by observation with either eye patched. The clinician can also hold the infant and spin in a circle, which stimulates the vestibulo-ocular reflex and helps demonstrate full abduction.

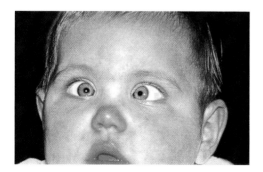

Figure 8-1 Infantile esotropia. *(Reproduced from Archer SM. Esotropia.* Focal Points: Clinical Modules for Ophthalmologists. *San Francisco: American Academy of Ophthalmology; 1994, module 12.)*

Asymmetry of monocular horizontal smooth pursuit is normal in infants up to age 6 months, with the nasal-to-temporal direction less well developed than the temporal-to-nasal. Patients with infantile esotropia have persistent smooth pursuit asymmetry throughout their lives. Fusion maldevelopment nystagmus syndrome (also known as *latent* and *manifest latent nystagmus*) is also a commonly associated motility anomaly. Cycloplegic refraction characteristically reveals low hyperopia (1.00–2.00 diopters [D]).

A severe form of infantile esotropia, referred to as *Ciancia syndrome,* consists of large-angle esotropia (>50Δ), abducting nystagmus, and mild abduction deficits. Children with this syndrome uniformly use cross-fixation.

Management

Because accommodative esotropia can occur as early as age 4 months, significant hyperopic refractive error should be corrected by prescribing the full cycloplegic refraction. A small-angle esotropia that is variable or intermittent may be more likely to respond to hyperopic correction than would a large-angle or a constant esotropia.

Ocular alignment is rarely achieved without surgery in early-onset esotropia. Previously, it was thought that concurrent amblyopia should be fully treated before surgery. However, it has recently been shown that successful postoperative alignment is as likely to occur in patients with mild to moderate amblyopia at the time of surgery as it is in those whose amblyopia has been fully treated preoperatively. When ocular alignment is achieved earlier, there may be the added benefits of better fusion, stereopsis, and long-term stability.

The goal of surgical treatment of infantile esotropia is to reduce the deviation to orthotropia or as close to it as possible. Ideally, this results in normal vision in each eye and the development of some degree of sensory fusion. Alignment within 8Δ–10Δ of orthotropia frequently results in the development of the monofixation syndrome, characterized by peripheral fusion, central suppression, and favorable appearance. This small-angle strabismus, also known as a *microtropia,* generally represents a stable, functional surgical outcome even though bifoveal fusion is not achieved; it is therefore considered a successful surgical result. In addition, the child's psychological and motor development may improve and accelerate after the eyes are straightened, and bonding between infant and parents may improve.

Most ophthalmologists in North America agree that surgery should be undertaken early. The belief is that the eyes should be aligned by age 24 months, preferably earlier, to optimize binocular cooperation. Surgery can be performed in healthy children as early as age 4 months. The Congenital Esotropia Observational Study showed that when patients with a constant esotropia of at least 40Δ present after 10 weeks of age, the deviations are unlikely to resolve spontaneously. Using this as a basis, some surgeons suggest even earlier surgery, with the aim of achieving a superior sensory outcome. Smaller angles can be monitored, as they may improve spontaneously. However, a European multicenter prospective study (ELISS) comparing early versus delayed strabismus surgery showed only a slight improvement in gross binocularity in the early-surgery group (lower amount of suppression), but a higher number of procedures were performed in the early-surgery group to achieve outcomes similar to those of the delayed-surgery group.

Various surgical approaches have been suggested for infantile esotropia. The most common initial procedure is recession of both medial rectus muscles. Recession of a medial rectus muscle combined with resection of the ipsilateral lateral rectus muscle is also effective. Two-muscle surgery spares the other horizontal rectus muscles for subsequent surgery should it be needed, which is not uncommon. For infants with large deviations (>50Δ–60Δ), some surgeons operate on 3 or even 4 horizontal rectus muscles at the time of the initial surgery, or they add botulinum toxin injection to the medial rectus muscle recession. Significant inferior oblique muscle overaction can be treated at the time of the initial surgery. Chapter 14 discusses surgical procedures in detail.

Botulinum toxin injection alone into the medial rectus muscles has also been used as primary treatment of infantile esotropia. Usually, 2–3 injections into each medial rectus muscle are required, and the average time to achieve alignment is longer with this form of treatment (17 months) than with surgery (2 months).

Birch EE, Stager DR, Everett ME. Random dot stereoacuity following surgical correction of infantile esotropia. *J Pediatr Ophthalmol Strabismus.* 1995;32(4):231–235.

Pediatric Eye Disease Investigator Group. The clinical spectrum of early-onset esotropia: experience of the Congenital Esotropia Observational Study. *Am J Ophthalmol.* 2002;133(1):102–108.

Simonsz HJ, Kolling GH, Unnebrink K. Final report of the early vs. late infantile strabismus surgery study (ELISSS), a controlled, prospective, multicenter study. *Strabismus.* 2005;13(4):169–199.

Accommodative Esotropia

Accommodative esotropia is defined as a convergent deviation of the eyes associated with activation of the accommodative reflex. All accommodative esodeviations are acquired and have the following characteristics:

- onset typically between 6 months and 7 years of age, averaging 2½ years of age (can be as early as age 4 months)
- usually intermittent at onset, becoming constant
- often hereditary
- sometimes precipitated by trauma or illness
- frequently associated with amblyopia
- diplopia possible (especially with onset at an older age) but usually disappears with development of a facultative suppression scotoma in the deviating eye

Types of accommodative esotropia are listed in Table 8-1 and discussed below.

Pathogenesis and Types of Accommodative Esotropia

Refractive accommodative esotropia

The mechanism of refractive accommodative esotropia involves 3 factors: uncorrected hyperopia, accommodative convergence, and insufficient fusional divergence. Uncorrected hyperopia forces the patient to accommodate to focus the retinal image. With accommodation come the other components of the near triad, namely convergence and miosis. If the patient's fusional divergence mechanism is insufficient to compensate for the increased convergence tonus, esotropia results. The angle of esotropia is generally between 20Δ and 30Δ and approximately equal at distance and near fixation. Patients with refractive accommodative esotropia have an average of +4.00 D of hyperopia.

High accommodative convergence/accommodation ratio esotropia

In patients with a *high accommodative convergence/accommodation (AC/A) ratio,* excess convergence tonus for the amount of accommodation required to focus is present when the proper full cycloplegic refraction is used. In this entity, the deviation is present only at near or is much larger at near.

The refractive error in high AC/A esotropia averages +2.25 D. However, this form of esotropia can occur in patients with high or normal degrees of hyperopia, emmetropia, or even myopia.

Partially accommodative esotropia

Patients with partially accommodative esotropia show a reduction in the angle of esotropia when wearing glasses but have a residual esotropia despite treatment of amblyopia and provision of the full hyperopic correction. This is more likely to occur if there is a long delay in refractive correction. Sometimes, partially accommodative esotropia results from decompensation of a pure refractive accommodative esotropia; in other instances, an initial nonacccommodative esotropia subsequently develops an accommodative component.

Evaluation

Vision of the 2 eyes can be equal, or amblyopia can be present. Versions and ductions may be normal, or overelevation in adduction or dissociated strabismus (discussed in Chapter 11) may be present. The deviation should be measured using an accommodative target at distance and at near. Alternate cover testing on initial examination typically reveals an intermittent comitant esotropia that is larger at near than at distance.

Management

Refractive accommodative esotropia

Treatment of refractive accommodative esotropia consists of correction of the full amount of hyperopia, as determined under cycloplegia. Significant delay in initiating treatment following the onset of the esotropia increases the likelihood that a portion of the esodeviation will fail to respond to spectacle correction. If binocular fusion is maintained, the refractive correction can later be decreased to 1.00–2.00 D less than the full cycloplegic refraction. This is thought to possibly aid in emmetropization. Amblyopia, if present, may respond to spectacle correction alone, but treatment with occlusion or penalization may be needed if the amblyopia persists after a period of spectacle wear.

Parents must understand not only that full-time wear of the glasses is important but also that the refractive correction can only help control the strabismus, not cure it. The esotropia, without glasses, may increase initially after the correction is worn. Discussing these issues with parents at the time the prescription is given is helpful.

Strabismus surgery may be required when a patient with presumed refractive accommodative esotropia fails to achieve an ocular alignment within the fusion range (8Δ–10Δ) with correction (partially accommodative esotropia). The ophthalmologist should recheck the cycloplegic refraction before proceeding with surgery in order to rule out latent uncorrected hyperopia. Refractive surgery, though still deemed experimental for this condition, can also be considered for older patients who continue to need refractive correction to maintain good ocular alignment.

Brugnoli de Pagano OM, Pagano GL. LASIK for treatment of refractive accommodative esotropia. *Ophthalmology.* 2012;119(1):159–163.

High AC/A esotropia

A high AC/A ratio can be managed optically, pharmacologically, or surgically; it can also be observed.

- *Bifocals.* Plus spectacle lenses for hyperopia reduce accommodation and therefore reduce accommodative convergence. Bifocals further reduce or eliminate the need to accommodate for near fixation. If bifocals are employed, they should initially be prescribed in the executive or 35-mm flat-top style with the lowest plus power needed (up to +3.00 D) to achieve ocular alignment at near fixation without cycloplegia. The top of the segment should bisect the pupil, and the vertical height of the bifocal should not exceed that of the distance portion of the lens. Detailed instructions concerning the bifocal should be given to the optician. Progressive bifocal lenses have been used successfully in older children who know how to properly use bifocal spectacles. If progressive bifocals are used, they should be fitted higher than they are in adult lenses (at about 4 mm). An ideal response to bifocal glasses is restoration of normal binocular function (fusion and stereopsis) at both distance and near fixation. An acceptable response is fusion at distance with less than 10Δ of residual esotropia through the bifocal at near (signifying the potential for fusion). While some children improve spontaneously with time, others can be slowly weaned from bifocals. The process of reducing the bifocal power in 0.50–1.00 D steps can be started at about age 7 or 8 and should be completed by age 10–12 years. If a child cannot be weaned from bifocals, surgery can be considered.
- *Long-acting cholinesterase inhibitors.* Long-acting cholinesterase inhibitors (eg, echothiophate iodide) decrease accommodative convergence. These drugs act directly on the ciliary body, facilitating transmission at the myoneural junction. They reduce the central demand for accommodative innervation and thus reduce the amount of convergence induced by accommodation. In the past, echothiophate was sometimes used to treat patients with high AC/A esotropia. This agent, which is associated with some systemic and ophthalmic complications (eg, development of iris cysts, cataracts; increased response to depolarizing muscle relaxants), is no longer commercially sold in the United States and is now used only rarely.
- *Surgery.* Surgical management of high AC/A esotropia is controversial. Some ophthalmologists advocate surgery (medial rectus muscle recessions with or without posterior fixation or pulley fixation) to normalize the AC/A ratio, which may allow for discontinuation of bifocals and use of contact lenses. The risk of overcorrection at distance is small (<10%). Prism adaptation for the near deviation, the preoperative use of prisms to determine the maximum deviation, is used by some ophthalmologists.

- *Observation.* Many patients show a decrease in the near deviation with time and ultimately develop binocular vision at both distance and near fixation. Some ophthalmologists observe the near deviation as long as the distance alignment allows for the development of peripheral fusion.

For the long-term management of both refractive and high AC/A accommodative esotropia, it is important to remember that measured hyperopia usually increases until age 5–7 years before it starts to decrease. Therefore, if the esotropia with glasses increases, the cycloplegic refraction should be repeated and the full correction prescribed.

If glasses or medication corrects all or nearly all of the esotropia and if some degree of sensory binocular cooperation or fusion is present, the clinician may begin to reduce the strength of the glasses to create a small esophoria, which is thought to stimulate fusional divergence. An increase in the fusional divergence combined with the natural decrease of both the hyperopia and the high AC/A ratio may enable the patient to eventually maintain straight eyes without bifocals or glasses altogether.

Partially accommodative esotropia

Treatment of partially accommodative esotropia consists of strabismus surgery for the deviation that persists while the patient wears the full hyperopic correction. It is important that the patient and parents understand before surgery that its purpose is to produce straight eyes with glasses—not to allow the child to discontinue wearing glasses altogether. In older patients, refractive surgery can be considered to both reduce the hyperopic refractive error and improve the ocular alignment. Results of these procedures for partially accommodative esotropia are not as impressive as those for pure refractive accommodative esotropia.

Acquired Nonaccommodative Esotropias

Basic Acquired Nonaccommodative Esotropia

Comitant esotropia that develops after age 6 months and that is not associated with an accommodative component is called *basic acquired nonaccommodative esotropia*. As in infantile esotropia, the amount of hyperopia is not significant, and the deviation is similar at distance and near. Acquired esotropia may be acute in onset. In such cases, the patient immediately becomes aware of the deviation and may have diplopia. A careful motility evaluation is important to rule out an accommodative or paretic component. Temporary but prolonged disruption of binocular vision—such as may result from a hyphema, preseptal cellulitis and mechanical ptosis, or prolonged patching for amblyopia—is a known precipitating cause of acquired nonaccommodative esotropia. In patients with acquired nonaccommodative esotropia, fusion is thought to be tenuous, so this temporary disruption of binocular vision upsets the balance, resulting in esotropia.

Because the onset of nonaccommodative esotropia in an older child may be a sign of an underlying neurologic disorder, neuroimaging and neurologic evaluation may be indicated when other symptoms or signs of neurologic abnormality are present, such as lateral incomitance, deviation greater at distance than near, abnormal head position, diplopia, or concomitant headache. Many patients with acquired nonaccommodative esotropia have a history of normal binocular vision; thus, the prognosis for restoration of single binocular vision with prisms and/or surgery is good. Therapy consists of amblyopia treatment, if needed, and surgical correction or botulinum toxin injection as soon as possible after the onset of the deviation. The Prism Adaptation Study showed a smaller undercorrection rate (approximately 10% less) with surgery based on the prism-adapted angle.

Jacobs SM, Green-Simms A, Diehl NN, Mohney BG. Long-term follow-up of acquired nonaccommodative esotropia in a population-based cohort. *Ophthalmology*. 2011;118(6): 1170–1174. Epub 2011 Jan 26.

Repka MX, Connett JE, Scott WE. The one-year surgical outcome after prism adaptation for the management of acquired esotropia. *Ophthalmology*. 1996;103(6):922–928.

Cyclic Esotropia

Cyclic esotropia is rare, with an estimated incidence of 1:3000–1:5000 strabismus cases. Onset typically occurs during the preschool years. The esotropia is comitant and occurs intermittently, usually every other day (48-hour cycle). Variable intervals and 24-hour cycles have also been documented.

Fusion and binocular vision are usually absent or defective on the strabismic day, with marked improvement or normalization on the orthotropic day. Diplopia on strabismic days can occur and is more often a prominent symptom in patients whose onset of esotropia occurred at a relatively older age and who are unable to develop suppression. Occlusion therapy may convert the cyclic deviation into a constant one.

Surgical treatment of cyclic esotropia is usually effective. The amount of surgery is based on the maximum angle of deviation present when the eyes are esotropic.

Sensory Esotropia

Monocular vision loss from various causes (eg, cataract, corneal clouding, optic nerve or retinal disorders) may cause sensory (deprivation) esotropia.

Obstacles preventing clear and focused retinal images and symmetric visual stimulation must be identified and remedied promptly, if possible. When marked abnormalities such as total unilateral congenital cataract are present, animal and clinical data indicate that restoration of the best-possible visual input must be accomplished at an early age if irreversible amblyopia is to be avoided. If surgery or botulinum toxin injection is indicated for strabismus, it is generally performed only on the eye with a significant deficit.

Divergence Insufficiency

The characteristic finding of divergence insufficiency is an esodeviation that is greater at distance than at near. The deviation is comitant in vertical and horizontal gaze, and fusional divergence is reduced. Divergence paralysis may represent a more severe form of divergence insufficiency. Because true paralysis of divergence cannot generally be documented, the term *divergence insufficiency* is preferred. Divergence insufficiency can be divided into a primary, isolated form and a secondary form associated with neurologic abnormalities, including pontine tumors, increased intracranial pressure, or severe head trauma. In these secondary cases, the divergence insufficiency is probably due to sixth nerve paresis that is so mild that the abduction deficit has not yet become clinically evident. A thorough clinical evaluation can frequently distinguish between the 2 forms of divergence insufficiency. Primary, isolated divergence insufficiency is a benign condition that predominantly occurs in patients older than 50 years; symptoms sometimes resolve within several months. Patients with secondary divergence insufficiency require neuro-imaging to rule out treatable intracranial lesions. Treatment of the underlying neurologic disorder (eg, corticosteroids for temporal arteritis, treatment of intracranial hypertension) may relieve symptoms. Management of diplopia consists of base-out prisms, botulinum toxin injection of the medial rectus muscles, and strabismus surgery.

Spasm of the Near Reflex

Spasm of the near reflex (also known as *ciliary spasm* or *convergence spasm*) is a spectrum of abnormalities of the near response. Patients present with varying combinations of ex-cessive convergence, accommodation, and miosis. The etiology is generally thought to be functional, related to psychological factors such as stress and anxiety. In rare cases, it can be associated with organic disease. Patients may present with acute esotropia alternating at other times with orthotropia. Substitution of a convergence movement for a gaze move-ment on horizontal versions is characteristic. Monocular abduction is normal in spite of marked abduction limitation on version testing. Pseudomyopia may occur.

Treatment consists of cycloplegic agents such as atropine or homatropine, hyperopic correction for patients with significant hyperopia, and bifocals. Counseling to address underlying issues that are triggering this response may be helpful. Botulinum toxin injec-tions of the medial rectus muscles and strabismus surgery can be considered with caution if the spasm cannot be broken.

Kaczmarek BB, Dawson E, Lee JP. Convergence spasm treated with botulinum toxin. *Strabismus.* 2009;17(1):49–51.

Consecutive Esotropia

Esotropia following a history of exotropia is called *consecutive esotropia.* It can be a spon-taneous event or it can develop after surgery for exotropia. Spontaneous consecutive eso-tropia is rare and almost always occurs in the face of neurologic disorders, such as cerebral palsy, or with very poor vision in 1 eye. Postsurgical consecutive esotropia, on the other hand, is not uncommon. Fortunately, it often resolves over time. In fact, an initial small overcorrection is desirable after surgery for exotropia, as it is associated with an improved long-term success rate. Treatment options for consecutive esotropia, whether spontane-ous or persistent postoperatively, include base-out prisms, hyperopic correction, alternat-ing occlusion, botulinum injection, and strabismus surgery. In postsurgical consecutive esotropia, unless the deviation is very large or a slipped or lost muscle is suspected, sur-gery or botulinum toxin injection should be postponed for several months because of the possibility of spontaneous improvement.

A slipped or lost lateral rectus muscle produces varying amounts of esotropia, depend-ing on the amount of slippage, and should be suspected in consecutive esotropia following lateral rectus recession surgery if a significant abduction deficit is present. However, if the ipsilateral medial rectus muscle was resected at the time of the lateral rectus recession, the consecutive esotropia could be due to a tight medial rectus muscle. Forced-duction testing helps differentiate between these two causes. In cases of a slipped or lost lateral rectus muscle, surgical exploration is required. Transposition procedures may be necessary when lost muscles cannot be found. For slipped muscles, the true muscle should be identified and secured with a suture, the pseudotendon attached to the sclera resected, and the true muscle advanced and secured back to the sclera at the proper position. (See Chapter 14, Fig 14-1, and the accompanying text discussion.)

Nystagmus and Esotropia

Several types of nystagmus are associated with esotropia. *Fusion maldevelopment nystagmus syndrome (FMNS;* also known as *latent* and *manifest latent nystagmus*) is a feature of infantile esotropia. Ciancia syndrome (discussed earlier in this chapter) is a severe form of infantile esotropia associated with an abducting nystagmus. Nystagmus blockage syndrome occurs in children with congenital nystagmus who use convergence to "damp," or decrease the amplitude or frequency of, their nystagmus. See also Chapter 13.

Incomitant Esotropia

The term *incomitant esotropia* is used when the esodeviation varies in size in different positions of gaze.

Sixth Nerve Palsy

Palsy of the sixth cranial nerve (abducens) occurring within the first 2 months of life is not common and is usually transient. Most cases of suspected congenital sixth nerve palsy are actually infantile esotropia with cross-fixation. Congenital sixth nerve palsy may be difficult to differentiate from esotropic Duane retraction syndrome in young infants (see Chapter 12), as the unique retraction feature of this syndrome may not be evident in an infant who has shallow orbits and who may not track well to extreme side gaze. Esotropic Duane retraction syndrome is a much more frequent cause of persistent abduction deficit in infants than is sixth nerve palsy. A distinguishing characteristic is that for an equal amount of abduction deficit, the deviation in primary position is usually much larger in sixth nerve palsy than it is in esotropic Duane retraction syndrome.

See BCSC Section 5, *Neuro-Ophthalmology,* for further discussion of sixth nerve palsy.

Pathogenesis
Congenital sixth nerve palsy is usually benign and transient. Some surmise that it is caused by the increased intracranial pressure associated with the birth process. In any case, it usually resolves spontaneously. Sixth nerve palsy occurs much more frequently in childhood than in infancy. Approximately one-third of cases in older children are associated with intracranial lesions and may have other associated neurologic findings. Other cases may be related to infectious or immunologic processes that involve cranial nerve VI. Isolated transient sixth nerve palsy is thought to be caused most commonly by a virus in a child or a microvascular occlusive event in an adult.

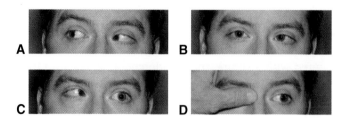

Figure 8-2 Sixth nerve palsy, left eye. **A,** Right gaze. **B,** Esotropia in primary position. **C,** Limited abduction, left eye. **D,** Still incomplete but further abduction of left eye when fixating, a finding important in the plan for surgical correction. *(Courtesy of Edward L. Raab, MD.)*

Evaluation

Older patients may report diplopia and often have a compensatory head turn toward the side of the paralyzed lateral rectus muscle, which they have adopted to relieve the diplopia. If the child presents soon after onset, vision in the eyes is usually equal. The esotropia increases in gaze toward the paralyzed lateral rectus muscle. Saccadic velocities show slowing of the affected lateral rectus muscle, and active force generation tests document weakness of that muscle. Versions show limited or no abduction of the affected eye (Fig 8-2).

A careful history should be taken, including antecedent infections, head trauma, hydrocephalus, hypertension and diabetes mellitus in adults, or other possible inciting factors for sixth cranial nerve weakness. In light of the high prevalence of associated intracranial lesions in children with sixth nerve palsy, neurologic evaluation and gadolinium-enhanced magnetic resonance imaging of the head and orbit are usually indicated, even in the absence of other focal neurologic findings.

Management

Patching may be necessary to prevent or treat amblyopia if the child is not using a compensatory head posture or if the child is very young. Press-on prisms are sometimes used to correct diplopia in primary position. Correction of a significant hyperopic refractive error may help prevent the development of an associated accommodative esotropia. Botulinum toxin injection of the ipsilateral medial rectus muscle is sometimes used to decrease the esotropia and prevent secondary contracture. If the deviation does not resolve after 6 months of treatment, surgery may be indicated. Options include horizontal rectus muscle surgery if abduction is at least partially preserved or vertical rectus muscle transposition surgery if abduction is absent (see Chapter 14).

Other Forms of Incomitant Esotropia

Medial rectus muscle restriction may result from thyroid eye disease, medial orbital wall fracture, excessive medial rectus muscle resection, or congenital fibrosis of the extraocular muscles. Duane retraction syndrome and Möbius syndrome begin as paralytic disorders, and secondary restriction of the medial rectus may develop later. Patients with high myopia may develop esotropia due to displacement of the posterior globe between the lateral and superior rectus muscles (see Chapter 12).

For further discussion of these special forms of strabismus, see Chapter 12 of this volume and BCSC Section 5, *Neuro-Ophthalmology.*

CHAPTER 9

Exodeviations

An exodeviation is a manifest or latent divergent strabismus. The frequency of exodeviations varies among different ethnic groups. In Europeans and North and South Americans, exodeviations are the second most common form of strabismus, occurring approximately one-third as often as esodeviations, whereas in Asians, exodeviations are more common than esodeviations. Risk factors for exotropia include maternal smoking during pregnancy, premature birth, family history of strabismus, and uncorrected refractive errors.

Pseudoexotropia

The term *pseudoexotropia* refers to an appearance of exodeviation when in fact the eyes are properly aligned. Pseudoexotropia is much less common than pseudoesotropia (see Chapter 8). It may result from the following:

- wide interpupillary distance
- positive angle kappa without other ocular abnormalities (See the discussions of angle kappa in Chapter 7 and in BCSC Section 3, *Clinical Optics.*)
- positive angle kappa together with ocular abnormalities such as temporal dragging of the macula in retinopathy of prematurity

Exophoria

Exophoria is an exodeviation controlled by fusion under normal viewing conditions. An exophoria is detected when binocular vision is interrupted, as during an alternate cover test. Exophoria is fairly common and is often asymptomatic if the angle of strabismus is small and fusional convergence amplitudes are adequate. Prolonged, detailed visual work may bring about asthenopia. Breakdown of an exophoria to an exotropia may occur transiently during a serious illness or after ingestion of sedatives or alcohol. Treatment is usually not necessary unless an exophoria progresses to intermittent exotropia or it causes asthenopic symptoms.

Intermittent Exotropia

Intermittent exotropia is the most common type of exodeviation that clinicians encounter.

Clinical Characteristics

The onset of intermittent exotropia usually occurs before age 5 years. Intermittent exotropia may develop during the first year of life, in which case it must be differentiated from (a) the intermittent strabismus that is common in the first 1–2 months of life and that spontaneously resolves; and (b) constant infantile exotropia (discussed later in this chapter). Because proper eye alignment with intermittent exotropia requires that compensatory fusional factors be active, the deviation often becomes manifest during times of visual inattention, fatigue, or stress. Parents of affected children often report that the exotropia occurs late in the day or during illness, daydreaming, or drowsiness on awakening. Exposure to bright light often causes a reflex closure of 1 eye (which is why strabismus is sometimes referred to as a "squint").

Exodeviations are usually larger when the patient views distant targets, and they may be difficult to elicit at near. Because most parental interactions with young children occur at near, parents of a child with an exodeviation may not notice it initially. Intermittent exotropias can be associated with small hypertropias, A and V patterns, and overelevation and underelevation in adduction.

Untreated intermittent exotropia may progress toward constant exotropia. During this progression, tropic episodes occur at lower levels of fatigue and last for longer periods. Children younger than 10 years usually do not experience diplopia when they are tropic, because of suppression. However, normal retinal correspondence and good binocular function remain when the eyes are straight. Amblyopia is uncommon unless the intermittent exotropia progresses to constant or nearly constant exotropia at an early age or unless another amblyogenic factor, such as anisometropia, is present.

Evaluation

The clinical evaluation begins with a history, including the age of onset of the strabismus, whether the exotropia is becoming more frequent, and the circumstances under which the deviation is manifest. During the examination, an assessment is made of the patient's control of the exodeviation, which can be categorized as follows:

- *Good control:* Exotropia manifests only after cover testing, and the patient resumes fusion rapidly without blinking or refixating.
- *Fair control:* Exotropia manifests after fusion is disrupted by cover testing, and the patient resumes fusion only after blinking or refixating.
- *Poor control:* Exotropia manifests spontaneously and may remain manifest for an extended time.

Some ophthalmologists use the Newcastle Control Score to quantitatively grade the control exhibited by patients with intermittent exotropia.

Prism and alternate cover testing should be used to evaluate the exodeviation at fixation distances of 6 m and 33 cm. A far distance measurement at 30 m or greater (eg, at the end of a long hallway or out a window) may uncover a latent deviation or bring out an even larger one. The deviation at near fixation is often less than the deviation at distance fixation. This difference is usually due to *tenacious proximal fusion,* a slow-to-dissipate fusion mechanism at near, but it may also be due to a high accommodative convergence/accommodation (AC/A) ratio; however, a high AC/A ratio occurs much less commonly in exotropia than in esotropia (see Chapter 8). For patients with significantly more exodeviation at distance than at near, a near alternate cover test, administered after 30–60 minutes of monocular occlusion to eliminate the effects of tenacious proximal fusion, may help distinguish between a truly high AC/A ratio and a distance–near disparity due to tenacious proximal fusion (a pseudo-high AC/A ratio). A patient with a pseudo-high AC/A ratio has roughly equal distance and near measurements after occlusion, whereas a patient with a truly high AC/A ratio continues to have significantly less exodeviation at near. Testing with +3.00 D lenses at near or −2.00 D lenses at distance can confirm the abnormality of the AC/A ratio.

Haggerty H, Richardson S, Hrisos S, Strong NP, Clarke MP. The Newcastle Control Score: a new method of grading the severity of intermittent distance exotropia. *Br J Ophthalmol.* 2004;88(2):233–235.

Kushner BJ, Morton GV. Distance/near differences in intermittent exotropia. *Arch Ophthalmol.* 1998;116(4):478–486.

Classification

Intermittent exotropia may be classified based on the difference between prism and alternate cover test measurements at distance and at near and the change in near measurement produced by monocular occlusion or +3.00 D lenses:

- *Pseudodivergence excess exotropia* is the most common form of intermittent exotropia. Patients initially have larger deviations at distance than at near fixation, but this difference becomes minimal after monocular occlusion or with +3.00 D lenses at near.
- *Basic exotropia* is present when the exodeviation is approximately the same at distance and near fixation.
- *True divergence excess exotropia* is the least common form of intermittent exotropia. It is present when the distance deviation is greater than the near deviation, and the deviation does not equalize after monocular occlusion or with +3.00 D lenses at near.
- *Convergence weakness exotropia* is present when the exodeviation is greater at near than at distance. This type is discussed later in the chapter.

Sensory testing usually reveals excellent stereopsis with normal retinal correspondence when the eyes are aligned and suppression when the exodeviation is manifest. Uncommonly, patients may manifest diplopia when the eyes are exotropic.

Treatment

There are no firm guidelines for determining when patients with intermittent exotropia require treatment. Opinions vary widely regarding the timing of surgery and the use of nonsurgical methods to delay or possibly prevent the need for surgical intervention.

Nonsurgical management

Correction of refractive errors Corrective lenses should be prescribed for significant myopic, astigmatic, and hyperopic refractive errors. Correction of even mild myopia may improve control of the exodeviation. Mild to moderate degrees of hyperopia are not routinely corrected in children with intermittent exotropia because of concern about worsening the deviation. However, children with marked hyperopia (>+4.00 D or >+1.50 D hyperopic anisometropia) may be unable to sustain accommodation, and this results in a blurred retinal image and manifest exotropia. Optical correction may improve retinal image clarity and help control the exodeviation in these patients.

Some ophthalmologists use additional minus lenses, usually 2.00–4.00 D beyond the actual refractive error, to stimulate accommodative convergence to help control the exodeviation. This therapy may cause asthenopia in school-aged children, however. It can be effective as a temporizing measure to promote fusion and delay surgery while the visual system is immature. For patients in whom the initial overrcorrection results in control, the prescription can be gradually tapered and surgery may be avoided.

Occlusion therapy Patching of patients with amblyopia may improve control of exotropic deviations. For patients without amblyopia, part-time patching of the dominant (nondeviating) eye or alternating daily patching in the absence of a strong ocular preference can be an effective treatment for small- to moderate-sized deviations, particularly in young children. The improvement is often temporary, however, and many patients eventually require surgery.

Active orthoptic treatments Antisuppression therapy/diplopia awareness and fusional convergence training can be used alone or in combination with patching, minus lenses, and surgery. For deviations of 20 prism diopters (Δ) or less, orthoptic treatment alone has been reported by some authors to have a long-term success rate comparable to that of surgery. Others, finding this treatment to be of no benefit, recommend surgery for any poorly controlled deviation. A potential risk of antisuppression orthoptic therapy is the loss of ability to suppress diplopia, which may be quite bothersome.

Prisms Although they can be used to promote fusion in intermittent exotropia, base-in prisms are seldom chosen for long-term management because they can cause a reduction in fusional vergence amplitudes.

Surgical treatment

Surgery is customarily performed when there is documented progression toward constant exotropia, as evidenced by a manifest deviation occurring more frequently, decreased control, or decreased distance stereoacuity. No consensus exists regarding specific indications; however, the best sensory outcomes are probably achieved with motor alignment before age 7 or with strabismus duration of fewer than 5 years, or while the deviation is still intermittent. Many surgeons use a manifest deviation occurring more than 50% of the time as a criterion for surgery.

For pseudodivergence excess exotropia, symmetric recession of both lateral rectus muscles is the most common surgical procedure. Patients with basic intermittent exotropia may do better with combined lateral rectus muscle recession and medial rectus muscle resection, or larger lateral rectus muscle recessions than those used for patients with pseudodivergence excess. For patients with smaller exodeviations, unilateral lateral rectus muscle recessions may be performed.

Some surgeons believe that the usual quantity of surgery (see Chapter 14) may result in overcorrection if the exotropia in each side gaze is less than that in primary position by at least 10Δ. Thus, if lateral rectus muscle recessions are planned for such patients, these surgeons might reduce the amount of surgery on each side by 1 mm. Other surgeons consider such alignment measurements to be an artifact.

Patients with true divergence excess exotropia have an increased risk of developing near esodeviations after lateral rectus muscle recessions and may require bifocal glasses if the near esodeviation is associated with a high AC/A ratio (see the Evaluation section).

Botulinum toxin may also be used to treat intermittent exotropia, although multiple injections are commonly needed.

Kushner BJ. Selective surgery for intermittent exotropia based on distance/near differences. *Arch Ophthalmol.* 1998;116(3):324–328.

Postoperative alignment A small-angle esotropia in the immediate postoperative period is desirable, because it is associated with a decreased risk of recurrent exotropia. Patients may experience diplopia during the time they are esotropic, and they should be advised of this possibility. An esotropia that persists beyond 3–4 weeks or that develops after 1–2 months in patients who were initially well-aligned postoperatively usually requires additional treatment such as base-out prisms or patching. Corrective lenses may be considered if significant hyperopia is present. Bifocals can be used for a high AC/A ratio. Unless deficient ductions suggest a slipped or lost muscle, a delay of a few months is recommended before reoperation, because spontaneous improvement is common. If the esotropia persists, surgical options include unilateral or bilateral recession of the medial rectus muscle, advancement of the recessed lateral rectus muscles, or injection of botulinum toxin.

Mild to moderate residual exodeviation is often treated with observation alone if fusional control is good. However, persistent exotropia commonly worsens over time. Base-in prisms, patching, and optical management may be used for such patients. If the deviation progresses, surgical options include re-recession of the lateral rectus muscles, resections of the medial rectus muscles, or injections of botulinum toxin.

Some patients develop monofixational exotropia (a constant exodeviation <8Δ) after treatment of intermittent exotropia. These patients have decreased stereopsis, as occurs in patients with the more common monofixational esotropia (see Chapter 8).

Over time, patients with small-angle esotropias following surgery are less likely to develop recurrent exotropia. However, conversion to monofixation, with subnormal stereopsis, may occur in these patients. For this reason, some ophthalmologists prefer to delay surgery in young children in whom good preoperative visual acuity and stereopsis might be exchanged for a small-angle esotropia and decreased stereopsis postoperatively. However, other ophthalmologists worry that delaying surgery too long could allow permanent suppression to develop and decrease long-term stability following surgical correction.

Convergence Weakness Exotropia

Convergence weakness exotropia is present when the near deviation is greater than the distance deviation. There are 2 main types of convergence weakness exotropia: convergence insufficiency (CI), in which there is usually no distance deviation, and convergence weakness associated with exotropia at both distance and near fixation, but greater at near.

The presentation and management of CI differ from those of other types of exotropia. Patients typically have minimal or no deviation at distance. They are usually older, often teenagers or adults. CI is seen more commonly in patients with Parkinson disease than in age-matched controls. Symptoms of CI include asthenopia, blurred near vision, and diplopia, and they are most noticeable during reading. Evaluation reveals poor near fusional convergence amplitudes and a remote near point of convergence. In rare cases, accommodative spasms may occur if accommodation and convergence are stimulated in an effort to overcome the CI.

Treatment of CI typically involves orthoptic exercises. Base-out prisms can be used to stimulate fusional convergence during reading. Stereograms, "pencil push-ups," and other near-point exercises are often employed. Also, computer-based convergence training programs are available. If these exercises fail, base-in prism reading glasses may be used. Surgical treatment, usually medial rectus muscle resections, may be indicated in patients whose problems persist despite medical therapy.

The second type of convergence weakness is present when there are manifest deviations at distance and near, but greater at near. Some patients with this type have had previous medial rectus muscle recessions and may show underaction of these muscles. Advancement of the previously recessed medial rectus muscles, with or without recession of the lateral rectus muscles, is commonly used to treat these patients. For patients with convergence weakness who have not had previous surgery, a procedure in which the standard amount of lateral rectus muscle recession and medial rectus resection (see Chapter 14) are reversed may be useful.

Kraft SP, Levin AV, Enzenauer RW. Unilateral surgery for exotropia with convergence weakness. *J Ped Ophthalmol Strabismus.* 1995;32(3):183–187.

Constant Exotropia

Constant exotropia is encountered most often in older patients with sensory exotropia or patients with long-standing intermittent exotropia that has decompensated.

Surgical treatment of constant exotropia usually consists of either bilateral lateral rectus muscle recessions or unilateral lateral rectus muscle recession combined with medial rectus muscle resection. For patients with very large (>50Δ) deviations, surgery on 3 or 4 muscles is sometimes performed.

Some patients have an enlarged field of peripheral vision because they have large areas of nonoverlapping fields. These patients may notice a field constriction when the eyes are straightened.

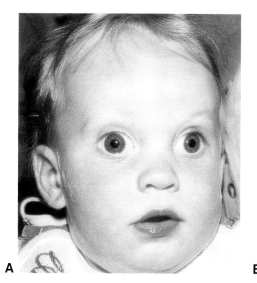 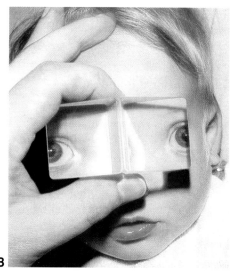

Figure 9-1 Infantile exotropia. **A,** This 10-month-old infant with infantile exotropia also shows developmental delay. **B,** Krimsky testing using 2 base-in prisms to measure the large exotropia. *(Reproduced from Wilson ME. Exotropia. Focal Points: Clinical Modules for Ophthalmologists. San Francisco: American Academy of Ophthalmology; 1995, module 11.)*

Infantile Exotropia

Infantile exotropia is much less common than infantile esotropia. It presents before age 6 months with a large-angle constant deviation (Fig 9-1). Although infants with constant exotropia may be otherwise healthy, they are at increased risk of having associated neurologic impairment or craniofacial disorders. A careful developmental history is important, and referral for neurologic assessment should be considered if there are indications of delay. Patients with constant infantile exotropia are operated on early in life, with outcomes being similar to those for infantile esotropia (see Chapter 8). Early surgery can lead to monofixation with gross binocular vision, but restoration of normal binocular function is rare. Patients may develop dissociated vertical deviations and overelevation in adduction (see Chapter 11).

Sensory Exotropia

Any condition that severely reduces vision in 1 eye—for example, anisometropia, corneal or lens opacities, optic atrophy or hypoplasia, retinal lesions, or amblyopia—can cause sensory exotropia. It is not known why some persons become esotropic and others exotropic after unilateral vision loss. Although both sensory esotropia and sensory exotropia occur in infants and young children, exotropia predominates in older children and adults. If the vision in the exotropic eye can be improved, peripheral fusion may sometimes be re-established after surgical realignment, provided the sensory exotropia has not been present for an extended period. Loss of fusional abilities, known as *central fusion disruption,* can lead to constant and permanent diplopia when adult-onset sensory exotropia has been present for several years before vision rehabilitation and realignment. In these patients, intractable diplopia may persist, even with well-aligned eyes.

Consecutive Exotropia

Exotropia that occurs after a period of esotropia is called *consecutive exotropia*. In rare cases, exotropia may spontaneously develop in a patient who was previously esotropic but who has not had surgery. Much more commonly, consecutive exotropia develops after previous surgery for esotropia (postsurgical exotropia), usually developing within a few months or years after the initial surgery. However, in some patients with infantile esotropia, the exotropia may not develop until adulthood. Treatment of postsurgical exotropia depends on many factors, including the type and amount of previous surgery, the presence of duction limitations, and lateral incomitance.

Other Forms of Exotropia

Exotropic Duane Retraction Syndrome

Duane retraction syndrome can present with exotropia, usually accompanied by deficient adduction and a head turn away from the affected eye. See Chapter 12 for further discussion.

Neuromuscular Abnormalities

A constant exotropia may result from third nerve palsy, internuclear ophthalmoplegia, or myasthenia gravis. These conditions are discussed in Chapter 12 and in BCSC Section 5, *Neuro-Ophthalmology.*

Dissociated Horizontal Deviation

Dissociated strabismus complex may include vertical, horizontal, and torsional components (see Chapter 11). When a dissociated abduction movement is predominant, the condition is called *dissociated horizontal deviation (DHD)*. Though not a true exotropia, DHD can be confused with a constant or intermittent exotropia. Dissociated vertical deviation and latent nystagmus often coexist with DHD (Fig 9-2). In rare cases, patients may manifest both DHD and intermittent esotropia. DHD must be differentiated from anisohyperopia associated with intermittent exotropia. In these patients, the exotropic deviation is present when the patient fixates with the normal eye but is absent during fixation with the hyperopic eye because of accommodation. Treatment of DHD usually consists of unilateral or bilateral lateral rectus recession in addition to any necessary oblique or vertical muscle surgery.

Convergence Paralysis

Convergence paralysis is a condition distinct from convergence insufficiency and usually secondary to an intracranial lesion. It is characterized by normal adduction and

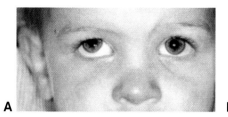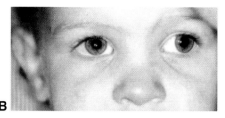

Figure 9-2 Dissociated strabismus complex. **A,** When the patient fixates with the left eye, a prominent dissociated vertical deviation is shown in the right eye. **B,** However, when the patient fixates with the right eye, a prominent dissociated horizontal deviation is shown in the left eye. *(Reproduced from Wilson ME. Exotropia.* Focal Points: Clinical Modules for Ophthalmologists. *San Francisco: American Academy of Ophthalmology; 1995, module 11.)*

accommodation, with exotropia and diplopia present at attempted near fixation only. Convergence paralysis is most commonly associated with dorsal midbrain syndrome (see BCSC Section 5, *Neuro-Ophthalmology*). Patients appearing to have convergence paralysis due to malingering or lack of effort may be distinguished by the absence of a pupillary reaction when they are instructed to focus at near.

Treatment of convergence paralysis is difficult and often limited to use of base-in prisms at near to alleviate the diplopia. Plus lenses may be required if accommodation is limited. Monocular occlusion is indicated if diplopia cannot be otherwise treated.

CHAPTER 10

Pattern Strabismus

Pattern strabismus is present when a horizontal deviation changes in magnitude between upgaze and downgaze. The most common type is a *V pattern,* in which the horizontal deviation is more divergent (less convergent) in upgaze than in downgaze. An *A pattern* is present when the horizontal deviation is more divergent (less convergent) in downgaze compared with upgaze. An A or V pattern is found in 15%–25% of horizontal strabismus cases. Less common variations of pattern strabismus include Y, X, and λ (lambda) patterns.

Etiology

Ophthalmologists have considered each of the following conditions to be a cause of A and V patterns, but this issue remains unsettled:

- *Dysfunction of oblique muscles.* Apparent inferior oblique muscle overaction is associated with V patterns (Figs 10-1, 10-2), and superior oblique muscle overaction with A patterns (Figs 10-3, 10-4), reflecting the ancillary abducting action in upgaze and downgaze, respectively, attributed to these muscles. Whether a true primary overaction of the oblique muscles exists, especially with respect to their vertical actions, is controversial (see Chapter 11). Because the terms *overelevation*

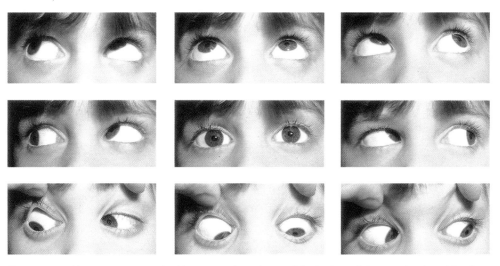

Figure 10-1 V-pattern esotropia. Note overelevation and limitation of depression in adduction.

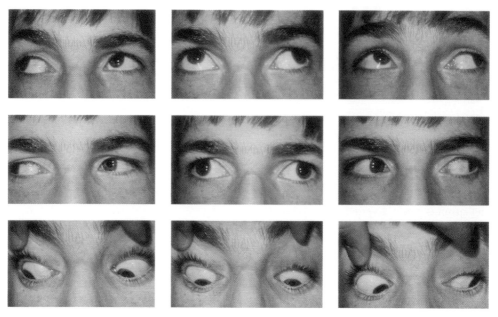

Figure 10-2 V-pattern exotropia with moderate overelevation in adduction. In this patient, there is no apparent underaction of either superior oblique muscle.

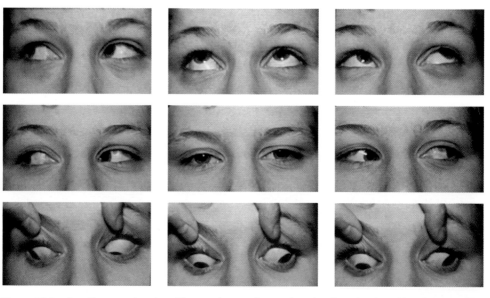

Figure 10-3 A-pattern exotropia with overdepression and underelevation in adduction. *(Modified with permission from Levin A, Wilson T, eds. The Hospital for Sick Children's Atlas of Pediatric Ophthalmology and Strabismus. Philadelphia: Lippincott Williams & Wilkins; 2007:11.)*

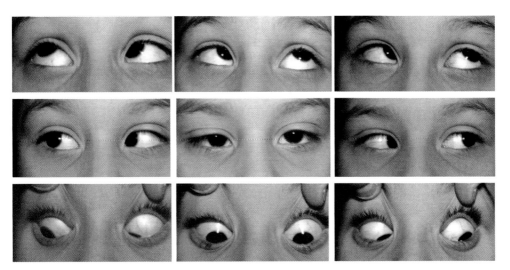

Figure 10-4 A-pattern esotropia with bilateral overdepression and underelevation in adduction, left eye greater than right. *(Courtesy of Edward L. Raab, MD.)*

in adduction (OEAd) and *overdepression in adduction (ODAd)* accurately describe the abnormality without implying an etiology, they have been suggested as alternatives to the traditional terminology.

- *Abnormalities of the orbital pulley system.* Abnormalities (heterotopia) of the orbital pulley system (see Chapter 3) have been described as a cause of simulated oblique muscle overactions and of altered rectus muscle pathways and functions, which can result in A or V patterns. These pulley effects may help explain the observation that patients with upward- or downward-slanting palpebral fissures (Fig 10-5) may show A and V patterns because of an underlying variation in orbital configuration reflected in the orientation of the fissures. Similarly, patients with craniofacial anomalies (see Chapter 18) may have a V-pattern strabismus with marked elevation of the adducting eye as a manifestation of exaggerated altered muscle pathways.
- *Dysfunction of horizontal rectus muscles.* One early school of thought attributed A and V patterns to varying effectiveness of the lateral rectus muscles in the upper half of the vertical gaze field, and of the medial rectus muscles in the lower half of this field. According to this concept, increases in lateral rectus or medial rectus

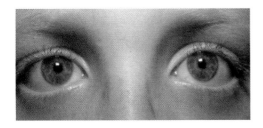

Figure 10-5 Downward slant of the palpebral fissures, often associated with a V-pattern horizontal deviation. *(Courtesy of Edward L. Raab, MD.)*

muscle action produce a V pattern; decreased action of these muscles produces an A pattern. Although, empirically, horizontal rectus muscle surgery that includes displacement of the insertions may effectively treat the underlying deviation, there is no convincing evidence that innervation of these muscles varies in vertical gazes.

- *Selective innervation of horizontal rectus muscles.* This is a possible contributing factor and is under investigation (see Chapter 3).
- *Dysfunction of vertical rectus muscles.* Increases or decreases in the tertiary adducting action of these muscles may result in a less convergent or more divergent alignment in upgaze or downgaze and a corresponding pattern.

Clinical Features and Identification

A and V patterns are determined by measuring alignment while the patient fixates on an accommodative target at distance, with fusion prevented, in primary position and in straight upgaze and downgaze, approximately 25° from the primary position. Proper refractive correction is necessary during measurement because an uncompensated accommodative component can introduce exaggerated convergence in downgaze.

An A pattern is considered clinically significant when the difference in measurement between upgaze and downgaze is at least 10 prism diopters (Δ); for a V pattern, the difference must be at least 15Δ. The difference is larger for a V pattern because normally there is some physiologic convergence in downgaze.

Most, but not all, patients with pattern strabismus have apparent overaction of the oblique muscles (OEAd or ODAd).

V Pattern

The most common type of pattern strabismus, V pattern occurs most frequently in patients with infantile esotropia. Usually, the pattern is not present when the esotropia first develops but becomes apparent during the first year of life or later. V patterns also may occur in patients with superior oblique palsies, particularly if they are bilateral, and in patients with craniofacial malformations.

A Pattern

The second most common type of pattern strabismus, A patterns occur most frequently in patients with exotropia. A patterns are more common than V patterns in patients with infantile strabismus associated with craniofacial malformations, trisomy 21, and myelomeningocele.

Y Pattern

Patients with Y patterns (pseudo-overaction of the inferior oblique) have normal ocular alignment in primary position and downgaze but diverge in upgaze. They appear to have overacting inferior oblique muscles, but the deviation actually results from aberrant innervation of the lateral rectus muscles in upgaze. Clinical characteristics that help identify this form of strabismus include the following: (1) the overelevation is not seen when the eyes are moved directly horizontally, but it becomes manifest when the eyes are moved medially and slightly elevated; (2) there is no fundus torsion; (3) there is no difference in vertical deviation with head tilts; and (4) there is no superior oblique muscle underaction.

> Kushner BJ. Pseudo inferior oblique overaction associated with Y and V patterns. *Ophthalmology.* 1991;98(10):1500–1505.

X Pattern

An X pattern is present when the deviation in primary position increases in both upgaze and downgaze. This pattern is usually associated with overelevation and overdepression in adduction when the eye moves slightly above or below direct side gaze. X patterns are most commonly seen in patients with large-angle exotropia, and the apparent overaction results from contracture of the lateral rectus muscle, with slippage of the globe as the eye adducts.

λ Pattern

This rare pattern is a variant of A-pattern exotropia. It is present when the deviation is the same in primary position and upgaze and increases in downgaze. The λ pattern is usually associated with ODAd.

Management

Clinically significant patterns typically are treated surgically, in combination with correction of the underlying horizontal deviation.

General Principles

The following are guidelines for planning surgical correction of pattern deviations. See Chapter 14 for further discussion of some of the procedures and concepts mentioned here.

1. For patients with patterns associated with apparent overaction of the oblique muscles (OEAd, ODAd), weakening of the oblique muscles is performed.
2. For patients with no apparent overaction of the oblique muscles or a pattern inconsistent with oblique dysfunction, vertical transposition of the horizontal muscles is performed. The muscles are transposed from one-half of the width to the full width of the insertion. The medial rectus muscles are always moved toward the "apex" of the pattern (ie, upward in A patterns and downward in V patterns). The lateral rectus muscles are moved toward the open end or "empty space" (ie, upward in V patterns and downward in A patterns). A useful mnemonic is MALE: *M*edial rectus muscle to the *a*pex, *l*ateral rectus muscle to the *e*mpty space. These rules apply whether the horizontal rectus muscles are weakened or tightened (Fig 10-6).

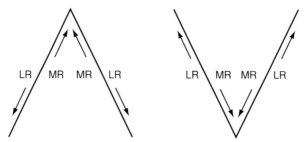

Figure 10-6 Direction of displacement of medial rectus (MR) and lateral rectus (LR) muscles in operations to treat A-pattern *(left)* and V-pattern *(right)* deviations. A useful mnemonic is MALE: *m*edial rectus muscle to the *a*pex, *l*ateral rectus muscle to the *e*mpty space. *(Reprinted with permission from von Noorden GK, Campos EC.* Binocular Vision and Ocular Motility: Theory and Management of Strabismus. *6th ed. St Louis: Mosby; 2002:388.)*

3. When horizontal rectus muscle recession-resection surgery is the preferred choice because of other pertinent factors (eg, prior surgery, unimprovable vision in 1 eye), displacement of the rectus muscle insertions should be in mutually opposite directions, according to the rules stated previously. Unlike what occurs when both horizontal rectus muscles of an eye are moved in the same direction, this displacement has little, if any, vertical effect in the primary position.

4. Some surgeons adjust the amount of horizontal surgery because of the potential effect of oblique muscle weakening on the horizontal deviation, particularly for superior oblique muscle surgery, but this is controversial. Some believe that bilateral superior oblique weakening causes a change of 10Δ–15Δ toward convergence in primary position and suggest modifying the amount of horizontal surgery to compensate for this expected change. For inferior oblique muscle weakening procedures, the amount of horizontal rectus muscle surgery does not need to be altered, because the inferior oblique muscle weakening does not substantially change primary position alignment.

5. Surgery on the vertical rectus muscles (eg, temporal displacement of the superior rectus muscles for A-pattern esotropia or temporal displacement of the inferior rectus muscles for V-pattern esotropia) is rarely employed, because the horizontal rectus muscle operations required for the underlying esotropia or exotropia can correct the pattern with appropriate displacement of the muscles.

Treatment of Specific Patterns

Table 10-1 summarizes the surgical treatment of pattern strabismus (see also Chapter 14).

V pattern

For V-pattern exotropia or esotropia associated with OEAd, weakening of the inferior oblique muscles is performed, usually either a myectomy or recession. This corrects up to 15Δ–20Δ of V pattern. For patients who also have dissociated vertical deviation (DVD), anterior transposition of the inferior oblique muscle may improve both the V pattern and the DVD. Because patients with V-pattern infantile esotropia who are younger than

Table 10-1 Surgical Treatment of Pattern Strabismus

Type of Pattern	Most Common Clinical Association	Treatment		
		With OEAd or ODAd	Without OEAd or ODAd	Other
V Pattern	Infantile esotropia	Weakening of inferior oblique muscle	Vertical transposition of horizontal rectus muscles	If DVD present, anterior transposition of inferior oblique muscles
A Pattern	Exotropia	Weakening of superior oblique muscle	Vertical transposition of horizontal rectus muscles	Trisomy 21: Vertical transposition of horizontal rectus muscles
Y Pattern	Pseudo-inferior oblique overaction			Superior transposition of lateral rectus muscles
X Pattern	Large-angle exotropia (pseudo-overaction due to contracture of lateral rectus muscles)			Recession of lateral rectus muscle
λ Pattern	Variant of A-pattern exotropia	Weakening of superior oblique muscle		

ODAd = overdepression in adduction; OEAd = overelevation in adduction.

2 years are at risk of developing DVD, anterior transposition of the inferior oblique may be considered in this group to preemptively address the DVD.

For patients without OEAd, appropriate vertical transposition of the horizontal rectus muscles is performed (see Fig 10-6).

A pattern

For A-pattern exotropia or esotropia associated with ODAd, weakening of the superior oblique muscles is performed. Tenectomy of the posterior 7/8 of the insertions is an effective method for treating approximately 20Δ of A pattern, with no significant effect on torsion. Lengthening of the tendon by recession, insertion of a spacer, or a Z-lengthening procedure may also be used. Bilateral superior oblique tenotomy is a very powerful procedure that may correct up to 40Δ–50Δ of A pattern. There is a risk of induced torsional imbalance with this procedure, which may cause problems for patients with fusional ability.

For patients without OEAd, appropriate vertical transposition of the horizontal rectus muscles is performed (see Fig 10-6).

Patients with trisomy 21 associated with early-onset esotropia may develop A-pattern strabismus with ODAd. The pattern in these patients is usually due to orbital abnormalities associated with trisomy 21. Vertical transposition of the horizontal rectus muscles is employed for such patients.

Y pattern

Because Y patterns are not due to overaction of the inferior oblique muscles, weakening these muscles is not an effective treatment. Superior transposition of the lateral rectus muscles is generally used for patients with this pattern.

X pattern

X patterns are usually due to pseudo-overaction of the oblique muscles caused by contracture of the lateral rectus muscles in patients with large-angle exotropia. Recession of the lateral rectus muscles alone usually improves the pattern.

λ pattern

These patterns are typically associated with ODAd. Appropriate superior oblique weakening procedures may be used in patients with this pattern.

CHAPTER 11

Vertical Deviations

A vertical deviation can be a heterotropia or a heterophoria (see Chapter 2). A vertical tropia is described according to the resting position of the deviating nonfixating eye. Thus, if the right eye is higher than the left and the left eye is fixating, the deviation is termed a *right hypertropia*. If the right eye is lower than the fixating left eye, it is called a *right hypotropia*. If the ability to alternately fixate is present, the deviation is usually named for the hyperdeviating eye. In the case of a vertical heterophoria, the deviation is, by convention, termed according to the hyperdeviating eye. Thus, a vertical phoria in which the right eye is higher than the left eye is termed a *right hyperphoria*.

Surgical treatment of these conditions is discussed in Chapter 14.

A Clinical Approach to Vertical Deviations

In diagnosing a vertical deviation, a useful first step is to analyze the relationship between the elevators and the depressors of the 2 eyes. In the case of a right hyperdeviation, 1 of 4 situations can arise when the left eye is covered and the right eye is forced to fixate, depending on the innervational relationship between the eyes. The specific scenario is determined by the final position of the nonfixating left eye once the cover is removed:

1. The innervation to the depressors of the right eye is matched in the left eye, leading to a left hypotropia of a magnitude similar to that of the original right hypertropia. This is termed a "true" vertical tropia.
2. The left eye does not adopt a lower position but remains in the same position. This may reflect a violation of Hering's law of motor correspondence (see Chapter 5), confirming the presence of a unilateral (right) *dissociated vertical deviation (DVD)*. (DVD is discussed in more detail later in this chapter.)
3. The left eye rises under the cover, leading to a left hyperdeviation when the cover is removed. This situation also seems to violate Hering's law and represents a bilateral DVD, also termed a *double hyperphoria*.
4. The left eye adopts a hypotropic position under the cover but not to the same degree as the original hypertropia of the right eye. This can represent a combination of a true vertical tropia and a dissociated component (DVD) or, alternatively, a primary versus secondary deviation due to a restriction or palsy (see Chapter 5).

To simplify the discussion, the combined form (situation 4) is not addressed in this chapter. If the patient has a true hypertropia, a few principles aid in confirming the diagnosis:

1. A hyperdeviation that is incomitant in the horizontal plane suggests an oblique muscle disorder, while a comitant one is more consistent with a vertical rectus problem.
2. Deviations can be caused by innervational disorders (overaction or underaction of muscles) or mechanical problems (bone, muscle, or soft-tissue abnormalities within the orbit).
3. Whether it is an innervational or mechanical problem, one of the most common causes of a true vertical tropia is fourth nerve (superior oblique) palsy. Thus, the clinical examination must rule out this possibility.
4. If the deviation is incomitant in the horizontal plane or is long-standing and comitant, a head-tilt test (see Chapter 7, Fig 7-10) should be performed to determine whether an oblique muscle palsy may be the cause.
5. In a case of superior oblique palsy, the clinician must assume the palsy is bilateral until it is proven otherwise, especially when the patient has a history of trauma or a lesion of the central nervous system.

Incomitant Vertical Tropias

Incomitant vertical tropias commonly feature a hypertropia that is significantly worse on gaze to one side. They are often, but not exclusively, associated with oblique muscle abnormalities.

Overelevation and Overdepression in Adduction

There are several causes of overelevation in adduction (OEAd) and overdepression in adduction (ODAd) (Tables 11-1, 11-2). These include true overaction and underaction of the oblique muscles (see later in this chapter), as well as several conditions that can simulate oblique muscle overactions. These cases have also been labeled *oblique muscle pseudo-overactions*.

DVD can lead to an overelevation in adduction when the line of sight of the involved eye is blocked by the nose. There are circumstances, such as with large-angle exotropia and thyroid eye disease, in which clinical examination of ocular rotations indicates apparent overaction of both the superior and the inferior oblique muscles. In such cases, elevation or depression of the vertical rectus muscle of the opposite, abducting eye is restricted in the lateral portion of the bony orbit. The clinical findings can be explained as an attempt by the vertical rectus muscle to overcome this restriction through extra innervation, which, according to Hering's law (see Chapter 5), is distributed to the yoke oblique muscle as well. Alternatively, overelevation may be due to slippage of a tight lateral rectus as the eye adducts and rises above or below the midline (see Chapter 10). Unless it is severe, this condition does not require that the surgical plan include weakening of the oblique muscle.

Table 11-1 **Causes of Overelevation in Adduction**

Inferior oblique muscle overaction (primary or secondary)
Dissociated vertical deviation
Large-angle exotropia
Rectus muscle pulley heterotopia
Orbital dysmorphism (eg, craniofacial syndromes)
Duane retraction syndrome
Anti-elevation syndrome after contralateral inferior oblique muscle anterior transposition
Contralateral inferior rectus muscle restriction (eg, after orbital floor fracture, in thyroid eye
   disease)
Skew deviation

Table 11-2 **Causes of Overdepression in Adduction**

Superior oblique muscle overaction (primary or secondary)
Large-angle exotropia
Rectus muscle pulley heterotopia
Orbital dysmorphism (eg, craniofacial syndromes)
Duane retraction syndrome
Brown syndrome
Contralateral superior rectus muscle contracture (eg, after muscle resection)
Skew deviation

What appears to be an overaction may actually be due to abnormal function of a different extraocular muscle. Magnetic resonance imaging (MRI) studies have found connective tissue pulleys where the path of the inferior oblique muscle crosses that of the inferior rectus muscle. This arrangement is said to lead to a dynamic interaction of these muscles during vertical rotation that could give the appearance of overaction (see Chapter 3). In addition, malpositioning of the vertical rectus pulleys can lead to anomalous vertical actions that can simulate oblique muscle overactions. This can be seen in craniofacial syndromes. For example, an inferiorly displaced lateral rectus muscle can cause the normally positioned medial rectus muscle to act as an elevator in adduction; this causes an overelevation in adduction and a V-pattern deviation that simulate an inferior oblique muscle overaction. Conversely, a superiorly displaced lateral rectus muscle can produce an overdepression in adduction—simulating a superior oblique overaction—along with an A-pattern deviation. Lateral and medial malpositioning of vertical rectus muscles can also create pseudo-overactions of oblique muscles. One treatment implication is that large A and V patterns associated with these anomalous pulley positions respond poorly to oblique muscle surgery; it is more effective to relocate rectus muscle positions.

Other causes of OEAd and ODAd include the upshoots and downshoots of Duane retraction syndrome (see Chapter 12), restrictions of the superior or inferior rectus muscles (causing overinnervation of contralateral oblique muscles), skew deviation (see BCSC Section 5, *Neuro-Ophthalmology*), limitation of elevation in abduction after inferior oblique muscle anterior transposition (anti-elevation syndrome; see Chapter 14), and severe Brown syndrome (see Chapter 12).

Inferior oblique muscle overaction

Overaction of the inferior oblique muscle is one cause of OEAd. It is termed *primary* when it is not associated with superior oblique muscle palsy. It is called *secondary* when it accompanies palsy of the superior oblique muscle or the contralateral superior rectus muscle. The eye is elevated in adduction, both on horizontal movement and in upgaze (Fig 11-1).

One explanation of primary overaction relates to vestibular factors governing postural tonus of the extraocular muscles. Some observers have questioned the possibility of a true primary inferior oblique overaction, preferring to describe the movement merely as overelevation in adduction.

Clinical features Primary inferior oblique muscle overaction has been reported to develop between ages 1 and 6 years in up to two-thirds of patients with infantile strabismus (esotropia or exotropia). It also occurs, less frequently, in association with acquired esotropia or exotropia and, occasionally, in patients with no other strabismus. Bilateral overaction can be asymmetric; this is usually seen when vision is poor in 1 eye, leading to greater overaction in that eye.

With the eyes in lateral gaze, alternate cover testing shows that the higher (adducting) eye refixates with a downward movement and that the lower (abducting) eye refixates with an upward movement. When inferior oblique muscle overaction is bilateral, the higher and lower eyes reverse their direction of movement in the opposite lateral gaze. These features differentiate inferior oblique overaction from DVD (see discussion later in this chapter), in which neither eye refixates with an upward movement, whether adducted, abducted, or in primary position. A V-pattern horizontal deviation (see Chapter 10) and extorsion are common with overacting inferior oblique muscles.

Management In all but the mildest cases, a procedure to weaken the inferior oblique muscle (recession, disinsertion, myectomy, marginal myotomy, or anterior transposition) is indicated. Some surgeons grade the weakening procedure depending on the severity of the overaction (see also Chapter 14). Variations in the structure or path of this muscle may affect the surgical result.

Some observers believe that a modest recession actually functions as an anterior transposition, an operation that is useful for correcting marked overaction of the inferior oblique muscle and DVD—particularly when both are present simultaneously. Extorsion can also be improved by this procedure. Results vary according to the new location of the anterior and posterior fibers of the reinserted inferior oblique muscle. A spread-out

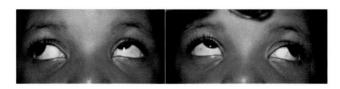

Figure 11-1 Bilateral inferior oblique muscle overaction. Overelevation in adduction, seen best in the upper fields. *(Courtesy of Edward L. Raab, MD.)*

reinsertion, especially if closer to the limbus than the inferior rectus muscle, can restrict elevation, especially when the eye is abducted (anti-elevation syndrome). In general, weakening of the inferior oblique muscles has an insignificant effect on horizontal alignment in primary position.

Kushner BJ. Restriction of elevation in abduction after inferior oblique anteriorization. *J AAPOS.* 1997;1(1):55–62.

Superior oblique muscle overaction

Superior oblique muscle overaction is one of several causes of overdepression in adduction (ODAd).

Clinical features A vertical deviation in primary position often occurs with unilateral or asymmetric bilateral overaction of the superior oblique muscles. The lower eye contains the overacting superior oblique muscle in unilateral overaction and the more prominently overacting superior oblique muscle in bilateral overaction. The overacting superior oblique muscle causes a hypotropia of the adducting eye, which is accentuated in the lower field (Fig 11-2). A horizontal deviation, most often exotropia, may be present and may lead to an A pattern (see Chapter 10). Intorsion is common with superior oblique muscle overaction. Most cases of bilateral superior oblique overaction are primary overactions.

Management In a patient with a clinically significant hypertropia or hypotropia or an A pattern, a procedure to weaken the superior oblique tendon (recession, tenotomy, tenectomy, or lengthening by insertion of a silicone spacer or nonabsorbable suture or by Z-lengthening) is appropriate (see Chapter 14). Significant intorsion will also be reduced with any of these procedures. Many surgeons are reluctant to perform superior oblique tendon weakening in patients with single binocular vision because the resulting, sometimes asymmetric, torsional and/or vertical effects can cause diplopia in these patients. As with inferior oblique muscle overaction, the horizontal deviation can be corrected during the same operative session. Some surgeons, anticipating a convergent effect in primary position, adjust their surgical amounts for horizontal rectus muscles when simultaneously weakening the superior oblique muscles.

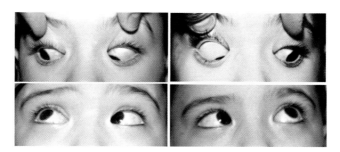

Figure 11-2 *Top row,* Bilateral superior oblique muscle overaction. Overdepression in adduction, seen best in the lower fields. *Bottom row,* Associated bilateral inferior oblique muscle underaction. *(Courtesy of Edward L. Raab, MD.)*

Superior Oblique Muscle Palsy

The most common paralysis of a single cyclovertical muscle is fourth nerve palsy, which involves the superior oblique muscle. It can be congenital or acquired; if the latter, it is usually a result of closed head trauma or, less commonly, vascular problems of the central nervous system, diabetes mellitus, or a brain tumor. Direct trauma to the tendon or the trochlear area is an occasional cause of unilateral superior oblique muscle palsy. One study showed that most patients with congenital superior oblique palsy had absent ipsilateral trochlear nerves and varying degrees of superior oblique muscle hypoplasia, while a minority had normal nerves and muscle bulks.

The same clinical features can result from a congenitally lax, attenuated, or even absent superior oblique tendon; from an unusual course of the muscle; or from functional consequences of malpositioned orbital pulleys—although strictly speaking, these are not paralytic entities. Superior oblique muscle underaction can also occur in several craniofacial abnormalities (see Chapter 18).

To differentiate congenital from acquired superior oblique muscle palsy, the clinician can examine childhood photographs to detect a compensatory head tilt. Facial asymmetry from long-standing head tilting and large vertical fusional amplitudes also indicate chronicity. The distinction is important because recently diagnosed palsy that cannot be attributed to known trauma suggests the possibility of a serious intracranial lesion and the need for neurologic investigation. Diagnostic evaluation for isolated nontraumatic fourth nerve palsy usually uncovers ischemic or idiopathic etiologies. Lack of signs of recovery by 3 months after onset should prompt neuroimaging. It should be noted that congenital superior oblique muscle palsy may not manifest until the child is older, but a large vertical fusional amplitude is typically present with no associated neurologic disorders. In this case, neuroimaging may not be necessary.

Neurologic aspects of superior oblique muscle palsy are discussed in BCSC Section 5, *Neuro-Ophthalmology*.

Yang HK, Kim JH, Hwang JM. Congenital superior oblique palsy and trochlear nerve absence: a clinical and radiological study. *Ophthalmology.* 2012;119(1):170–177. Epub 2011 Sep 15.

Clinical features

Either the normal or the affected eye can be preferred for fixation. Examination of versions usually reveals underaction of the involved superior oblique muscle and overaction of its antagonist inferior oblique muscle; however, the action of the superior oblique muscle can appear normal. In a unilateral palsy, the hyperdeviation is typically incomitant, especially in the acute stages. Over time, contracture of the ipsilateral superior rectus or contralateral inferior rectus muscle can lead to a "spread of comitance," with the result that there is minimal difference in the magnitude of the hypertropia when the patient looks from one side to the other. If depression cannot be evaluated because of the eye's inability to adduct (eg, in third nerve palsy), superior oblique muscle function can be evaluated by observing whether the eye intorts, as judged by the movement of surface landmarks or examination of the fundus, when the patient attempts to look downward and inward from primary position. Loss of strength of the superior oblique muscle leads to extorsion of the eye. If the degree of extorsion is large enough, subjective incyclodiplopia, in which the patient describes the image as appearing to tilt inward, can occur.

The diagnosis of unilateral superior oblique muscle palsy is further established by results of the 3-step test (Fig 11-3; see also Chapter 7, Fig 7-10) and the double Maddox rod test to measure torsional imbalance (see Chapter 7). However, the results of the 3-step test can be confounded by DVD, entities involving restriction, and some cases of skew deviation. During the double Maddox rod test or ophthalmoscopy, intorsion of the higher eye—instead of the expected extorsion—signifies skew deviation, especially when there are associated neurologic findings. In addition, if the patient is placed supine, the vertical tropia typically does not change in superior oblique palsy, while it decreases significantly in skew deviation. Some ophthalmologists document serial changes in the deviation by means of the Hess screen or the Lancaster red-green test or by plotting the field of single binocular vision (see Chapter 7).

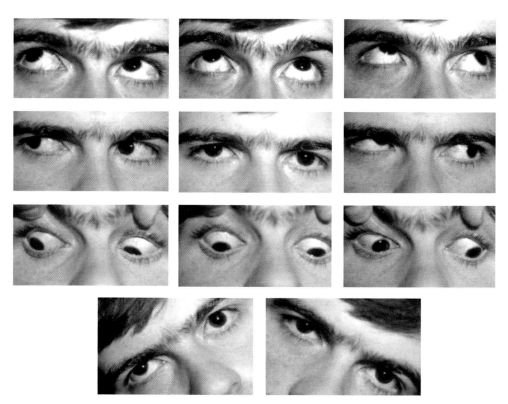

Figure 11-3 Right superior oblique muscle palsy. There is a right hypertropia in primary position that increases in left gaze and with head tilt to the right. Note accompanying overaction of the right inferior oblique muscle. *(Courtesy of Edward L. Raab, MD.)*

To differentiate bilateral from unilateral superior oblique muscle palsy, the following criteria are used:

- *Unilateral cases* usually show little if any V pattern (see Chapter 10) and less than 10° of extorsion in downgaze. Subjective incyclodiplopia is uncommon, unless the palsy is severe. The 3-step test yields positive results for the involved side only. Abnormal head positions—usually a tilt toward the shoulder opposite the side of the weakness—are common. Finally, the oblique muscle dysfunction is confined to the involved eye.
- *Bilateral cases* usually show a V pattern. Extorsion is 10° or more in downgaze; more than 20° of extorsion is highly suggestive of bilateral involvement. Subjective incyclodiplopia is common in acquired bilateral cases. The Bielschowsky head-tilt test yields positive results on tilt to each side—that is, right head tilt reveals a right hypertropia and left head tilt a left hypertropia. There is bilateral oblique muscle dysfunction. Patients may exhibit a chin-down head posture. Markedly asymmetric bilateral palsies that initially appear to be unilateral are called *masked bilateral palsies*. Signs of masked bilateral palsy include bilateral objective fundus extorsion, esotropia in downgaze, and even the mildest degree of oblique muscle dysfunction on the presumedly uninvolved side. Masked bilateral palsies are more common in patients with closed head trauma. They must be distinguished from situations in which the initial palsy is overcorrected, leading to a postoperative oblique muscle abnormality in the fellow eye.

Management

In small, symptomatic deviations that lack a prominent torsional component—especially those that have become comitant—prisms that compensate for the hyperdeviation in primary position may be used to overcome diplopia. Abnormal head position, significant vertical deviation, diplopia, and asthenopia are indications for surgery. Common operative strategies are discussed in the following sections (see also Chapter 14).

Unilateral superior oblique muscle palsy The approach to surgical treatment of a unilateral palsy depends on several factors:

- comitance or incomitance of the hyperdeviation
- size of the hyperdeviation in primary position
- diagnostic gaze positions in which the hyperdeviation is largest
- presence of cyclodiplopia or significant extorsion
- degree of laxity of the superior oblique tendon

When the deviation is incomitant, the surgeon can weaken the antagonist inferior oblique muscle if the hyperdeviation is worse in contralateral upgaze or strengthen the weak superior oblique muscle if the hyperdeviation is worse in contralateral downgaze. If the superior oblique muscle is lax, as in some cases of congenital superior oblique palsy, the tendon should be tightened; the most common procedure choice is tendon tucking. Laxity can be confirmed at surgery by a forced-duction test in which the globe is pushed (translated) posteriorly into the orbit while it is simultaneously extorted, thus tensing the superior oblique tendon. The presence of cyclodiplopia or significant extorsion also indicates that a superior oblique tendon strengthening procedure should be considered for inclusion in the surgical plan; options include tendon tucking and the various forms of the Harada-Ito procedure (see Chapter 14).

If the deviation is no greater than 15Δ in primary position, one of these options alone may be effective. When the inferior oblique muscle is weakened, the amount of deviation in primary position that is corrected by any weakening technique is proportional to the degree of preoperative overaction of the muscle. This procedure is not performed in skew deviation because inferior oblique muscle weakening would aggravate the intorsion of the higher eye.

If the hyperdeviation is incomitant and measures greater than 15Δ in primary position, it usually is also large in the ipsilateral (secondary) gaze field. In this situation, recession of the ipsilateral superior rectus muscle or the contralateral (yoke) inferior rectus muscle should be added to the oblique muscle surgery. The choice depends on whether the hyperdeviation is worse in downgaze or upgaze, as well as the tightness of these muscles on forced-duction testing. Either muscle can be recessed with an adjustable suture.

If the deviation has become comitant, vertical rectus muscle surgery is generally preferred. For deviations of less than 15Δ–20Δ, recession of 1 vertical rectus muscle should suffice; for larger hyperdeviations, both may have to be weakened.

In the unusually severe case with a vertical deviation greater than 35Δ in primary position, 3-muscle surgery is usually required. In this situation, most surgeons favor recession of the overacting antagonist inferior oblique muscle, plus either the ipsilateral superior rectus or contralateral inferior rectus muscle or both, as dictated by forced-duction test results. Ipsilateral superior oblique tendon tucking may have to be included if the tendon is lax.

On version testing, Hering's law may cause the superior oblique muscle to overact in the normal eye. If the surgeon is misled and performs superior oblique tenotomy on the normal eye, thereby converting a unilateral superior oblique palsy to a bilateral one, disabling torsional diplopia can result.

Whatever the approach, it is important to avoid overcorrection of a long-standing unilateral superior oblique muscle palsy in adult patients. Overcorrection can worsen with time and can cause disabling diplopia.

Bilateral superior oblique muscle palsy Surgical planning for treatment of bilateral superior oblique muscle palsy can be complex as surgery on both eyes is required and any asymmetry of the paralysis must be taken into account. The plan depends on several factors:

- magnitude of inferior oblique overaction and superior oblique weakness
- degree of laxity of the superior oblique tendons
- magnitude of cyclodiplopia and extorsion
- presence and size of a hyperdeviation in primary position
- size of the V pattern

If the palsies are symmetric and both inferior oblique muscles are significantly over-acting, weakening of both muscles is appropriate but may not be completely effective on its own. If the superior oblique muscles are lax or weak and cyclodiplopia or sizable extorsion is present, these muscles should be strengthened, using either tendon tucking or one of the variations of the Harada-Ito procedure.

If the paralysis is asymmetric, a hyperdeviation is usually present in primary position and the hyperdeviations on right and left gaze differ. There are several options for correcting this asymmetry, including symmetric oblique muscle surgery with a unilateral vertical rectus recession and asymmetric oblique muscle surgery tailored to correct more oblique muscle function in the eye with the worse palsy.

There are other, less common approaches to treating bilateral superior oblique palsy, including bilateral inferior rectus muscle recessions, which serve to add extra innervational drive on downgaze to help overcome the superior oblique deficits.

Any of these approaches should collapse a large V pattern, but if there is concern that some of the pattern may persist after one of the options is chosen, additional surgery may be necessary (see Chapter 10).

Inferior Oblique Muscle Palsy

Whether inferior oblique muscle palsy actually exists has been questioned. Most cases are congenital or posttraumatic. Some cases could be explained by a highly localized orbital lesion, but this is rare. It has recently been suggested that at least some cases, especially those with a history of head trauma or with additional neurologic findings, are a form of skew deviation, even if the diagnosis of inferior oblique muscle palsy is supported by results of the 3-step test (Fig 11-4). Other cases are thought to be explained by demonstrable abnormalities of the muscle.

In inferior oblique muscle palsy, the hypotropic eye is intorted, which may lead to subjective excyclodiplopia (image appears to tilt outward); in skew deviation, the hypotropic eye is extorted, a finding incompatible with the diagnosis of inferior oblique muscle palsy. These phenomena are analogous to those described in regard to superior oblique palsy. Cases in which the results of the 3-step test are not clear may represent asymmetric or unilateral primary superior oblique muscle overaction with secondary underaction of the inferior oblique muscle.

Clinical features

As with Brown syndrome (see Chapter 12), elevation is deficient in the adducted position of the eye. The features that distinguish inferior oblique muscle palsy from congenital Brown syndrome are listed in Table 11-3.

Management

Indications for treatment of inferior oblique muscle palsy are abnormal head position, vertical deviation in primary position, and diplopia. Management consists of weakening either the ipsilateral superior oblique muscle or the contralateral superior rectus muscle. The former procedure will aggravate the existing extorsion of the hypotropic eye if an undetected skew deviation is the true underlying abnormality.

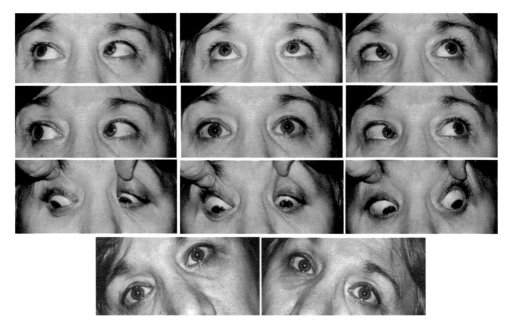

Figure 11-4 Right inferior oblique muscle palsy. There is a small left hypertropia in primary position that increases in left gaze and with head tilt to the left, the 3-step pattern consistent with this diagnosis. This patient had no abnormal neurologic findings. Note convergence in straight upgaze, an important point of differentiation from Brown syndrome. *(Courtesy of Edward L. Raab, MD.)*

Table 11-3 Comparison of Inferior Oblique Muscle Palsy and Congenital Brown Syndrome

	Inferior Oblique Muscle Palsy	Congenital Brown Syndrome
Forced-duction testing	Negative	Positive
Strabismus pattern	A pattern	None or V pattern
Superior oblique muscle overaction	Usually significant	None or minimal
Torsion	Intorsion	None
Head-tilt test	Positive	Negative

Other Incomitant Vertical Tropias

Several other hypertropias are not oblique muscle disorders yet may present with incomitance. These include innervational problems, such as the upshoots and downshoots seen in Duane retraction syndrome and partial third nerve palsy; and mechanical disorders, such as Brown syndrome, thyroid eye disease, orbital tumors, and orbital implants (eg, glaucoma drainage devices, scleral buckles). These topics are discussed elsewhere in this volume and in other BCSC Sections.

Comitant Vertical Tropias

Comitant vertical tropias commonly exhibit a hypertropia or a hypotropia that does not change significantly when gaze is shifted from one side to the other.

Monocular Elevation Deficiency

Monocular elevation deficiency (previously termed *double-elevator palsy*) involves a limitation of upward gaze with a hypotropia that is similar in adduction and abduction. This motility pattern may be caused by restriction of the inferior rectus muscle or by an innervational deficit (weakness of 1 or both elevator muscles or a monocular supranuclear gaze disorder). Patients may have a combination of a restriction and elevator muscle deficit.

Clinical features

Monocular elevation deficiency features a hypotropia of the involved eye that increases in upgaze, a chin-up position with fusion in downgaze, and ptosis or pseudoptosis (Fig 11-5).

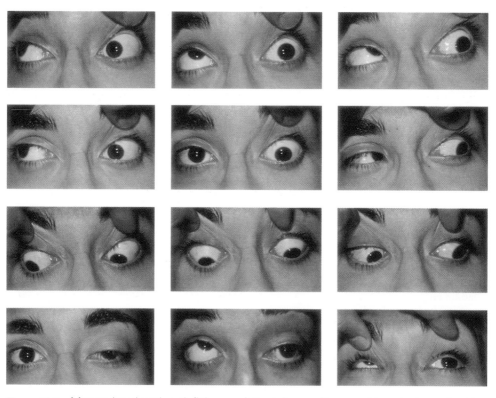

Figure 11-5 Monocular elevation deficiency of the left eye. *Top row,* No voluntary elevation of the left eye above horizontal. *Second row,* Hypotropia of the left eye across the horizontal fields of gaze. *Third row,* Depression of the left eye is unaffected. *Bottom left,* Ptosis (true and pseudo-) of the left upper eyelid during fixation with the right eye (in the top 3 rows, the left upper eyelid is elevated manually). *Bottom center,* Persistence of ptosis and marked secondary overelevation of the right eye during fixation with the left eye. *Bottom right,* A partial Bell phenomenon, with the left eye elevating above the horizontal on forced eyelid closure.

True ptosis is present in 50% of patients. If any other feature of third nerve palsy is present, that condition should be suspected rather than monocular elevation deficiency.

Clinical features of the 3 forms of monocular elevation deficiency are as follows:

- restriction

  - positive forced duction on elevation
  - normal elevation force generation and elevation saccadic velocity (no muscle paralysis)
  - often an extra or deeper lower eyelid fold on attempted upgaze
  - poor or absent Bell phenomenon

- elevator muscle innervational deficit

  - free forced duction on elevation
  - reduced elevation force generation and saccadic velocity
  - preservation of Bell phenomenon (indicating a supranuclear cause) in many cases

- combination

  - positive forced duction on elevation
  - reduced elevation force generation and saccadic velocity

In support of this classification, studies using MRI have shown either focal thickening of the inferior rectus muscle, supporting a restrictive etiology, or normal ocular motor nerves, suggesting a central unilateral disorder of upgaze.

Management

Indications for treatment include a large vertical deviation in primary position, with or without ptosis, and an abnormal chin-up head position. If restriction originating from below the eye is present, the inferior rectus muscle should be recessed, using an adjustable suture if possible. If there is no restriction, the medial and lateral rectus muscles can be transposed toward the superior rectus muscle *(Knapp procedure)*. Alternatively, the surgeon can recess the ipsilateral inferior rectus and either recess the contralateral superior rectus muscle or resect the ipsilateral superior rectus muscle. Ptosis surgery should be deferred until the vertical deviation has been corrected and the pseudoptosis component removed.

Kim JH, Hwang JM. Congenital monocular elevation deficiency. *Ophthalmology.* 2009;116(3): 580–584.

Orbital Floor Fractures

Clinical features and management of orbital floor fractures are discussed in Chapter 27 and in BCSC Section 7, *Orbit, Eyelids, and Lacrimal System.* The discussion in this chapter focuses on motility abnormalities in patients with these fractures.

Clinical features

Diplopia in the immediate postinjury stage is to be expected and is not necessarily an indication for urgent intervention. Depending on the site of the bony trauma, muscles can be either entrapped and restricted or paralyzed due to nerve damage. Palsy of a muscle may resolve over several months. If the fracture requires surgery, the range of eye movements may improve. On the other hand, fibrosis after trauma may cause restriction to persist even after successful repair of the fracture.

Management

Treatment of strabismus is usually needed when diplopia persists in primary position or downgaze or there is an associated compensatory head position. Some mild limitations of eye movements can be managed with prisms.

Planning of eye muscle surgery depends on the fields where diplopia is present and on the relative contributions of muscle restriction and paresis. For a nonresolving hypotropia in primary position (Fig 11-6), recession of the ipsilateral inferior rectus muscle can be effective, especially if the muscle is tight on forced-duction testing. Similarly, an incomitant esotropia (with diplopia on side gaze) due to restriction on the medial side may be improved by recession of the ipsilateral medial rectus muscle.

Initially, a hypertropia due to weakness of the inferior rectus muscle without entrapment is managed with observation, because the weakness may improve with time. If recovery is not complete within 6–12 months of the injury and there is at least a moderate degree of active force, resection of the affected muscle can be performed. If the hypertropia is large, the procedure can be combined with recession (with or without an adjustable suture) of the ipsilateral superior rectus muscle. Alternatively, recession of the contralateral inferior rectus muscle, with or without the addition of a posterior fixation suture *(fadenoperation),* can be used to limit the fellow eye's downgaze movement and match the duction deficiency of the injured eye. A substitute to match the infraduction limitation

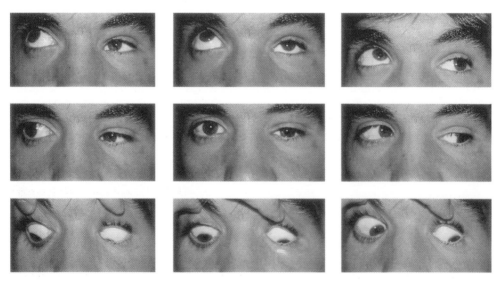

Figure 11-6 Old left orbital floor fracture with inferior rectus muscle entrapment. Note limitation of elevation of the left eye and pseudoptosis from enophthalmos. The eyelids are elevated manually in the bottom row.

is a combined recession and resection of the contralateral inferior rectus muscle. Transposition of the ipsilateral medial and lateral rectus muscles to the inferior rectus muscle (inverse Knapp procedure) may be necessary for treatment of complete chronic inferior rectus muscle palsy. Whether or not prior orbital surgery has been performed to release entrapped tissues, partial restriction persists in many cases even though imaging studies may show no residual entrapment. This restriction can limit the success of surgery.

Other Comitant Vertical Tropias

Other disorders that feature a hypertropia that does not change significantly from right to left gaze include innervational problems, such as superior division (partial) palsy of the third cranial nerve; and mechanical disorders such as thyroid eye disease, congenital fibrosis of the extraocular muscles, and orbital tumors. A long-standing superior oblique palsy may also develop a spread of comitance. These topics are discussed elsewhere in this volume and in other BCSC Sections.

Dissociated Vertical Deviation

Dissociated vertical deviation (DVD) is an innervational disorder found in more than 50% of patients with infantile strabismus (esotropia or exotropia). There are 2 explanations for the origin of DVD. One theory is that it is the result of mechanisms to compensate for latent nystagmus, with the oblique muscles playing the principal role. An alternative theory suggests that deficient fusion allows the primitive dorsal light reflex, which is prominent in other species, to emerge.

Brodsky MC. Dissociated vertical divergence: a righting reflex gone wrong. *Arch Ophthalmol.* 1999;117(9):1216–1222.

Guyton DL. Ocular torsion reveals the mechanisms of cyclovertical strabismus: the Weisenfeld lecture. *Invest Ophthalmol Vis Sci.* 2008;49(3):847–857.

Clinical Features

DVD usually presents by age 2 years, whether or not the horizontal deviation has been surgically corrected. Either eye slowly drifts upward and outward, with simultaneous extorsion, when occluded or during periods of visual inattention (Fig 11-7). Some patients attempt to compensate by tilting the head, for reasons that still have not been conclusively identified.

In bilateral or unilateral DVD, the vertical movement usually predominates, but sometimes the principal dissociated movement is one of abduction (*dissociated horizontal deviation* or *DHD*). DVD is usually bilateral but is frequently asymmetric. It may occur spontaneously (manifest DVD) or only when 1 eye is occluded (latent DVD). In addition to DHD, latent nystagmus and horizontal strabismus are often associated with DVD. These entities are manifestations of deficient binocular vision.

Measurement of DVD is difficult and imprecise. In one method, a base-down prism is placed in front of the upwardly deviating eye while it is behind an occluder. The occluder

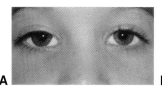 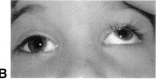 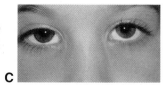

Figure 11-7 Dissociated vertical deviation, left eye. **A,** Straight eyes during binocular viewing conditions. **B,** Large left hyperdeviation immediately after the eye is covered and then uncovered. **C,** Left eye drifts back down toward midline. Note that the right eye does not adopt a hypotropic position when the left eye drifts back to the midline.

is then switched to the fixating lower eye. The prism power is adjusted until the deviating eye shows no downward movement to refixate. Results are similar when a red Maddox rod is used to generate a horizontal line for the dissociated higher eye while the other eye fixates on a small light; vertical prism power is adjusted to eliminate the separation of the light and the line. Each eye is tested separately in cases of bilateral DVD.

Management

Treatment of DVD is indicated if the deviation is noticeable (generally more than 6Δ–8Δ) and occurs frequently during the day. Changing fixation preference using optical penalization is effective mostly in unilateral or highly asymmetric bilateral DVD. Since DVD is a cause of OEAd, distinguishing it from overaction of the inferior oblique muscles is important because the surgical approaches to these 2 conditions are different in most cases.

Surgery on the vertical muscles often improves the condition but rarely eliminates it. Recessions of the superior rectus muscle, ranging from 6 to 10 mm according to the size of the hypertropia, can be effective. Bilateral surgery is performed whenever both eyes can fixate; asymmetric recessions are an option if the DVD is asymmetric. If there is residual DVD after superior rectus muscle recession, inferior rectus muscle resection or plication can be performed, with careful dissection to minimize lower eyelid advancement. Inferior oblique muscle anterior transposition is also effective in treating DVD, especially if it is accompanied by inferior oblique muscle overaction.

Related Videos

The following videos contain additional information on topics covered in this chapter and are available at www.aao.org/bcscvideo. Mobile-device users can scan the QR code below to access the videos.

- Inferior Oblique Weakening Procedures (9 min, 17 sec)
- Superior Oblique Tucking (4 min, 9 sec)
- Superior Oblique Muscle Tenotomy (3 min, 38 sec)
- Oblique Muscle Forced-Duction Testing (1 min)

CHAPTER 12

Special Forms of Strabismus

The BCSC *Master Index* and BCSC Section 5, *Neuro-Ophthalmology,* should be consulted for additional discussion of several entities covered in this chapter. See Chapter 14 for discussion of some of the surgical procedures mentioned in this chapter.

Congenital Cranial Dysinnervation Disorders

Congenital cranial dysinnervation disorders (CCDDs) are a group of strabismus entities that have in common a developmental defect of one or more cranial nerve nuclei and, as a result, hypoplasia or absence of the nerves themselves. These anomalies lead to various patterns of abnormal innervation of the eye muscles, which often result in secondary abnormal structural changes to the affected muscles, usually stiffening or contractures. Onset of the innervation anomalies can be as early as the first trimester in utero. Included in this group are Duane retraction syndrome, congenital fibrosis of the extraocular muscles (CFEOM), Möbius syndrome, and some cases of congenital fourth nerve palsy (see Chapter 11). Recent work suggests that congenital Brown syndrome may also be a form of CCDD.

> Engle EC. The genetic basis of complex strabismus. *Pediatr Res.* 2006;59(3):343–348.
> Engle EC. Oculomotility disorders arising from disruptions in brainstem motor neuron development. *Arch Neurol.* 2007;64(5):633–637.
> Traboulsi EI. Congenital cranial dysinnervation disorders and more. *J AAPOS.* 2007;11(3): 215–217.

Duane Retraction Syndrome

Duane retraction syndrome is a spectrum of ocular motility disorders characterized by anomalous co-contraction of the medial and lateral rectus muscles on actual or attempted adduction of the involved eye or eyes; this co-contraction causes the globe to retract. Horizontal eye movement can be limited to various degrees in both abduction and adduction. An upshoot or downshoot often occurs when the affected eye is innervated to adduct; vertical slippage of a tight lateral rectus muscle by 1–2 mm, which has been demonstrated by magnetic resonance imaging (MRI) studies, has been proposed as the cause. An alternative theory is that anomalous vertical rectus muscle activity is responsible for upshoots and downshoots, but this is less common.

Although most affected patients have Duane retraction syndrome alone, many associated systemic defects have been observed, such as Goldenhar syndrome (hemifacial microsomia, ocular dermoids, ear anomalies, preauricular skin tags, and eyelid colobomas) and Wildervanck syndrome (sensorineural hearing loss and Klippel-Feil anomaly with fused cervical vertebrae). A defect in development occurring between the fourth and sixth weeks of gestation appears to be the cause of Duane retraction syndrome, according to studies of patients prenatally exposed to thalidomide.

Most cases of Duane retraction syndrome are sporadic, but approximately 5%–10% show autosomal dominant inheritance. Instances of links to more generalized disorders have been reported. Discordance in monozygotic twins raises the possibility that the intrauterine environment may be important in the development of this syndrome. A higher prevalence in females is reported in most series, and there is a predilection for the left eye.

In most anatomical and imaging studies, the nucleus of the sixth cranial nerve is absent or hypoplastic and an aberrant branch of the third cranial nerve innervates the lateral rectus muscle. Results of electromyographic studies have been consistent with this finding. Although Duane retraction syndrome is considered an innervational anomaly, tight and broadly inserted medial rectus muscles and fibrotic lateral rectus muscles, with corresponding forced-duction abnormalities, are often encountered during surgery.

Clinical features

The most widely used classification of Duane retraction syndrome defines 3 groups, but they may represent differences only in the severity of horizontal rotation limitations: type 1 refers to poor abduction, frequently with primary position esotropia (Fig 12-1); type 2 refers to poor adduction and exotropia (Fig 12-2); and type 3 refers to poor abduction

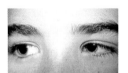 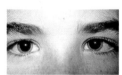 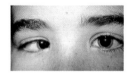 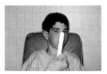

Figure 12-1 Type 1 Duane retraction syndrome with esotropia, left eye, showing limitation of abduction, almost full adduction, and retraction of the globe on adduction. *Far right,* Compensatory left head turn. *(Courtesy of Edward L. Raab, MD.)*

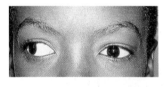 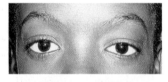 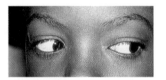

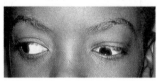 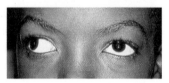

Figure 12-2 Type 2 Duane retraction syndrome, left eye. *Top row,* Full abduction and marked limitation of adduction. *Bottom row,* Variable upshoot and downshoot of the left eye with extreme right gaze effort. The typical primary position exotropia is not present in this patient. *(Courtesy of Edward L. Raab, MD.)*

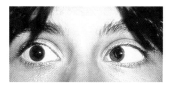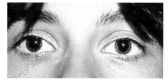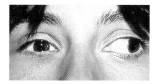

Figure 12-3 Type 3 Duane retraction syndrome, right eye. Severe limitation of abduction and adduction, with palpebral fissure narrowing even though adduction cannot be accomplished. There is no deviation in primary position. *(Courtesy of Edward L. Raab, MD.)*

and adduction, with esotropia, exotropia, or no primary position deviation (Fig 12-3). Approximately 15% of cases are bilateral; the type may differ between the 2 eyes. The spectrum of dysinnervation among cases means that classification of patients based on these categories can be arbitrary in some situations, especially in deciding between type 1 and type 3.

Type 1 Duane retraction syndrome (with esotropia and limited abduction) is the most common form, accounting for 50%–80% of cases in several series. Affected individuals or their caregivers often incorrectly believe that the normal eye is turning in excessively, not realizing that the involved eye is failing to abduct. Observation of globe retraction on adduction obviates the need for neurologic investigation for sixth nerve palsy, from which it must be differentiated; however, retraction can be difficult to appreciate in an infant. Another indicator that the condition is not sixth nerve palsy is the lack of correspondence between the absent or typically modest primary position esotropia (usually <30Δ) and the usually profound abduction deficit (a comparison useful in ruling out paralysis in other entities as well). A further point of differentiation is that even in esotropic Duane retraction syndrome, a small-angle exotropia is frequently present on gaze to the side opposite the affected eye, a finding not present in lateral rectus muscle paralysis. Finally, examination at the slit lamp can help confirm the diagnosis in mild cases: if the vertical slit-lamp beam cast from the cornea onto the lower eyelid is disrupted by globe retraction when the eye adducts, Duane retraction syndrome is present.

Management

No surgical approach will normalize rotations. Surgery is reserved for cases with a primary position deviation, a head turn, marked globe retraction, or large upshoots or downshoots. Since Duane retraction syndrome is a spectrum of motility disorders, the surgical plan has to be individualized for the patient. In many patients with this syndrome, the eyes are properly aligned in at least 1 position of gaze, allowing the development of binocular vision. The main goals of surgery are to centralize and expand the field of single binocular vision.

For type 1 Duane retraction syndrome, recession of the medial rectus muscle on the involved side has been the procedure most often used to correct the primary position deviation and eliminate the head turn. Adding recession of the opposite medial rectus (bilateral surgery) has been recommended for deviations larger than 20Δ in primary position. These operations do not usually improve abduction significantly. Primary position overcorrection due to excessive medial rectus recession can occur, and the resulting exotropia will worsen when the involved eye is adducted. Recession of the lateral rectus muscle of the uninvolved eye can offset this effect.

Because of the likelihood that globe retraction will worsen, most surgeons do not favor resection of the lateral rectus muscle for type 1 Duane retraction syndrome, but there are occasional exceptions. Partial or full lateral transposition of both of the vertical rectus muscles or the superior rectus alone, with or without posterior scleral fixation (myopexy) has been found to improve abduction.

The most commonly recommended surgery for type 2 Duane retraction syndrome is recession of the lateral rectus muscle on the involved side in proportion to the size of the exotropia; resection of the medial rectus muscle is avoided. Some surgeons recess both lateral rectus muscles if a large-angle exotropia is present.

Patients with type 3 Duane syndrome often have straight eyes in or near the primary position and little, if any, head turn. Severe globe retraction may be lessened by recession of both the medial and the lateral rectus muscles, which also may benefit the induced anomalous vertical movements. This is also an option for treating retraction in type 1 and type 2 Duane retraction syndrome. The lateral recession must be very large to improve the retraction. Procedures to address the upshoot or downshoot include large lateral rectus recession, splitting of the lateral rectus muscle in a Y configuration, retroequatorial fixation of the lateral rectus muscle, and, more recently, disinsertion of the lateral rectus muscle and reattachment to the lateral periosteum of the orbit.

Rosenbaum AL. Costenbader lecture. The efficacy of rectus muscle transposition surgery in esotropic Duane syndrome and VI nerve palsy. *J AAPOS.* 2004;8(5):409–419.

Congenital Fibrosis of the Extraocular Muscles

Congenital fibrosis of the extraocular muscles (CFEOM), or congenital fibrosis syndrome, is a group of rare congenital disorders in which extraocular muscle (EOM) restriction is present and fibrous tissue replaces these muscles. Some forms have been noted to be inherited, usually as an autosomal dominant trait but occasionally in an autosomal recessive fashion. Cases of CFEOM involve developmental defects of cranial nerve nuclei and of the nerves themselves, resulting in dysinnervation and abnormal structure of the EOMs.

Heidary G, Engle EC, Hunter DG. Congenital fibrosis of the extraocular muscles. *Semin Ophthalmol.* 2008;23(1):3–8.

Clinical features

There are several variations of CFEOM. Generalized fibrosis is the most severe form, affecting all the EOMs of both eyes, including the levator palpebrae superioris. Congenital unilateral fibrosis is nonfamilial.

A variant that involves the inferior rectus muscle alone may be unilateral or bilateral and sporadic or familial. This condition is commonly inherited as an autosomal dominant trait.

Strabismus fixus involves the horizontal rectus muscles, usually the medial rectus muscles, causing severe esotropia. The condition is usually sporadic and can be acquired late.

Vertical retraction syndrome affects the superior rectus muscle and causes inability to depress the eye.

Diagnosis of CFEOM depends on finding limited voluntary motion with restriction, which is usually severe and can be confirmed with forced-duction testing. The congenital onset is important in distinguishing the syndrome from thyroid eye disease.

Management

Surgery for CFEOM is difficult and requires release of the restricted muscles (ie, weakening procedures). Fibrosis of the adjacent tissues may be present as well. A good surgical result aligns the eyes in primary position, but full ocular rotations cannot be restored and the outcome is unpredictable.

Yazdani A, Traboulsi EI. Classification and surgical management of patients with familial and sporadic forms of congenital fibrosis of the extraocular muscles. *Ophthalmology.* 2004;111(5): 1035–1042.

Möbius Syndrome

Clinical features

Möbius syndrome (or "sequence"; see Chapter 15) is a rare condition characterized by the association of both sixth and seventh nerve palsies, the latter causing masklike facies. Patients may also manifest gaze palsies that can be attributed to abnormalities in the paramedian pontine reticular formation or the sixth cranial nerve nucleus. Many patients also have limb, chest, and tongue defects, and some geneticists think that Möbius syndrome is one of a family of syndromes in which hypoplastic limb anomalies may be associated with orofacial and cranial nerve defects. Poland syndrome (absent pectoralis muscle) is another variant.

Patients with Möbius syndrome exhibit 1 of 3 patterns of motility involvement, probably related to the severity and timing of the in utero insult:

1. Orthotropia in primary position with marked deficits in abduction and adduction (Fig 12-4) (40% of cases)
2. Esotropia with cross-fixation and sparing of convergence and adduction (50% of cases)
3. Large exotropia with absence of convergence (10% of cases)

Some patients appear to have palpebral fissure changes on adduction or vertical EOM involvement.

Management

Medial rectus muscle recession has been advocated for patients with large-angle esotropia, but caution should be exercised in the presence of a significant limitation of adduction. Some surgeons have undertaken to improve abduction by performing vertical rectus muscle transposition procedures after medial rectus muscle restriction has been relieved.

Carta A, Mora P, Neri A, Favilla S, Sadun AA. Ophthalmologic and systemic features in Möbius syndrome: an Italian case series. *Ophthalmology.* 2011;118(8):1518–1523. Epub 2011 Apr 3.

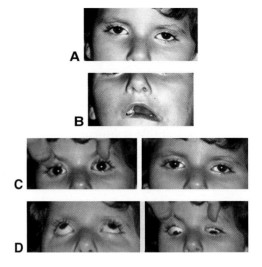

Figure 12-4 Möbius syndrome. **A,** Straight eyes in primary position. **B,** The patient cannot smile because of bilateral seventh nerve palsy. **C,** Bilaterally absent adduction and severely limited abduction. **D,** Vertical movements are not affected. *(Courtesy of Edward L. Raab, MD.)*

Miscellaneous Special Forms of Strabismus

Brown Syndrome

Although it is included in most lists of vertical deviations (see Chapter 11), Brown syndrome is best considered a special form of strabismus. The characteristic restriction of elevation in adduction was originally thought to be caused by shortening of the supposed sheath of the superior oblique tendon. It is now attributed to various abnormalities of the tendon–trochlea complex (see Chapter 3), and recent evidence indicates that structural problems within the orbit but remote from the superior oblique tendon, including instability of the lateral rectus pulley, can present an identical clinical picture *(pseudo–Brown syndrome)*. Recent work suggests that congenital Brown syndrome may be a form of CCDD.

Most cases are congenital. Prominent causes of the acquired form include trauma in the region of the trochlea, iatrogenic causes such as scleral buckles and glaucoma drainage devices, orbital tumors, and systemic inflammatory conditions such as rheumatoid arthritis. The latter often result in intermittent Brown syndrome, which may resolve spontaneously. Sinusitis has also led to Brown syndrome; thus, patients with acute-onset presentation of Brown syndrome of undetermined cause should undergo imaging of the orbits and paranasal sinuses to investigate this possibility. The condition is bilateral in approximately 10% of cases. Resolution of congenital Brown syndrome has been thought to be unusual, but a recent report describes spontaneous improvement in 75% of cases, often over many years.

> Dawson E, Barry J, Lee J. Spontaneous resolution in patients with congenital Brown syndrome. *J AAPOS.* 2009;13(2):116–118. Epub 2008 Dec 12.

Clinical features

Well-recognized clinical features of Brown syndrome include deficient elevation in adduction that improves in abduction but often not completely (Fig 12-5). Several findings

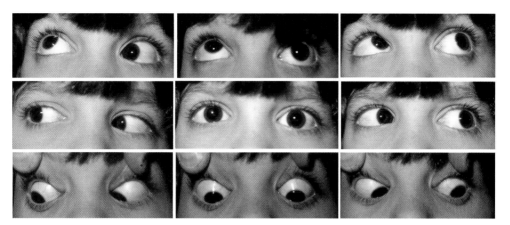

Figure 12-5 Brown syndrome, left eye. No elevation of the left eye when adducted; left eye is depressed instead. Elevation is also severely limited in straight-up gaze and moderately so even in up-and-left gaze. Note the characteristic divergence in straight-up gaze and lack of ipsilateral superior oblique overaction. *(Courtesy of Edward L. Raab, MD.)*

differentiate Brown syndrome from inferior oblique muscle paralysis (see Chapter 11, Table 11-3).

An unequivocally positive forced-duction test demonstrating restricted passive elevation in adduction is essential for the diagnosis. Retropulsion of the globe during this test stretches the superior oblique tendon and accentuates the restriction. In restrictions involving the inferior rectus muscle or its surrounding tissues, by contrast, the limitation of passive elevation is accentuated by forceps-induced proptosis of the eye rather than by retropulsion.

Attempts at elevation straight upward usually cause divergence (V pattern) due to lateral diversion of the globe as it meets resistance from the tight superior oblique tendon (see Fig 12-5). This finding is an important point of distinction from inferior oblique muscle paralysis, which usually exhibits an A pattern (see Chapter 11, Table 11-3). In adduction, the palpebral fissure widens, and a downshoot of the involved eye occurs on gaze to the opposite side in severe cases. The overdepression in adduction seen in Brown syndrome (see Chapter 11, Table 11-2) can be distinguished from that of true superior oblique muscle overaction because downshoot in the latter occurs less abruptly as adduction is increased. In mild Brown syndrome, no hypotropia is present in primary position. Severe cases of Brown syndrome exhibit both a downshoot in adduction and a primary position hypotropia, often accompanied by a chin-up head posture or a head turn away from the affected eye. Moderate cases have findings between these extremes.

Management

Observation alone is appropriate for mild congenital Brown syndrome. When Brown syndrome is secondary to rheumatoid arthritis or other systemic inflammatory diseases, resolution may occur as systemic treatment brings the underlying disease into remission or when corticosteroids are injected near the trochlea.

Surgery is indicated for more severe congenital cases. Sheathectomy, originally advocated by Harold Brown, has been abandoned in favor of ipsilateral superior oblique tenotomy nasal to the superior rectus muscle. However, iatrogenic superior oblique muscle paresis occurs in a significant minority of patients after this procedure. Careful handling of the intermuscular septum during surgery and avoidance of complete tenotomy as a sole procedure can reduce the incidence of this sequela. Options used currently include insertion of an inert spacer or suture between the cut ends of the superior oblique tendon, a Z-plasty of the tendon on the medial side, and partial (80%) tenectomy of the posterior portion of the tendon on the temporal side. Using any of these procedures, the surgeon should repair the intermuscular septum to prevent contact of the spacer or suture with nearby structures and therefore avoid a downgaze restriction due to adhesions to the upper nasal quadrant of the globe. To reduce the consequences of superior oblique muscle palsy after tenotomy, some surgeons perform simultaneous ipsilateral inferior oblique muscle weakening.

Wright KW. Brown's syndrome: diagnosis and management. *Trans Am Ophthalmol Soc.* 1999; 97:1023–1109.

Third Nerve Palsy

In children, third nerve palsy can be congenital (40%–50% of cases) or can be caused by conditions such as trauma, inflammation, or viral infection. It can also occur as a manifestation of ophthalmoplegic migraine, after vaccination, or (infrequently) as a result of a neoplastic lesion. In adults, the usual causes are intracranial aneurysm, microvascular infarction, inflammation, trauma, infection, or tumor. See BCSC Section 5, *Neuro-Ophthalmology,* for detailed discussion of the causes and manifestations of third nerve palsy. This section is concerned primarily with the principles of treatment of the disturbed motility.

Clinical features

The location of the lesion along the central and peripheral pathway of the third cranial nerve determines the presenting features. Ischemic causes may spare the pupil, whereas compressive lesions, such as tumors or aneurysms, typically cause mydriasis. Complete paralysis results in limited adduction, elevation, and depression of the eye, causing exotropia and often hypotropia. These findings are expected because the remaining unopposed muscles are the lateral rectus (abductor) and the superior oblique (abductor and depressor), except when the cause of the paralysis involves the nerves supplying these muscles as well. Upper eyelid ptosis is usually present, often with pseudoptosis due to the depressed position of the involved eye (Fig 12-6).

The clinical findings and treatment may be complicated by misdirection (aberrant regeneration) of the damaged nerve, presenting as anomalous eyelid elevation, pupil constriction, or vertical excursion of the globe—any or all of which can occur on attempted rotation into the field of action of the EOMs supplied by the injured nerve. A miotic pupil is sometimes seen in congenital cases, irrespective of whether there is aberrant regeneration. Affected adults report incapacitating diplopia unless the involved eye is occluded by ptosis or other means.

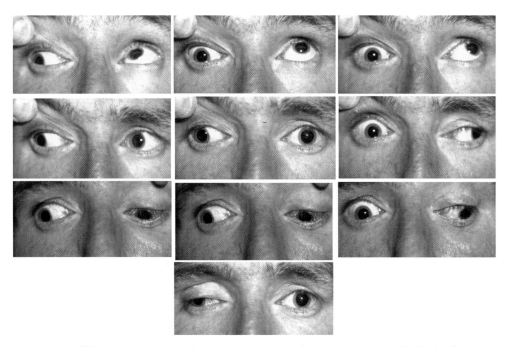

Figure 12-6 Third nerve palsy, right eye, with ptosis *(bottom photo)* and limited adduction, elevation, and depression (upper eyelid elevated manually in top 9 photos). *(Courtesy of Edward L. Raab, MD.)*

Management

Except in congenital cases, it is advisable to wait at least 6 months, and even up to 12 months, for spontaneous recovery before proceeding with surgical correction. Patients with at least partial recovery are much better candidates for good functional and cosmetic results. Because the visual system is still developing in pediatric patients, amblyopia is a common finding that must be treated aggressively.

Surgical elevation of the upper eyelid and incomplete realignment without useful single binocular fields may reinforce the incapacitating diplopia in adult patients with previously good binocular visual function. Prism adaptation testing has shown that adult patients who can achieve single binocular vision with prisms of any power before surgery are most likely to do well. The incidence of diplopia in patients younger than 8 years is low because of suppression (see Chapter 6).

Third nerve palsy presents difficult surgical challenges because multiple EOMs, including the levator muscle, are involved. Replacing all of the lost rotational forces on the globe is impossible; therefore, the goal of surgery is adequate alignment for binocular function in primary position and in slight downgaze for reading.

Selection of the surgical procedure is dictated by the number and condition of the involved muscles and the presence or absence of noticeable paradoxical rotations. In a case of incomplete paralysis, a large recession-resection of the horizontal rectus muscles to correct the exodeviation, with supraplacement of both to correct the hypotropia, is effective.

For complete paralysis, a large lateral rectus muscle recession combined with fixation of the globe to the nasal orbital periosteum is one suggested approach. Disinsertion of the lateral rectus muscle and reattachment to the lateral orbital periosteum can maximize inactivation of the muscle. Some surgeons correct hypotropia with concurrent superior oblique tenotomy. Transfer of the superior oblique tendon to the upper nasal quadrant of the globe also has been employed; however, anomalous eye movements can result from this procedure. Most surgeons reserve correction of ptosis for a subsequent procedure, which allows for more accurate positioning of the upper eyelid.

Sixth Nerve Palsy

Paralysis of the sixth cranial (abducens) nerve is less common in children than in adults. This entity is discussed in Chapter 8. See BCSC Section 5, *Neuro-Ophthalmology,* for additional discussion.

Thyroid Eye Disease

Thyroid eye disease affects the eye and the orbit in a variety of ways. Only motility disturbances are covered in this volume.

Edema, inflammation, and fibrosis of the EOMs due to lymphocytic infiltration occur in this disease. Not only do these pathologies restrict motility, but the massively enlarged muscles can cause compressive optic neuropathy. Detection of muscle enlargement by orbital imaging helps confirm the diagnosis.

The myopathy is not caused by thyroid dysfunction. Rather, both conditions probably result from a common autoimmune disease. Thyroid-stimulating immunoglobulins (TSIs) likely mediate thyroid eye disease and may be regarded as a functional biomarker for this condition. Some patients also have myasthenia gravis (discussed later in this chapter), complicating the clinical findings. An association between severity of thyroid eye disease and smoking has recently become apparent; the hazard ratio for strabismus surgery is almost double in patients with thyroid disease who smoke.

Clinical features

The muscles affected in thyroid eye disease, in decreasing order of severity and frequency, are the inferior rectus, medial rectus, superior rectus, and lateral rectus. The condition is most often bilateral and is often asymmetric. Forced-duction test results are almost always positive in one or more directions.

Most often, the patient presents with some degree of upper eyelid retraction, proptosis, hypotropia, and esotropia (Fig 12-7). Thyroid eye disease is a common cause of acquired vertical deviation in adults (see Chapter 11), especially women, but it is rare in children.

Management

Diplopia and abnormal head position are the principal indications for strabismus surgery. The operation may eliminate diplopia in primary gaze but rarely restores normal motility because of the restrictive myopathy, the need for large recessions in some cases to place the eye in primary position, and the ongoing underlying disease.

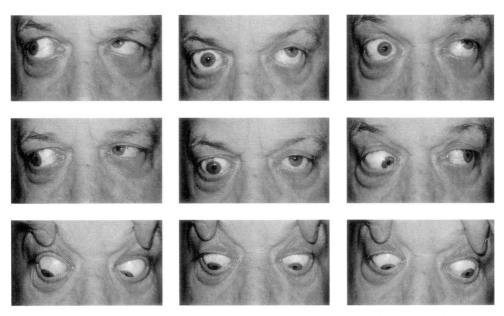

Figure 12-7 Thyroid eye disease. Note right upper eyelid retraction and restrictive right hypotropia with very limited elevation. Other rotations are not affected.

It is best to perform surgery after strabismus measurements and thyroid function tests have stabilized; waiting for at least 6 months and even 12 months is recommended. In the meantime, prisms may alleviate diplopia. Botulinum toxin may reduce the severity of fibrosis when injected into tight muscles in the acute phase. Performance of surgery before stability is achieved has been studied in patients with severe head positions. The results were favorable, but half the patients required further surgery.

Recession of the affected muscles is the preferred surgical treatment, addressing the tight muscles in 1 or both eyes. Strengthening procedures usually worsen restriction, but in carefully selected cases they may be helpful as part of the surgical plan. Adjustable sutures can be helpful in these difficult cases. Slight initial undercorrection is desirable, because late progressive overcorrection is common, especially with large inferior rectus muscle recessions. Limited depression of the eyes after inferior rectus muscle recessions can interfere with patients' bifocal use. Proptosis can become worse after EOM recessions.

If the need for orbital decompression is foreseeable, it is usually preferable to postpone strabismus surgery until decompression has been accomplished. Likewise, eyelid surgery is usually postponed until the strabismus is treated because upper eyelid retraction may improve once the patient no longer strains to elevate the eye.

Large recessions of very tight inferior rectus muscles can cause lower eyelid retraction severe enough to require subsequent correction. Severing the lower eyelid retractors as part of the strabismus surgery has led to some success at preventing this complication. If necessary, a spacer of banked sclera or synthetic material can be placed to vertically lengthen the lower eyelid tarsus.

Thomas SM, Cruz OA. Comparison of two different surgical techniques for the treatment of strabismus in dysthyroid ophthalmopathy. *J AAPOS.* 2007;11(3):258–261.

Chronic Progressive External Ophthalmoplegia

Clinical features

Chronic progressive external ophthalmoplegia (CPEO) is a rare form of mitochondrial cytopathy that can affect various body systems. It usually begins in childhood with ptosis and slowly progresses to total paralysis of the eyelids and EOMs. CPEO may be sporadic or familial. Although a true pigmentary retinal dystrophy is usually absent, constricted visual fields and electrodiagnostic abnormalities can occur. The diagnosis of CPEO is confirmed when muscle biopsy results show ragged red fibers or specific alterations of mitochondrial DNA are detected. *Kearns-Sayre syndrome* consists of retinal pigmentary changes, CPEO, and cardiomyopathy (especially heart block).

See BCSC Section 2, *Fundamentals and Principles of Ophthalmology,* Section 5, *Neuro-Ophthalmology,* and Section 12, *Retina and Vitreous,* for additional information on these and other mitochondrial disorders.

Management

It is important to ensure that the patient's cardiac status is evaluated, because life-threatening arrhythmias can occur in Kearns-Sayre syndrome. Treatment options for the ocular motility disorder are limited; small surgical series report a high rate of long-term undercorrections. Cautious surgical elevation (suspension) of the upper eyelids can lessen a severe chin-up head posture.

Myasthenia Gravis

Myasthenia gravis is a disorder in which antibodies directed against acetylcholine receptors cause muscle dysfunction. Onset in childhood is uncommon. A transient neonatal form, caused by the placental transfer of acetylcholine receptor antibodies of mothers with myasthenia gravis, exists but usually subsides rapidly. Another variety is not immune mediated and exhibits a familial predisposition.

The disease may be purely ocular. In its most severe form, it frequently occurs as part of a major systemic disorder that involves other skeletal muscles, especially in patients who have not received immunosuppressive therapy. Generalization to systemic myasthenia is less common in childhood-onset ocular myasthenia than in the adult-onset form.

BCSC Section 5, *Neuro-Ophthalmology,* discusses both the ocular and the systemic aspects of myasthenia gravis in depth. Additional information is available on the website of the Myasthenia Gravis Foundation of America, Inc (www.myasthenia.org).

Clinical features

The principal ocular manifestation of myasthenia gravis is weakening of the EOMs, including the levator muscle. Most cases (90%) exhibit both ptosis and limited ocular rotations. The ocular signs can resemble any unilateral or bilateral ophthalmoplegia, even the extremely rare isolated paralysis of the inferior rectus muscle.

Affected muscles fatigue rapidly, so ptosis typically worsens when the patient is required to look upward for 30 seconds. In the sleep test, the patient rests in a dark room with the eyelids closed for 20–30 minutes; ptosis often subsequently resolves in patients with myasthenia gravis. The presence of the *Cogan lid-twitch sign,* an overshoot of the eyelid when the patient looks straight ahead after looking down for several minutes, is also highly suggestive.

External application of ice over the involved eyelids for 2–5 minutes improves function of the levator palpebrae superioris and other affected EOMs, providing a rapid and reliable method of establishing this diagnosis without the need for drug administration.

The classic edrophonium test can establish the diagnosis (Fig 12-8). Neostigmine, an alternative test medication, has the advantage of allowing more time to measure changes in alignment, as the effect of this agent begins later than that of edrophonium and is prolonged.

Electromyography shows decreased electrical activity of involved muscles after prolonged voluntary innervations and increased activity (including faster saccadic velocity) after administration of edrophonium or neostigmine. Documentation of abnormalities by single-fiber electromyography or the presence of circulating anti–acetylcholine receptor or anti–muscle-specific kinase antibodies confirms the diagnosis, but a negative result does not rule it out.

Table 12-1 compares the features of thyroid eye disease with those of CPEO and myasthenia gravis.

Ortiz S, Borchert M. Long-term outcomes of pediatric ocular myasthenia gravis. *Ophthalmology.* 2008;115(7):1245–1248. Epub 2007 Dec 26.

Management

A full discussion of treatment of the various forms of myasthenia gravis is beyond the scope of this chapter. In adults, the ocular manifestations are frequently resistant to the usual systemic myasthenia treatment. However, pediatric ocular myasthenia is often successfully managed with pyridostigmine alone. In adults and children in whom the ocular deviation has stabilized, standard eye muscle surgery can help restore binocular function in at least some gaze positions. Ptosis occasionally requires upper eyelid surgery.

Esotropia and Hypotropia Associated With High Myopia

In highly myopic patients, extremely increased axial length can cause the elongated globe to herniate between the superior and lateral rectus muscles. High-resolution MRI studies

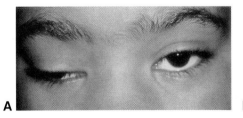 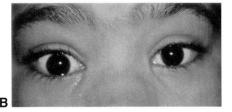

A   **B**

Figure 12-8 Myasthenia gravis. **A,** Bilateral ptosis (right more than left) with right hypotropia and exotropia. **B,** Following edrophonium injection, the eyes show orthotropia, normal eyelid position, and the lacrimation that frequently accompanies edrophonium injection.

Table 12-1 Differentiation of Conditions Producing Ptosis and Extraocular Muscle Involvement

	Thyroid Eye Disease	Chronic Progressive External Ophthalmoplegia (CPEO)	Myasthenia Gravis
Age	Rare in children	Any age	Any age
Muscle preferentially involved	Inferior rectus muscles, medial rectus muscles	Levator palpebrae, all ocular motor muscles	Levator palpebrae, any ocular motor muscles
Fatigability	No, unless coexistent with myasthenia gravis	No	Yes
Response to edrophonium	No, unless coexistent with myasthenia gravis	No	Yes
Other eye signs	External eye signs	Pigmentary retinopathy, optic neuropathy	No
Forced ductions	Restriction	Restriction if long-standing	Normal
Clinical course	May resolve or progress	Slowly progresses	Fluctuates; may involve generalized weakness
Eyelids	Retraction	Ptosis	Ptosis
Diplopia	Yes	No	Yes
Other signs and symptoms	Tachycardia, arrhythmia, tremor, weight loss, diarrhea, heat intolerance	Heart block, retinopathy (manifestations of Kearns-Sayre syndrome)	Dysphagia, jaw weakness, limb weakness, dyspnea

have shown stretching and dehiscence of the intermuscular septum between these 2 muscles. They also demonstrated inferior slippage of the lateral rectus pulley and other supporting tissues, along with medial displacement of the inferior rectus. These anomalies cause a progressively worsening hypotropia and esotropia. The medial rectus is often tight, exacerbating the severity of the esotropia.

Various surgical procedures have been devised to overcome the defect by stabilizing the position of the lateral rectus muscle. An effective option is a joining of the superior and lateral rectus muscles, usually with a nonabsorbable suture, to reposition the globe. Recession of the medial rectus muscle may also be needed if the muscle is tight.

Yamaguchi M, Yokoyama T, Shiraki K. Surgical procedure for correcting globe dislocation in highly myopic strabismus. *Am J Ophthalmol.* 2010;149(2):341–346. Epub 2009 Nov 24.

Internuclear Ophthalmoplegia

The anatomical and functional features of the *medial longitudinal fasciculus (MLF)* are discussed in BCSC Section 5, *Neuro-Ophthalmology.* The MLF integrates the nuclei of the cranial nerves governing ocular motility and has major connections with the vestibular nuclei. An intact MLF is essential for the production of conjugate eye movements. Lesions of the MLF result in a typical pattern of disconjugate movement called *internuclear ophthalmoplegia (INO).* Abnormalities of this pathway are frequently seen in patients with demyelinating disease, but they may also occur in patients who have had cerebrovascular accidents or brain tumors.

Clinical features

On horizontal versions, the eye ipsilateral to the MLF lesion adducts slowly and incompletely or not at all, whereas the abducting eye exhibits a characteristic horizontal jerk nystagmus (see Chapter 13). Both eyes adduct normally on convergence. Skew deviation may be present, in addition to exotropia.

Management

If exotropia persists, medial rectus muscle resection and unilateral or contralateral lateral rectus muscle recession (to limit exotropia in lateral gaze) can help eliminate diplopia, particularly in bilateral cases.

Ocular Motor Apraxia

Ocular motor apraxia, also known as *saccadic initiation failure,* is a rare supranuclear disorder of ocular motility, sometimes including strabismus. The congenital form may be familial, most commonly autosomal dominant.

This condition has been associated with premature birth and developmental delay. Bilateral lesions of the frontoparietal cortex, agenesis of the corpus callosum, hydrocephalus, and Joubert syndrome (abnormal eye movements, developmental delay, microcephaly, hypoplasia of the cerebellar vermis, and retinal dysplasia, among several anomalies) also have been associated with the condition, as have type 3 Gaucher disease and ataxia-telangiectasia. Several case reports have identified mass lesions of the cerebellum that compress the rostral part of the brainstem. Neurodevelopmental evaluation and imaging of the brain are advisable for assessment of children with ocular motor apraxia, especially if there is an associated vertical apraxia.

Clinical features

In ocular motor apraxia, normal voluntary horizontal saccades cannot be generated. Instead, changes in horizontal fixation are accomplished by a head thrust that overshoots the target, followed by a rotation of the head back in the opposite direction once fixation is established. The initial thrust serves to break fixation; an associated blink serves the same purpose. Vertical saccades and random eye movements are intact, but horizontal vestibular and optokinetic nystagmus are impaired. The head thrust may improve in late childhood.

The differential diagnosis of acquired ocular motor apraxia includes conditions that affect the generation of voluntary saccades, including metabolic and degenerative diseases such as Huntington chorea. (See also BCSC Section 5, *Neuro-Ophthalmology.*)

Superior Oblique Myokymia

Superior oblique myokymia is a rare entity whose cause is poorly understood. Some evidence indicates that it is caused by aberrant regeneration of fourth cranial nerve fibers. Another suggested etiology is vascular compression of the nerve, which can be confirmed by MRI.

Clinical features

In superior oblique myokymia, there are abnormal torsional movements of the eye that cause diplopia and monocular oscillopsia. Usually, patients are otherwise neurologically normal. Recurrences may persist indefinitely.

Management

Treatment is not necessary if the patient is not disturbed by the visual symptoms. Various systemic medications (such as carbamazepine, phenytoin, propranolol, baclofen, gabapentin) and topical timolol have produced inconsistent results but have been advocated as first-line treatment, since some patients will benefit, at least in the short term. Effective surgical treatment requires that the superior oblique muscle be disconnected from the globe by generous tenectomy. This typically results in a superior oblique palsy, so some surgeons perform simultaneous inferior oblique muscle weakening.

Williams PE, Purvin VA, Kawasaki A. Superior oblique myokymia: efficacy of medical treatment. *J AAPOS*. 2007;11(3):254–257. Epub 2007 Feb 5.

Strabismus Associated With Other Ocular Surgery

Refractive surgery that creates monovision to facilitate visual clarity at distance and near without optical aids (performed mainly in adults of presbyopic age; see BCSC Section 13, *Refractive Surgery*) can result in dissimilar sensory input to the 2 eyes. The dissimilarity can be sufficient to cause loss of motor control of the EOMs and disruption of fusion in predisposed patients.

Surgery for retinal detachment can lead to restricted rotations, because of scarring from dissection of the EOMs and the application of devices (such as a scleral buckle) required to bring about reattachment (see BCSC Section 12, *Retina and Vitreous*). Corrective surgery can be extremely difficult, especially if these elements must be removed. Consultation with a retina surgeon is valuable. Macular translocation surgery can cause torsional diplopia and other binocular sensory disturbances.

Glaucoma drainage devices are another potential source of scarring and interference with ocular rotations (see BCSC Section 10, *Glaucoma*). Treatment may require removal or relocation or substitution of the device, which creates a dilemma if it has been functioning well.

The EOMs can be damaged from retrobulbar injections, either by direct injury to the muscle or from a toxic effect of the injected material. Because of the usual placement of these injections, the vertical rectus muscles are the most vulnerable.

Injection of botulinum toxin into the eyelids can result in diffusion of this substance and a transient paralyzing effect on any of the EOMs.

Laceration or inadvertent excision of an entire section of the medial rectus muscle is one of several serious ocular and orbital complications of pterygium removal or endoscopic sinus surgery. Restoration of function can be an extremely difficult surgical challenge.

Kushner BJ, Kowal L. Diplopia after refractive surgery: occurrence and prevention. *Arch Ophthalmol*. 2003;121(3):315–321.

CHAPTER 13

Childhood Nystagmus

The prevalence of nystagmus in young children is approximately 0.35%. Nystagmus can be due to a motor defect that is compatible with relatively good vision, an ocular abnormality that impairs vision or fusion, or a neurologic abnormality. Distinguishing between these causes can be challenging. See BCSC Section 5, *Neuro-Ophthalmology,* for additional discussion of nystagmus.

General Features

Nystagmus is an involuntary, rhythmic oscillation of the eyes. In *pendular nystagmus,* the eyes oscillate with equal velocity in each direction. *Jerk nystagmus* denotes a movement of unequal speed. The fast component defines the direction of the nystagmus—for example, a right jerk nystagmus has a slow movement to the left and a fast movement (jerk) to the right.

The nystagmus movement can be further classified according to the frequency (number of oscillations per unit of time) and the amplitude (the angular distance traveled during the movement). The movements can be characterized as horizontal, vertical, or torsional or a combination of these. The characteristics of the nystagmus may change with gaze direction. For example, pendular nystagmus can become jerk nystagmus on extreme gaze.

Gaze position can affect the amplitude and frequency (intensity) of the nystagmus. This is especially true of jerk nystagmus, which can have a *null point* (or *null zone,* the gaze position in which the intensity of oscillations is diminished and the visual acuity improves), or which can decrease in intensity with gaze opposite the fast-phase component (analogous to Alexander's law for vestibular nystagmus). The abnormal head position that these patients assume in order to reduce nystagmus can be the most prominent manifestation of their condition.

Nomenclature

The National Eye Institute (NEI) has reclassified eye movement abnormalities, including nystagmus. For the discussion of nystagmus in this chapter, we use the traditional, familiar designations. The terminology recommended by the NEI-sponsored Committee for the Classification of Eye Movement Abnormalities and Strabismus (CEMAS) is indicated in parentheses throughout this chapter. The document produced by the CEMAS committee is available on the NEI website at www.nei.nih.gov/news/statements/cemas.pdf.

Evaluation

History

Many forms of nystagmus are inherited, either as a direct genetic abnormality or in association with other ocular conditions (Table 13-1). Thus, a family history, including inherited ocular or systemic diseases, is an important part of the initial evaluation. Although many cases of congenital motor nystagmus are sporadic, autosomal dominant, autosomal recessive, and X-linked inheritance have been described. Examination of family members with nystagmus can provide valuable prognostic information.

Perinatal events can affect the developing visual system and, if severe enough, can result in nystagmus. For this reason, the history should also include questions about the labor and delivery, maternal infections, and prematurity. For children older than 3 months, parental observations about head tilts, head movements, gaze preference, and viewing distances can aid in diagnosis.

Table 13-1 Ocular Conditions Associated With Nystagmus

Anterior segment abnormalities
- Congenital cataract
- Congenital glaucoma
- Iridocorneal dysgenesis

Primary sensory retinal abnormalities
- Leber congenital amaurosis
- Achromatopsia
- Blue-cone monochromatism
- Congenital stationary night blindness (X-linked and autosomal recessive)

Vitreoretinal abnormalities
- Cicatricial retinopathy of prematurity
- Coloboma involving macula
- Familial exudative vitreoretinopathy
- Norrie disease
- Retinal dysplasia
- Congenital retinoschisis
- Retinoblastoma

Foveal hypoplasia
- Albinism
- Aniridia
- Isolated

Optic nerve disorders
- Optic nerve hypoplasia
- Optic nerve coloboma
- Optic atrophy

Infectious diseases
- Congenital toxoplasmosis
- Cytomegalovirus
- Rubella
- Lymphocytic choriomeningitis virus
- Syphilis

Generalized central nervous system disorder
- Aicardi syndrome

Ocular Examination

Visual acuity

The level of visual function can be helpful for determining the cause of nystagmus. Patients with nystagmus and nearly normal visual acuity usually have congenital motor nystagmus (see the section "Congenital motor nystagmus" later in the chapter), which is a benign entity. Markedly decreased visual acuity usually implies either retinal or optic nerve abnormalities. Monocular visual acuity should be tested with fogging because monocular occlusion may increase nystagmus intensity. Binocular visual acuity should be measured at distance and near, with any desired head position permitted, to assess the child's true functional vision. Near visual acuity is usually better than distance. Children with distance acuity of less than 20/400 can sometimes read at the 20/40–20/60 level at near.

In preverbal children, the *optokinetic nystagmus (OKN)* drum can be used to estimate visual acuity. If vertical rotation of an OKN drum elicits a vertical nystagmus superimposed on the child's underlying nystagmus, the visual acuity is usually 20/400 or better. Preferential looking tests such as Teller Acuity Cards II (described in Chapter 1) can also be used. The examiner should keep in mind that, in patients with a horizontal nystagmus, the response can be more easily observed with the card held vertically.

Pupils

Pupils should be assessed for direct reaction to light, afferent defect, reaction to darkness, and anatomical structure.

Sluggish or absent response to light or an afferent defect indicates an anterior visual pathway abnormality such as optic nerve or retinal dysfunction. Responses can be normal in mild abnormalities, such as foveal hypoplasia, achromatopsia, and primary motor nystagmus. The normal response to darkness is the immediate dilation of the pupil. If, instead of dilating, the pupils paradoxically constrict, optic nerve or retinal disease is present.

In addition to pupillary responses, iris structure should be assessed. Defects such as iris colobomas suggest that optic nerve or retinal colobomas may also be present. Iris transillumination can be a sign of albinism. Aniridia and albinism are associated with foveal hypoplasia, poor vision, and nystagmus.

Ocular motility

Patients with nystagmus may have strabismus for several reasons: (1) as a result of poor vision, if that is the cause of the nystagmus; (2) due to damping the nystagmus by converging; or (3) because of latent nystagmus secondary to strabismus. Children with manifest latent nystagmus *(fusion maldevelopment nystagmus syndrome)* often fixate with the preferred eye in adduction to maximize their visual acuity and turn their heads to cross-fixate (look to the right with the left eye, to the left with the right eye).

Fundus

Optic nerve hypoplasia and foveal hypoplasia are common causes of nystagmus. Although many of the retinal disorders associated with nystagmus exhibit visible abnormalities, in some, the fundus appears normal or there are only subtle retinal pigmentary

Table 13-2 Conditions Associated With Decreased Vision and Minimal Fundus Changes

Leber congenital amaurosis
Achromatopsia
Blue-cone monochromatism
Congenital stationary night blindness
Foveal hypoplasia

changes (Table 13-2). In patients with nystagmus and normal-appearing fundi, electrophysiologic testing may be necessary to identify the cause.

Types of Childhood Nystagmus

Many forms of nystagmus can occur as variants of congenital nystagmus in some patients, or they can be acquired in others. In this chapter, these forms are discussed according to the category in which they are most commonly seen in children. While the characteristics of the nystagmus may be indistinguishable, the distinction between congenital and acquired is important because of the greater implications for associated neuropathology in acquired forms.

Congenital Nystagmus

Congenital motor nystagmus

Congenital motor nystagmus (CMN; *infantile nystagmus syndrome*) is a binocular conjugate nystagmus with several distinctive features (Table 13-3). It is not associated with central nervous system abnormalities. Patients have nearly normal visual function. The plane of nystagmus is most often horizontal, and it remains so on upgaze and downgaze (uniplanar). When CMN has a jerk waveform, it shows an exponential increase in velocity of the slow phase (Fig 13-1). A null point may be present. If one is present but not in primary position, the patient may adopt an abnormal head position to improve vision by placing the eyes near the null point. This head position becomes more pronounced as the child approaches school age. Also, head bobbing or movement may be present initially but usually decreases with age. Oscillopsia is rare.

CMN is damped by convergence and therefore can be associated with esotropia. This combination of nystagmus and esotropia has been termed *nystagmus blockage syndrome,* a distinction from those cases in which esotropia and nystagmus happen to coexist. Patients with nystagmus blockage syndrome characteristically present with an esotropia that "eats up prism" on attempted measurement and exhibit an increased jerk nystagmus on attempted lateral gaze.

Approximately two-thirds of patients with CMN exhibit a paradoxical inversion of the OKN response. Normally, when a patient with right jerk nystagmus views an OKN drum rotating to the patient's left (eliciting a pursuit left, jerk right response), the intensity

Table 13-3 Features of Congenital Motor Nystagmus

Conjugate
Horizontal
Uniplanar
Worsens with attempted fixation
Improves with convergence
Null point often present with abnormal head position
"Inverted" OKN response in two-thirds of patients
Oscillopsia usually not present

OKN = optokinetic nystagmus.

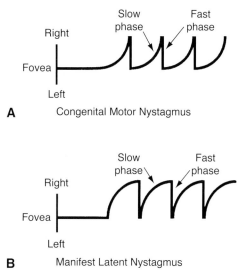

Figure 13-1 Left jerk nystagmus. **A,** Electronystagmographic evaluation of congenital motor nystagmus shows an exponential increase in velocity of the slow phase. **B,** An exponential decrease in velocity of the slow phase is the waveform characteristic of manifest latent nystagmus.

of the right jerk nystagmus increases. However, patients with CMN exhibit a damped right jerk nystagmus or possibly even a left jerk nystagmus. This paradoxical response occurs only in CMN.

Congenital sensory nystagmus

Congenital sensory nystagmus is secondary to a bilateral pregeniculate, afferent visual pathway abnormality. Inadequate image formation results in failure of development of the normal fixation reflex. If the visual pathway disorder is present at birth, the resulting nystagmus becomes apparent in the first 3 months of life. Its severity is somewhat correlated with the degree of vision loss. The waveform of sensory nystagmus can be pendular or jerk and cannot be distinguished from that of congenital motor nystagmus.

Searching, slow, wandering conjugate eye movements may also be observed. Searching nystagmus—defined as a roving or drifting, typically horizontal movement of the eyes without fixation—is usually seen in children whose visual acuity is worse than 20/200.

Pendular nystagmus occurs in patients with visual acuity of better than 20/200 in at least 1 eye. Jerk nystagmus is often associated with visual acuity between 20/60 and 20/100.

The associated bilateral pregeniculate afferent abnormality may be obvious, such as in children with bilateral cataracts or corneal opacities. The ocular abnormality may be more subtle, such as in children with optic nerve or foveal hypoplasia. A child with congenital sensory nystagmus as a result of a retinal dystrophy may have mild vascular attenuation, optic disc pallor, or a completely normal retinal appearance. An electroretinogram may be required for diagnosis. See Table 13-1 for a list of some ocular conditions that cause sensory nystagmus.

Periodic alternating nystagmus

Periodic alternating nystagmus (PAN; *central vestibular instability nystagmus*) is an unusual form of jerk nystagmus that can be congenital or acquired, especially with Arnold-Chiari malformation. The cause of congenital PAN is unknown, but it has been associated with oculocutaneous albinism. The nystagmus periodically changes direction. The motion typically starts with a jerk nystagmus in 1 direction; then the nystagmus slowly begins to damp, eventually leading to a period of no nystagmus lasting from 10 to 20 seconds. The nystagmus then jerks in the opposite direction in a cycle that repeats approximately every 4 minutes. Some children adopt an alternating head turn to take advantage of the changing null point.

Latent nystagmus

Another form of congenital nystagmus, latent nystagmus *(fusion maldevelopment nystagmus syndrome)* is a conjugate, horizontal jerk nystagmus that is a marker of fusion maldevelopment. Latent nystagmus occurs in children with decreased fusion, which results from either early-onset strabismus (infantile esotropia, most commonly) or decreased vision in 1 or both eyes. When 1 eye is occluded, a conjugate jerk nystagmus develops, with the fast phase directed toward the uncovered eye. Thus, a left jerk nystagmus occurs when the right eye is covered; a right jerk nystagmus, when the left eye is covered. This nystagmus is the only form that reverses direction with a change in fixation. Also, because the nystagmus damps when the fixating eye is in adduction, the head turn reverses with a change in fixation in order to use the fixating eye in adduction. Occlusion of the right eye induces a left jerk nystagmus with a left head turn, and occlusion of the left eye induces a right jerk nystagmus with a right head turn (Fig 13-2). Asymmetries in amplitude, frequency, and velocity of the nystagmus can also be present, depending on which eye is covered.

Because latent nystagmus is induced when an eye is covered, binocular visual acuity is better than monocular, and occlusion must be avoided during monocular tests of vision. The examiner can do this by using polarizing lenses and a polarized chart, blurring the nontested eye with a +5.00 D lens, using a translucent occluder, or positioning the occluder several inches in front of the eye not being tested.

Latent nystagmus is damped by fusion and increased with disruption of fusion (as occurs with ocular occlusion). Latent nystagmus may become manifest (manifest latent nystagmus) when both eyes are open but only 1 eye is being used for vision (ie, the other eye is suppressed or amblyopic). Electronystagmographic evaluation of latent and manifest

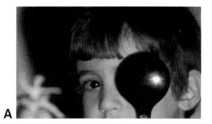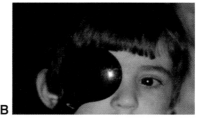

Figure 13-2 Latent nystagmus. **A,** There is a right head turn during fixation with the right eye. **B,** The head turn reverses during fixation with the left eye. The nystagmus damps with the fixating eye in adduction. *(Courtesy of Edward L. Raab, MD.)*

latent nystagmus shows similar waveforms with a slow phase of exponentially decreasing velocity (see Fig 13-1).

> Richards M, Wong A, Foeller P, Bradley D, Tychsen L. Duration of binocular decorrelation predicts the severity of latent (fusion maldevelopment) nystagmus in strabismic macaque monkeys. *Invest Ophthalmol Vis Sci.* 2008;49(5):1872–1878.

Acquired Nystagmus

Spasmus nutans

Spasmus nutans *(spasmus nutans syndrome)* is an idiopathic acquired nystagmus that manifests during the first 2 years of life, presenting as a triad of generally small-amplitude, high-frequency (shimmering) nystagmus; head nodding; and torticollis. The nystagmus is binocular but often asymmetric—sometimes to the point of appearing to be monocular— and can vary with gaze position. The nystagmus movement can be horizontal, vertical, or rotary (torsional) and is occasionally intermittent. The head nodding and torticollis appear to be compensatory movements that maximize vision. The natural history is for the abnormal head and eye movements to diminish by 3–4 years of age. Spasmus nutans is a benign disorder in most cases, but there is a high incidence of associated strabismus, amblyopia, and developmental delay.

Spasmus nutans–like nystagmus has been seen with chiasmal or suprachiasmal tumors and retinal dystrophies such as congenital stationary night blindness. Neuroradiologic investigation is therefore warranted with any evidence of optic nerve dysfunction (optic disc pallor, relative afferent pupillary defect) or any sign of neurologic abnormality. Because subtle optic disc pallor and relative afferent pupillary defects can be difficult to assess in children, some investigators believe that neuroimaging is indicated for all children with presumed spasmus nutans.

See-saw nystagmus

See-saw nystagmus is an unusual but dramatic type of nystagmus that has both vertical and torsional components. The name derives from the action of the familiar playground device. If 2 eyes were placed on a see-saw, one at either end, they would "roll down the plank" as the see-saw rose, with the high eye intorting and the low eye extorting. As the direction of the see-saw changed, so would that of the eye movement. Thus, the eyes make alternating movements of elevation and intorsion followed by depression and extorsion.

This type of nystagmus is often associated with a lesion in the rostral midbrain or the suprasellar area. In children, the most likely associated intracranial tumor is a cranio-pharyngioma. Confrontation visual fields may elicit a bitemporal defect. Neuroradiologic evaluation is necessary. A congenital form of see-saw nystagmus is seen with complete or partial achiasma.

Vertical nystagmus

Vertical nystagmus is uncommon. Congenital vertical nystagmus is sometimes seen in infants with inherited retinal dystrophies. Downbeat nystagmus, one form of vertical nystagmus, may occur as a congenital disorder associated with good vision and normal neurologic findings. This jerk nystagmus has a downward fast component and often a null point in upgaze. More commonly, vertical nystagmus is acquired and secondary to structural abnormalities such as the Arnold-Chiari malformation. Medications such as codeine, lithium, tranquilizers, and anticonvulsants may also cause this condition. Neurologic evaluation is usually indicated in patients with acquired vertical nystagmus.

Monocular nystagmus

Monocular nystagmus has been reported to occur in severely amblyopic and blind eyes (*Heimann-Bielschowsky phenomenon*). The oscillations are pendular, chiefly vertical, slow, variable in amplitude, and irregular in frequency.

Nystagmus-Like Disorders

Convergence-Retraction Nystagmus

Convergence-retraction nystagmus (*induced convergence-retraction*) is part of the dorsal midbrain syndrome, associated with paralysis of upward gaze, defective convergence, eyelid retraction, and pupillary light–near dissociation. In the pediatric age group, convergence-retraction nystagmus is commonly secondary to congenital aqueductal stenosis or a pinealoma. The nystagmus is best elicited on attempted upgaze saccades (eg, by asking the patient to track a downward-rotating OKN drum). Co-contraction of all horizontal extraocular muscles occurs, resulting in retraction of the globe. In addition, the medial rectus muscles overpower the lateral rectus muscles, causing the eyes to converge on attempted upgaze (hence the term *convergence-retraction*). However, voluntary convergence is minimal. The abnormal eye movements in convergence-retraction nystagmus are actually saccades. Therefore, convergence-retraction nystagmus is not a true nystagmus.

Opsoclonus

Opsoclonus is an eye movement disorder, not a true nystagmus. It consists of involuntary saccades that are rapid and multidirectional, often accompanied by somatic dyskinesias. Opsoclonus can occur intermittently and often presents as eye movements with very high frequency and large amplitude. Causes of opsoclonus in children include acute postinfectious cerebellar ataxia, viral encephalitis, and a paraneoplastic manifestation of neuroblastoma.

Treatment

Prisms

For the patient with nystagmus, use of prisms can improve head positions by shifting the retinal image toward the null point. Also, prisms can improve vision by inducing convergence. They can be used as the sole treatment of nystagmus or as a trial to predict surgical success. With powers ranging from 1Δ–40Δ, Fresnel press-on prisms, inexpensive plastic pieces that can be cut and then applied to glasses, can be used for both purposes, as powers of 10Δ–20Δ are often required. Ground-in prisms cause less distortion and are preferred for patients who require smaller amounts of prism.

To correct head positions, each prism is mounted with the apex pointing toward the null point. For example, for a patient with a left head turn and a null point in right gaze, the prism before the right eye should be oriented base-in, and the prism before the left eye should be oriented base-out. This shifts the image to the right and decreases the amount of head turn that the patient requires to gain the same visual benefit. If this technique improves the head position, strabismus surgery is also likely to be effective.

Prism spectacles may improve visual acuity by stimulating fusional convergence, which damps the nystagmus. In this situation, base-out prisms are placed in front of both eyes in amounts determined by trial and error.

Surgery for Nystagmus

Extraocular muscle surgery for nystagmus is indicated for correction of an abnormal head position, which is achieved by shifting the null point closer to the primary position. Surgery can also improve vision by decreasing nystagmus intensity (frequency times amplitude) and consequently foveation time. The types of surgery typically recommended are conjugate recessions in each eye *(Anderson procedure)*, a recession-resection on both eyes *(Kestenbaum procedure)*, or a recession of all 4 horizontal rectus muscles. See Chapter 14 for discussion of some of the surgical procedures mentioned in this chapter.

In a Kestenbaum or Anderson procedure, the eyes are surgically rotated toward the direction of the head turn and away from the null point or preferred gaze position. Each eye is operated on to move the eyes in the same direction. For example, if a patient with congenital nystagmus has a left head turn and null point in right gaze, the eyes are surgically rotated to the left by recession of the right lateral and left medial rectus muscles and by resection of the right medial and left lateral rectus muscles, thereby shifting the null point toward the primary position (Fig 13-3).

The amounts of recession-resection performed are listed in Table 13-4. The total amount of surgery for each eye (as measured in millimeters) is equal in order to rotate each globe an equal amount. For head turns of 30°, 40% augmentation is recommended; for turns of 45°, augmentation of 60% is employed. The augmented procedures may cause restriction of motility, which is usually necessary to achieve a satisfactory result.

If vertical torticollis is present with congenital nystagmus, chin-up or chin-down posturing may be ameliorated in some cases by vertical prism (again, apex toward the null point) or by surgery on the vertical rectus muscles or the oblique muscles. As with surgery

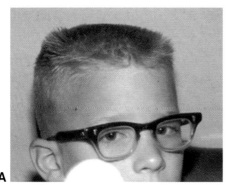 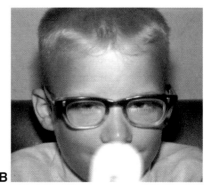

A   B

Figure 13-3   A, Congenital motor nystagmus with the null point in right gaze. **B,** Null point shifted by the Kestenbaum procedure, reducing the head turn. *(Courtesy of Edward L. Raab, MD.)*

Table 13-4 Amount of Surgery for Kestenbaum Procedure and Modifications*

Procedure	Kestenbaum, mm	40% Augmented, mm	60% Augmented, mm
Eye adducted in null point			
Recess medial rectus	5.0	7.0	8.0
Resect lateral rectus	8.0	11.0	12.5
Eye abducted in null point			
Recess lateral rectus	7.0	10.0	11.0
Resect medial rectus	6.0	8.5	9.5

*Amounts listed are for the original Kestenbaum procedure plus 2 modifications in which the amount of surgery is increased.

for horizontal nystagmus, the eyes are rotated away from the null point. Thus, if a chin-up, eyes-down head position is present, the inferior rectus muscles are recessed and the superior rectus muscles are resected. The amount of surgery is usually 8–10 mm of recession and resection of the vertical rectus muscles of each eye. Alternatively, combined weakening of a vertical rectus muscle and an oblique muscle in each eye can be used. For a chin-up head position, the inferior rectus and superior oblique muscles are weakened; for chin-down, the superior rectus and inferior oblique muscles are weakened. Improvement in the head position of nystagmus patients with a head tilt has been reported with torsional surgery involving the oblique muscles or transposition of the vertical rectus muscles.

When there is no eccentric null point and the Kestenbaum procedure is not indicated, recession of all the horizontal rectus muscles to a position posterior to the equator has been offered as an alternative. The amount of surgery is usually in the range of 8–10 mm of recession of both medial rectus muscles and 10–12 mm of recession of both lateral rectus muscles. Recent studies have found that merely disinserting and reattaching the horizontal rectus muscles, without recession or resection, produces similar results with presumably less risk of inducing new strabismus. This procedure results in improved foveation time on electronystagmography and secondary indicators of visual function such as recognition time; however, the effect on visual acuity is modest—an average improvement of about 1 line. Nystagmus surgery in the absence of abnormal head position is controversial.

Surgery for nystagmus blockage syndrome involves recession of the medial rectus muscles, usually with amounts that are larger than normal for the amount of esotropia. This may be combined with posterior fixation sutures (see Chapter 14).

For nystagmus patients with strabismus, surgery to shift the null point must be performed on the dominant fixating eye; surgery on the nondominant eye is then adjusted to account for the strabismus. For example, a patient who is right-eye dominant and has a right head turn and null point in left gaze would undergo a right medial rectus recession and right lateral rectus resection in the amounts indicated in Table 13-4. This would reduce esotropia or increase exotropia. Surgery on the nonpreferred eye is designed to correct the remaining deviation.

Hertle RW, Dell'Osso LF, FitzGibbon EJ, Thompson D, Yang D, Mellow SD. Horizontal rectus tenotomy in patients with congenital nystagmus: results in 10 adults. *Ophthalmology.* 2003;110(11):2097–2105.

Yang MB, Pou-Vendrell CR, Archer SM, Martonyi EJ, Del Monte MA. Vertical rectus muscle surgery for nystagmus patient with vertical abnormal head posture. *J AAPOS.* 2004;8(4): 299–309.

CHAPTER 14

Surgery of the Extraocular Muscles

While orthoptic exercises or prism spectacles are sufficient for some patients with strabismus, many require surgery in order to correct their alignment. Most often, this is achieved with incisional surgery. Historically, a variety of incisional procedures have been used, but chemodenervation, covered at the end of this chapter, has emerged as an alternative for some patients.

Evaluation

The history and a detailed motility evaluation, as part of a complete ocular examination, provide the information necessary for the surgeon to plan optimal strabismus surgery. Evaluation, tailored to the type of case, may include sensory binocularity testing, forced-duction testing, active force generation, saccadic velocity measurement, and simulation of the target postoperative alignment with prisms or an amblyoscope to assess the risk of diplopia and the opportunity for single binocular vision. (See Chapter 7 for discussion of these tests.) Preoperative discussions should address the expectations of the patient and family, as well as the risks and potential complications, especially if surgery on the only eye with good vision is considered.

Indications for Surgery

Surgery of the extraocular muscles (EOMs) is performed to improve visual function, appearance, or patient well-being or any combination of these. It may relieve asthenopia (a sense of ocular fatigue) in patients with heterophorias or intermittent heterotropias, or it may relieve the double vision that is often present in patients with adult-onset strabismus. Alignment of the visual axes can establish or restore fusion and stereopsis, especially if the preoperative deviation is intermittent or of recent onset. Correction of esotropia expands the binocular visual field. Some patients require an abnormal head position to relieve diplopia or to improve vision (eg, with nystagmus and an eccentric null point; see Chapter 13). For these patients, surgical treatment may not only increase the field of binocular vision but also shift it to a more useful, centered location. Correction of strabismus should be considered reconstructive rather than merely cosmetic, as it has many functional benefits.

Kraft SP. The functional benefits of adult strabismus treatment. *Am Orthoptic J.* 2008;58(1):2–9.

Planning Considerations

Visual Acuity

When a child has amblyopia, some surgeons prefer to treat the amblyopia before surgery, while others believe that the prognosis for binocular vision is better if surgery is not postponed. If a patient has dense amblyopia or permanent vision loss due to other causes, surgery is usually performed only on the eye with poor vision.

General Considerations

Symmetric surgery

The amount of surgery is based on the preoperative deviation. One commonly used set of guidelines for medial rectus muscle recession or lateral rectus muscle resection for esodeviations is given in Table 14-1 (also see the section Rectus Muscle Strengthening Procedures). Surgical options for infants with large-angle esotropia (>60Δ) include combined recession-resection of 3 or 4 rectus muscles or bilateral medial rectus muscle recessions of 7.0 mm. Augmentation of the latter with botulinum toxin has been advocated.

Surgical guidelines for exodeviation are provided in Table 14-2. Some surgeons employ bilateral lateral rectus muscle recessions of 9.0 mm or greater for deviations larger than 40Δ. Others prefer to limit lateral rectus recession to no more than 8.0 mm and add resection of 1 or both medial rectus muscles for larger-angle exotropias.

> Lueder GT, Galli M, Tychsen L, Yildirim C, Pegado V. Long-term results of botulinum toxin–augmented medial rectus recessions for large-angle infantile esotropia. *Am J Ophthalmol.* 2012;153(3):560–563.

Monocular recession-resection procedures

The figures given in Tables 14-1 and 14-2 may also be used in monocular recession-resection procedures, with the surgeon selecting the appropriate number of millimeters for each muscle. For example, for an esotropia of 30Δ, the surgeon would recess the medial rectus muscle 4.5 mm and resect the lateral rectus muscle 7.0 mm. For an exodeviation of 15Δ, the surgeon would recess the lateral rectus muscle 4.0 mm and resect the antagonist

Table 14-1 Surgical Amounts for Esodeviation

Angle of Esotropia, Δ	Recession MR OU, mm	or	Resection LR OU, mm
15	3.0		4.0
20	3.5		5.0
25	4.0		6.0
30	4.5		7.0
35	5.0		8.0
40	5.5		9.0
50	6.0		9.0

LR = lateral rectus; MR = medial rectus; OU = both eyes *(oculi uterque).*

Table 14-2 Surgical Amounts for Exodeviation

Angle of Exotropia, Δ	Recession LR OU, mm	or	Resection MR OU, mm
15	4.0		3.0
20	5.0		4.0
25	6.0		5.0
30	7.0		6.0
40	8.0		7.0

LR = lateral rectus; MR = medial rectus; OU = both eyes *(oculi uterque)*.

medial rectus muscle 3.0 mm. Monocular surgery for exotropia beyond these guidelines (ie, >50Δ) is likely to result in a limited rotation; thus, a 3- or 4-muscle procedure is preferable if there is at least moderately good vision in each eye.

Incomitance

When the size of the deviation varies in different gaze positions, the surgical plan should be designed with a goal of making the postoperative alignment more comitant.

Vertical incomitance of horizontal deviations

The treatment of horizontal deviations that change in magnitude in upgaze and downgaze—such as *A* or *V patterns*—is discussed in Chapter 10.

Horizontal incomitance

When the esodeviation or exodeviation changes significantly between right and left gaze, paralysis or restriction is suggested. In general, restrictions must be relieved for surgery to be effective, and the surgical amounts usually used to correct a misalignment of a given size may not be applicable.

When there is no restriction to account for an incomitant deviation, the deviation is treated as if it were caused by a weak muscle, whether from neurologic, traumatic, or other causes. If the weak muscle exhibits little or no force generation, transposition procedures are usually indicated. Otherwise, treatment consists of some combination of resection of the weak muscle (or advancement if it has been previously recessed) and weakening of its direct antagonist or yoke muscle.

In some cases, both restriction and paralysis are present, particularly in long-standing paretic strabismus, and a combination of treatment strategies is necessary. Forced-duction and active force generation testing are helpful in these cases.

Distance–near incomitance

Treatment of horizontal distance–near incomitance has classically consisted of medial rectus muscle surgery for deviations greater at near and lateral rectus muscle surgery for deviations greater at distance. Recent evidence suggests that, regardless of which muscles are operated on, the improvement in distance–near incomitance is similar.

Archer SM. The effect of medial versus lateral rectus muscle surgery on distance-near incomitance. *J AAPOS.* 2009;13(1):20–26.

Cyclovertical Strabismus

In many patients with cyclovertical strabismus, the deviation differs between right and left gaze and, on the side of the greater deviation, often between upgaze and downgaze as well. In general, surgery should be performed on those muscles whose field of action corresponds to the greatest vertical deviation unless results of forced-duction testing reveal contracture that requires a weakening procedure for a restricted muscle. For example, for a patient with a right hypertropia that is greatest down and to the patient's left, the surgeon should consider either strengthening the right superior oblique muscle or weakening the left inferior rectus muscle. (Strengthening and weakening of the oblique muscles are discussed later in this chapter.) If the right hypertropia is the same in left upgaze, straight left, and left downgaze, then any of the 4 muscles whose greatest vertical action is in left gaze may be chosen for surgery. In this example, the left superior rectus muscle or right superior oblique muscle could be strengthened, or the left inferior rectus muscle or right inferior oblique muscle could be weakened. Larger deviations may require surgery on more than 1 muscle.

Prior Surgery

In the surgical treatment of residual or recurrent strabismus after previous EOM surgery, EOMs that have not undergone prior surgery are technically easier and somewhat more predictable to operate on than those that have. Unfortunately, when previous surgery has resulted in muscle restriction or weakness with limited duction (due to excessive recession, slipped or lost muscle), reoperation on the involved muscle is usually necessary. If the restriction is a result of retinal detachment surgery, correction can usually be accomplished without removal of scleral explants. Consultation with the patient's retina surgeon is advisable in case such removal becomes necessary. For an eye that has previously undergone glaucoma surgery such as trabeculectomy or implantation of a glaucoma drainage device, strabismus surgery should be planned to minimize the risk of disrupting the filtering bleb.

Surgical Techniques for the Extraocular Muscles and Tendons

Step-by-step descriptions of each surgical procedure are beyond the scope of this volume. The references that follow are among several in which this information can be found.

Coats DK, Olitsky SE, eds. *Strabismus Surgery and Its Complications.* Berlin: Springer; 2007.
Wright KW. *Color Atlas of Strabismus Surgery.* 3rd ed. Irvine, CA: Wright; 2007.

Approaches to the Extraocular Muscles

Fornix incision

The fornix incision is made in either the superior or, more frequently, the inferior quadrants. The incision is located on bulbar conjunctiva, not actually in the fornix, 1–2 mm to the limbal side of the cul-de-sac, so that bleeding is minimized. The incision is made parallel to the fornix and is approximately 8–10 mm in length.

Bare sclera is exposed by incising the Tenon capsule deep to the conjunctival incision. Using this exposed bare sclera, the surgeon engages the muscle with a succession of muscle hooks. The conjunctival incision is pulled over the hook that has passed under the muscle. All 4 rectus muscles and both oblique muscles can be explored, if necessary, through inferotemporal and superonasal conjunctival incisions.

When properly placed, the 2-plane incision can be self-closing at the end of the operation by gentle massage of the tissues into the fornix, with the edges of the incision splinted by the overlying eyelid. Some surgeons prefer to close the incision with conjunctival sutures.

Limbal incision

The fused layer of conjunctiva and Tenon capsule is cleanly severed from the limbus. Some surgeons make the limbal incision (peritomy) 1–2 mm posterior to the limbus to spare limbal stem cells. A short radial incision is made at each end of the peritomy so that the flap of conjunctiva and Tenon capsule can be retracted to expose the muscle for surgery. At the completion of the operation, the flap is reattached, without tension, close to its original position with a single suture at each corner. If the conjunctiva is scarred from prior surgery and is tight, closure should be accomplished with recession of the anterior edge.

Rectus Muscle Weakening Procedures

Table 14-3 defines various rectus muscle weakening procedures and describes when each is used. The most common of these is simple recession, for which typical amounts of surgery for esotropia and exotropia are given in Tables 14-1 and 14-2. Because the conventional technique for rectus muscle recession involves passing sutures through thin sclera with the attendant risk of perforation, some surgeons prefer a *hang-back recession,* in which the recessed tendon is suspended by sutures that pass through the thicker stump of the original insertion. Although it is not known where the tendon reattaches to the sclera, there is empirical experience indicating that this method is usually reliable.

Rectus Muscle Strengthening Procedures

Strengthening procedures do not actually give the muscles more strength. Rather, they produce a tightening effect that tends to offset the opposite action of the antagonist muscle. Surgeons usually use the *resection* technique for this purpose, for which typical amounts of surgery for esotropia and exotropia are given in Tables 14-1 and 14-2. *Plication* of the tendon can be used as an alternative to produce a similar effect. A rectus muscle can also be tightened by *advancing* its insertion toward the limbus. This is an effective procedure when previous recession has resulted in an overcorrection.

Rectus Muscle Surgery for Hypotropia and Hypertropia

For reasonably comitant vertical deviations, recession and resection of vertical rectus muscles is appropriate. Recessions are generally preferred as a first procedure. A rough guideline is that approximately 3Δ of correction in primary position can be expected for

Table 14-3 Weakening Procedures Used in Strabismus Surgery

Procedure	Indications
Myotomy: cutting across a muscle *Myectomy:* removing a portion of muscle	Used by some surgeons to weaken the inferior oblique muscles
Marginal myotomy: cutting partway across a muscle, usually following a maximal recession	To weaken a rectus muscle further
Tenotomy: cutting across a tendon *Tenectomy:* removing a portion of tendon	Both used routinely to weaken the superior oblique muscle; silicone spacers have been interposed by some surgeons to control the weakening effect
Recession: removal and reattachment of a muscle (rectus or oblique) so that its insertion is closer to its origin	The standard weakening procedure for rectus muscles
Denervation and extirpation: the ablation of the entire portion of the muscle, along with its nerve supply, within the Tenon capsule	Used only on severely or recurrently overacting inferior oblique muscles
Recession and anteriorization: movement of the muscle's insertion anterior to its original position	Used primarily on the inferior oblique muscle, to reduce its elevation function; particularly useful with coexisting inferior oblique muscle overaction and dissociated vertical deviation
Posterior fixation suture (fadenoperation): attachment of a rectus muscle to the sclera 11–18 mm posterior to the insertion using a nonabsorbable suture; fixation to the muscle's pulley may be an alternative for medial rectus muscles	Used to weaken a muscle by decreasing its mechanical advantage; often used in conjunction with recession; sometimes used in high AC/A esotropia and in noncomitant strabismus

AC/A = accommodative convergence/accommodation.

every millimeter of vertical rectus muscle recession. For comitant vertical deviations of less than 10Δ that accompany horizontal deviations, displacement of the reinsertions of the horizontal rectus muscles in the same direction, by about one-half the tendon width (up for hypotropia, down for hypertropia), performed during a recession-resection procedure, is often sufficient. In order to use this option to correct a small vertical deviation, the surgeon may choose to do a recession-resection procedure in a situation where bilateral symmetric recessions would otherwise be preferred.

Adjustable Sutures

Some surgeons employ adjustable sutures to avoid an immediately obvious poor result or to increase the likelihood of success with 1 operation, but this modification does not ensure long-term satisfactory alignment. The surgeon completes the operation using externalized sutures and slipknots that allow the position of the surgical muscle to be altered during the early postoperative period. This technique can be used in children; however, a second general anesthesia is usually required.

Another alternative, used mainly in adults, is performance of surgery with the patient awake. Anesthetic agents that might affect ocular motility are avoided, and the patient's dynamic ocular motility and ocular alignment are observed and adjusted at the time of surgery. This technique can be difficult in patients with significant scarring, persons with thyroid eye disease, and children.

Isenberg SJ, Abdarbashi P. Drift of ocular alignment following strabismus surgery. Part 1: using fixed scleral sutures. *Br J Ophthalmol.* 2009;93(4):439–442.

Isenberg SJ, Abdarbashi P. Drift of ocular alignment following strabismus surgery. Part 2: using adjustable sutures. *Br J Ophthalmol.* 2009;93(4):443–447.

Oblique Muscle Weakening Procedures

Weakening the inferior oblique muscle

Table 14-3 lists the various inferior oblique muscle weakening procedures. These procedures are most commonly used for treatment of overelevation in adduction when it is believed to be due to inferior oblique muscle overaction. In all of these procedures, the surgeon must be sure that the entire inferior oblique muscle is weakened, since the distal portion and the insertion can be anomalously duplicated.

In cases that show marked asymmetry of the overactions of the inferior oblique muscles and no superior oblique muscle paralysis, unilateral surgery only on the muscle with the more prominent overaction is often followed by a significant degree of overaction in the fellow eye. Therefore, some surgeons recommend bilateral inferior oblique muscle weakening for asymmetric cases. A symmetric result is the rule and overcorrections are rare; however, inferior oblique muscles that are not overacting at all—even when there is overaction in the fellow eye—should not be weakened.

Secondary overaction of the inferior oblique muscle occurs in many patients who have superior oblique muscle paralysis. A weakening of that inferior oblique muscle typically corrects up to 15Δ of vertical deviation in primary position. The amount of vertical correction is roughly proportional to the degree of preoperative overaction (see Chapter 11).

Frequently, a weakening procedure is performed on each inferior oblique muscle for V-pattern strabismus. This is discussed in Chapter 10.

Moving the insertion of the inferior oblique muscle anteriorly to a point adjacent to the lateral border of the inferior rectus muscle *(inferior oblique anterior transposition, inferior oblique anteriorization)* weakens the normal actions of the inferior oblique. Because the neurofibrovascular bundle along the lateral border of the inferior rectus muscle can then serve as the effective origin for the distal portion of the muscle, anteriorization also allows the inferior oblique muscle to actively oppose elevation of the eye; that is, this muscle becomes an anti-elevator (see Chapter 3). This procedure has been found to be effective for treatment of dissociated vertical deviation (DVD) and is especially useful when DVD and inferior oblique muscle overaction coexist. See also Chapter 11.

Awadein A, Gawdat G. Bilateral inferior oblique myectomy for asymmetric primary inferior oblique overaction. *J AAPOS.* 2008;12(6):560–564.

Weakening the superior oblique muscle

Procedures to weaken the superior oblique muscle include tenotomy; tenectomy; Z-lengthening; placement of a spacer of silicone, fascia lata, or nonabsorbable suture loops between the cut edges of the tendon to functionally lengthen it; and recession. The purpose of spacers is to prevent an excessive gap between the cut edges, but they have the disadvantage of possible adhesion formation, which can alter motility. Unilateral weakening of a superior oblique muscle is not commonly performed except as the treatment for Brown syndrome (see Chapter 12) or for an isolated inferior oblique muscle weakness, which is rare. Unilateral superior oblique muscle weakening can affect not only vertical alignment but also torsion, potentially creating undesired extorsion. Many ophthalmologists favor a tenotomy of just the posterior 75%–80% of the tendon to preserve the torsional action, which is controlled by the most anterior tendon fibers.

Bilateral weakening of the superior oblique muscle can be performed for A-pattern deviations (see Chapter 10) and can be expected to cause an eso-shift in downgaze and almost no change in upgaze. In surgery on patients with normal binocularity, the possibility of creating diplopia from vertical or torsional strabismus must be considered.

Oblique Muscle Tightening (Strengthening) Procedures

Tightening the inferior oblique muscle

As mentioned previously, the actual effect of strengthening procedures is tightening of the muscle. Inferior oblique muscle tightening is seldom performed. To be effective, advancement of the inferior oblique muscle requires reinsertion more posteriorly and superiorly, which is technically difficult and exposes the macula to possible injury.

Tightening the superior oblique muscle

Tucking, plication, advancement, and resection of the superior oblique tendon are discussed in Chapter 11. Tucking the superior oblique tendon enhances both its vertical and torsional effect. Just the anterior half of the superior oblique tendon may be advanced temporally and somewhat closer to the limbus, a procedure known as the *Fells modification of the Harada-Ito procedure,* to reduce extorsion in patients with superior oblique muscle paralysis.

Stay Sutures

A stay (pull-over) suture is a temporary suture that is attached to the sclera at the limbus or under a rectus muscle insertion, brought out through the eyelids, and secured to periocular skin over a bolster to fix the eye in a selected position during postoperative healing. Some surgeons believe that this technique is particularly useful in cases with severely restricted rotations. Its disadvantages are that patients experience some discomfort and that the limbal attachment of the stay suture tends to be lost before the desired interval of 10–14 days after placement.

Transposition Procedures

Transposition procedures involve redirection of the paths of the EOMs. In the treatment of paralytic strabismus, Duane retraction syndrome, and monocular elevation deficiency, these procedures utilize the 2 muscles adjacent to the abnormal muscle to provide a tonic force vector. Vertical deviations are a possible complication of vertical rectus muscle transposition surgery. The effect of the transposition can be augmented by resecting the transposed muscles or by employing offset posterior fixation sutures (Foster modification). It has recently been suggested that transposition of only the superior rectus muscle, combined with recession of the medial rectus muscle, can also be effective.

Foster RS. Vertical muscle transposition augmented with lateral fixation. *J AAPOS*. 1997;1(1):20–30.

Mehendale RA, Dagi LR, Wu C, Ledoux D, Johnston S, Hunter DG. Superior rectus transposition and medial rectus recession for Duane syndrome and sixth nerve palsy. *Arch Ophthalmol*. 2012;130(2):195–201.

Posterior Fixation

Posterior fixation is a procedure in which a rectus muscle is sutured to the sclera far posterior to its insertion. The effect is weakening of the muscle in its field of action while having little, if any, effect on the alignment in primary position. This is a particularly useful procedure for treatment of incomitant strabismus. A similar effect may be achieved, at least for medial rectus muscles, by fixation to the muscle pulley.

Complications of Strabismus Surgery

Diplopia

Diplopia can occur after strabismus surgery, occasionally in older children but more often in adults. Surgery can move the fixated image out of a suppression scotoma. In the several months following surgery, various responses are possible:

- Fusion of the 2 images may occur.
- A new suppression scotoma may form, corresponding to the new angle of alignment. If the initial strabismus was acquired before age 10 years, the ability to suppress is generally well developed.
- Diplopia may persist.

Prolonged postoperative diplopia is uncommon. However, if strabismus was first acquired in adulthood, diplopia that was symptomatic before surgery is likely to persist unless comitant alignment and fusion are regained. Prisms that compensate for the deviation may be helpful during the preoperative evaluation to assess the fusion potential and the risk of bothersome postoperative diplopia.

A patient with unequal visual acuity can frequently be taught to ignore the dimmer, more blurred image. Further treatment is indicated for patients whose symptomatic diplopia persists more than 4–6 weeks after surgery, especially if it is severe and in the primary position. If vision in the eyes is equal or nearly so, temporary prisms should be tried and, if necessary, oriented to correct both vertical and horizontal deviations. The prism power can be changed periodically to address any residual diplopia. If this approach fails, additional surgery or botulinum toxin injection is a consideration. In some cases, intractable diplopia can be controlled only by occluding or blurring the less-preferred eye with a MIN lens (Fresnel, Bloomington, MN), Bangerter foil (Ryser, St Gallen, Switzerland), or transluscent tape.

Kushner BJ. Intractable diplopia after strabismus surgery in adults. *Arch Ophthalmol*. 2002;120(11):1498–1504.

Unsatisfactory Alignment

Unsatisfactory postoperative alignment—overcorrection, undercorrection, or development of an entirely new strabismus problem—is perhaps better characterized as one of several possible outcomes of strabismus surgery, albeit a disappointing one, rather than as a complication. Alignment in the immediate postoperative period, whether or not satisfactory, may not be permanent. Among the reasons for this unpredictability are poor fusion, poor vision, and contracture of scar tissue. Reoperations are often necessary.

Iatrogenic Brown Syndrome

Iatrogenic Brown syndrome can result from superior oblique muscle strengthening procedures. Taking care to avoid excessive tightening of the tendon when these procedures are performed minimizes the risk of this complication. When it occurs after superior oblique tucking, the tuck can sometimes be reversed if reoperation is undertaken soon after the original surgery. If not, then the standard superior oblique weakening procedures used in other forms of Brown syndrome can be employed (see Chapter 12).

Anti-Elevation Syndrome

Inferior oblique anteriorization can result in restricted elevation of the eye in abduction (*anti-elevation syndrome*). Reattaching the lateral corner of the muscle anterior to the spiral of Tillaux increases the risk; "bunching up" the insertion at the lateral border of the inferior rectus muscle may reduce the risk.

Kushner BJ. Restriction of elevation in abduction after inferior oblique anteriorization. *J AAPOS.* 1997;1(1):55–62.

Lost and Slipped Muscles

A rectus muscle that sustains trauma or that slips out of the sutures or instruments while unattached to the globe during an operation can become inaccessible posteriorly in the orbit. This consequence is most severe when it involves the medial rectus muscle, since it is the most difficult to recover. A lost muscle does not reattach to the globe but instead retracts through the Tenon capsule.

The surgeon should immediately attempt to find the lost muscle, if possible with the assistance of a surgeon experienced in this potentially complex surgery. Malleable retractors and a headlight are helpful. Minimal manipulation should be employed to bring into view the anatomical site through which the muscle and its sheath normally penetrate the Tenon capsule where, it is hoped, the distal end of the muscle can be observed and captured. If inspection does not reliably indicate that the muscle has been identified, sudden bradycardia when traction is exerted can often be confirmatory. Recovery of the medial rectus muscle has been achieved by using a transnasal endoscopic approach to the ethmoid sinus or by performing a medial orbitotomy. Transposition surgery may be required if the lost muscle is not found, but anterior segment ischemia may be a risk. Where to reattach the recovered muscle depends on several factors in the particular case and is largely a matter of judgment.

A *slipped muscle* is the result of inadequate suturing technique. The muscle recedes posteriorly within its capsule during the postoperative period. Clinically, the patient manifests a weakness of that muscle, with limited rotations and possibly decreased saccades in its field of action (Fig 14-1). Surgery should be performed as soon as possible in order to secure the muscle before further retraction and contracture take place. The surgeon can prevent slippage by making full-thickness locking bites that include muscle tissue, not merely capsule, before disinsertion. In reoperations for strabismus with deficient rotations, slippage or "stretched scar" should be suspected and the involved muscles explored.

Pulled-in-Two Syndrome

Dehiscence of a muscle during surgery has been termed *pulled-in-two syndrome (PITS)*. The dehiscence usually occurs at the tendon–muscle junction, and the inferior rectus may be the most frequently affected muscle. Advanced age, various myopathies, previous surgery, trauma, or infiltrative disease may predispose a muscle to PITS by weakening its structural integrity. Treatment is, when possible, re-anastomosis of the muscle using techniques similar to those employed for lost muscles (see previous section).

Perforation of the Sclera

During reattachment of an EOM, a needle may penetrate the sclera and pass into the suprachoroidal space or perforate the choroid and retina. Perforation can lead to retinal detachment or endophthalmitis (see BCSC Section 9, *Intraocular Inflammation and Uveitis*); in most cases, it results in only a small chorioretinal scar, with no effect on vision. Most perforations are unrecognized unless specifically looked for by ophthalmoscopy. If vitreous escapes through the perforation site, many surgeons apply immediate local cryotherapy or laser therapy. Topical antibiotics are generally given during the immediate postoperative period, even when vitreous has not escaped. Ophthalmoscopy during the postoperative period is an appropriate precaution, with referral to a retina consultant as needed.

Postoperative Infections

Intraocular infection is uncommon following strabismus surgery. Some patients develop mild conjunctivitis, which may be caused by allergy to suture material or postoperative

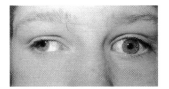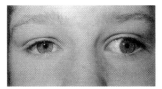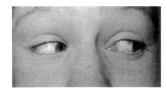

Figure 14-1 Slipped left medial rectus muscle. *Left,* Gaze right shows inability to adduct left eye. *Center,* Exotropia in primary position. *Right,* Gaze left shows full abduction. Note left palpebral fissure is wider than right.

medications, as well as by infectious agents. Preseptal and orbital cellulitis with proptosis, eyelid swelling, chemosis, and fever are rare (Fig 14-2). These conditions usually develop 2–3 days after surgery and generally respond well to systemic antibiotics. Patients should be warned of the signs and symptoms of orbital cellulitis and endophthalmitis so they will seek emergency consultation if necessary.

Foreign-Body Granuloma and Allergic Reaction

A foreign-body granuloma occasionally develops after EOM surgery, usually at the muscle's reattachment site. The granuloma is characterized by a localized, elevated, hyperemic, slightly tender mass (Fig 14-3). It may respond to topical corticosteroids. Surgical excision is necessary if the granuloma persists. Reactions to suture materials are now infrequent because gut suture is rarely used (Fig 14-4).

Epithelial Cyst

A noninflamed, translucent subconjunctival mass may develop if conjunctival epithelium is buried during muscle reattachment or incision closure (Fig 14-5). Occasionally, the cyst resolves spontaneously. Topical steroids may be helpful; persistent cases may require

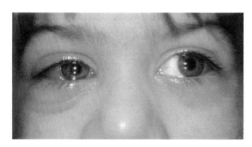

Figure 14-2 Orbital cellulitis, right eye, 2 days after bilateral recession of the lateral rectus muscles.

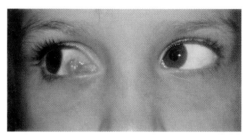

Figure 14-3 Severe postoperative granuloma over the right medial rectus muscle persisting 1 year after medial rectus recessions.

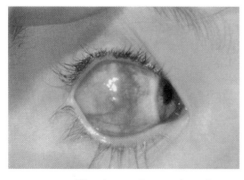

Figure 14-4 Allergic reaction to chromic gut. Allergic reactions are rarely seen with modern synthetic sutures such as polyglactin.

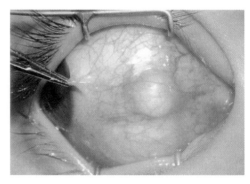

Figure 14-5 Postoperative epithelial cyst following right medial rectus muscle recession.

surgical excision. In some cases, the cyst is incorporated into the muscle tendon, so careful exploration is mandatory to identify this complication.

Conjunctival Scarring

Satisfaction from improved alignment may occasionally be overshadowed by unsightly scarring of the conjunctiva and the Tenon capsule. The tissues remain hyperemic and salmon pink instead of returning to their usual whiteness. This complication may result from the following:

- *Advancement of thickened Tenon capsule too close to the limbus.* In resection procedures, pulling the muscle forward may advance the Tenon capsule. The undesirable result is exaggerated in reoperations, when the Tenon capsule may be hypertrophied.
- *Advancement of the plica semilunaris.* During surgery on the medial rectus muscle using the limbal approach, the surgeon may mistake the plica semilunaris for a conjunctival edge and incorporate it into the closure. Though not strictly a conjunctival scar, the advanced plica, now pulled forward and hypertrophied, retains its fleshy color (Fig 14-6).

Treatment options include conjunctivoplasty with resection of scarred conjunctiva and transposition of adjacent conjunctiva; resection of subconjunctival fibrous tissue; recession of scarred conjunctiva; and amniotic membrane grafting.

Adherence Syndrome

Tears in the Tenon capsule with prolapse of orbital fat into the sub–Tenon space can cause formation of a fibrofatty scar that may restrict motility. Surgery involving the inferior oblique muscle is particularly prone to this complication because of the proximity of the fat space to the posterior border of the inferior oblique muscle. If recognized at the time of surgery, the prolapsed fat can be excised and the rent closed with absorbable sutures. Meticulous surgical technique usually prevents this serious complication.

Dellen

The term *dellen* (*delle,* singular) refers to shallow depressions and corneal thinning just anterior to the limbus; these occur when raised abnormal bulbar conjunctiva prevents the eyelid from adequately resurfacing the cornea with tear fluid during blinking (Fig 14-7).

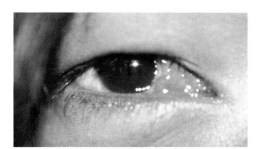

Figure 14-6 Hypertrophy involving the plica semilunaris. *(Courtesy of Scott Olitsky, MD.)*

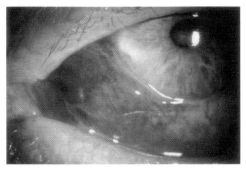

Figure 14-7 Corneal delle subsequent to post-operative subconjunctival hemorrhage.

Dellen are more apt to occur when the limbal approach to EOM surgery is used. They usually heal with time. Artificial tears or lubricants may be used until the chemosis subsides.

Anterior Segment Ischemia

The blood supply to the anterior segment of the eye is provided, in part, by the anterior ciliary arteries that travel with the 4 rectus muscles. Simultaneous surgery on 3 rectus muscles (as in a transposition procedure with simultaneous recession of an antagonist) or even 2 rectus muscles in patients with poor blood circulation may therefore lead to anterior segment ischemia (ASI). The earliest signs of this complication are cells and flare in the anterior chamber. More severe cases are characterized by corneal epithelial edema, folds in Descemet membrane, and an irregular pupil (Fig 14-8). This complication may lead to anterior segment necrosis and phthisis bulbi. No universally agreed-upon treatment exists for ASI. Because the signs of ASI are similar to those of typical uveitis, most ophthalmologists treat with topical, subconjunctival, or systemic corticosteroids, although there is no firm evidence supporting this approach.

It is possible to recess, resect, or transpose a rectus muscle while sparing its anterior ciliary vessels. Though difficult and time-consuming, this technique may be indicated in high-risk cases. Staging surgery, with an interval of several months between procedures, may be helpful. Because the anterior segment is partially supplied by the conjunctival circulation through the limbal arcades, using fornix instead of limbal incisions may provide some protection against the development of ASI.

Change in Eyelid Position

Change in the position of the eyelids is most likely to occur with surgery on the vertical rectus muscles. Pulling the inferior rectus muscle forward, as in a resection, advances the lower eyelid upward; recessing this muscle pulls the lower eyelid down, exposing sclera below the lower limbus (Fig 14-9). Surgery on the superior rectus muscle is less likely to affect upper eyelid position.

Changes in eyelid position can be obviated somewhat by careful dissection. In general, all intermuscular septum and fascial connections of the operated vertical rectus muscle must be severed at least 12–15 mm posterior to the muscle insertion, although doing this is contrary to the view of many surgeons that there should be minimal disturbance

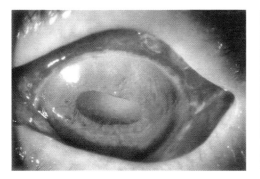

Figure 14-8 Superotemporal segmental anterior segment ischemia after simultaneous superior rectus muscle and lateral rectus muscle surgery following scleral buckling procedure.

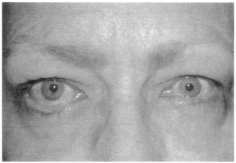

Figure 14-9 Patient treated for left hypertropia by recession of the right inferior rectus muscle, which pulled the right lower eyelid down, and resection of the left inferior rectus muscle, which pulled the left lower eyelid up.

of the Tenon capsule. Release of the lower eyelid retractors or advancement of the capsulopalpebral head is helpful to prevent lower eyelid retraction after inferior rectus muscle recession.

Refractive Changes

Changes in refractive error are most common when strabismus surgery is performed on 2 rectus muscles of an eye. An induced astigmatism of low magnitude usually resolves within a few months.

Anesthesia for Extraocular Muscle Surgery

Methods

In cooperative patients, topical anesthetic drops alone (eg, tetracaine 0.5%, proparacaine 0.5%, lidocaine 2%) are effective for most steps in an EOM surgical procedure. Lid blocks are not necessary if the eyelid speculum is not spread to the point of causing the patient pain. Topical anesthesia is not effective for control of the pain produced by pulling on or against a restricted muscle or for cases in which exposure is difficult.

Both local infiltration (peribulbar) and retrobulbar anesthesia make most EOM procedures pain free and should be considered in adults for whom general anesthesia may pose an undue hazard. The administration of a short-acting hypnotic by an anesthesiologist just before retrobulbar injection greatly improves patient comfort. Because injected anesthetics may influence alignment during the first few hours after surgery, suture adjustment is best delayed for at least half a day.

General anesthesia is necessary for children and is frequently used for adults as well, particularly those requiring bilateral surgery. Neuromuscular blocking agents such as succinylcholine, which are administered to facilitate intubation for general anesthesia, can temporarily affect the results of a traction test. Nondepolarizing agents, which do not have this effect, can be employed instead.

Postoperative Nausea and Vomiting

Nausea and vomiting formerly were common following eye muscle surgery. They now occur less frequently with the use of anesthetic agents and ancillary drugs such as droperidol, metoclopramide, diphenhydramine, ondansetron, and propofol.

Oculocardiac Reflex

The oculocardiac reflex is a slowing of the heart rate caused by traction on the EOMs, particularly the medial rectus muscle. In its most severe form, the reflex can produce asystole. The surgeon should be aware of the possibility of inducing the oculocardiac reflex when manipulating a muscle and should be prepared to release tension if the heart rate drops excessively. Intravenous atropine and other agents can protect against this reflex.

Malignant Hyperthermia

Malignant hyperthermia (MH) is important to pediatric ophthalmologists because of its association with strabismus, myopathies, ptosis, and musculoskeletal abnormalities. MH is a defect of calcium binding by the sarcoplasmic reticulum of skeletal muscle that can occur sporadically or be dominantly inherited with incomplete penetrance. When MH is triggered by inhalational anesthetics or the muscle relaxant succinylcholine, unbound intracellular calcium increases. This stimulates muscle contracture that results in massive acidosis. In its fully developed form, MH is characterized by extreme heat production, resulting from the hypermetabolic state.

MH can be fatal if diagnosis and treatment are delayed. The earliest sign is unexplained elevation of end-tidal carbon dioxide concentration. As soon as the diagnosis is made, surgery should be terminated, even if incomplete. Treatment is in the province of the anesthesiologist. See also BCSC Section 1, *Update on General Medicine*.

Chemodenervation Using Botulinum Toxin

Pharmacology and Mechanism of Action

Purified botulinum toxin type A is a protein drug produced from the bacterium *Clostridium botulinum*. This agent paralyzes muscles by blocking the release of acetylcholine at the neuromuscular junction. Botulinum toxin has a number of uses, but it was originally developed for the treatment of strabismus. Within 24–48 hours of injection, botulinum toxin is bound and internalized within local motor nerve terminals, where it remains active for many weeks. Paralysis of the injected muscle begins within 2–4 days after injection and lasts clinically for at least 5–8 weeks, in the case of EOM. This produces, in effect, a pharmacologic recession: the EOM lengthens while it is paralyzed by botulinum, and its antagonist contracts. These changes may produce long-term improvement in the alignment of the eyes. The recent introduction of bupivacaine injection into the antagonist muscle to provide a chemical resection effect may extend the durability of the correction and expand the range of deviations in which chemodenervation can be successfully employed.

Scott AB. Botulinum toxin injection of eye muscles to correct strabismus. *Trans Am Ophthalmol Soc.* 1981;79:734–770.

Scott AB, Miller JM, Shieh KR. Treating strabismus by injecting the agonist muscle with bupivacaine and the antagonist with botulinum toxin. *Trans Am Ophthalmol Soc.* 2009;107:104–109.

Indications, Techniques, and Results

When used to treat patients with strabismus, the toxin is injected directly, with a small-gauge needle, into selected EOMs. Injections into the EOMs are performed with the use of a portable electromyographic device, although experienced practitioners often dispense with electromyography. In adults, injections are performed with topical anesthetic; in children, general anesthesia is usually necessary.

Clinical trials using botulinum for the treatment of strabismus have shown this agent to be most effective in the following conditions:

- small- to moderate-angle esotropia and exotropia (<40Δ)
- postoperative residual strabismus (2–8 weeks following surgery or later)
- acute paralytic strabismus (especially sixth nerve palsy; sometimes fourth nerve palsy), to eliminate diplopia while the palsy resolves
- cyclic esotropia
- active thyroid eye disease (Graves disease) or inflamed or pre-phthisical eyes, when surgery is inappropriate
- as a supplement to medial rectus muscle recessions for large-angle infantile esotropia or lateral rectus muscle recessions for large-angle exotropia

Multiple injections may be required, particularly in adults. As with surgical treatment, results are best when there is fusion to stabilize the alignment. Botulinum injection is usually not effective in patients with large deviations, restrictive or mechanical strabismus (trauma, chronic thyroid eye disease), or secondary strabismus wherein a muscle has been overly recessed. Injection is ineffective in A and V patterns, dissociated vertical deviations, and chronic paralytic strabismus. The long-term recovery rate for patients with acute sixth nerve palsy treated with observation alone is similar to that of patients who receive botulinum.

Complications

The most common adverse effects of ocular botulinum treatment are ptosis, incomplete eyelid closure, dry eye, and induced vertical strabismus after horizontal muscle injection. These complications are usually temporary, resolving after several weeks. Rare complications include scleral perforation, retrobulbar hemorrhage, pupillary dilation, and permanent diplopia. Systemic botulism has been reported in animals and humans following massive injections of large muscle groups, but this has not been encountered in ophthalmologic use of botulinum toxin.

Gardner R, Dawson EL, Adams GG, Lee JP. Long-term management of strabismus with multiple repeated injections of botulinum toxin. *J AAPOS.* 2008;12(6):569–575.

Related Videos

The following videos contain additional information on topics covered in this chapter and are available at www.aao.org/bcscvideo. Mobile-device users can scan the QR code below to access the videos.

- 🎥 Limbal Incision (1 min, 13 sec)
- 🎥 Fornix Incision (1 min, 43 sec)
- 🎥 Recession of Medial Rectus Muscle (1 min, 13 sec; 2 min, 8 sec)
- 🎥 Resection of Lateral Rectus Muscle (3 min, 2 sec)

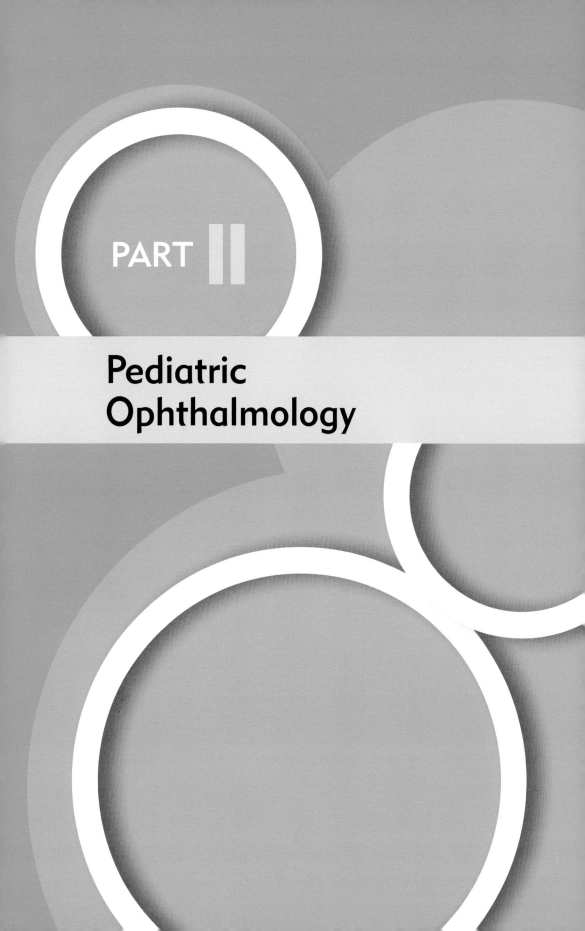

PART II

Pediatric
Ophthalmology

CHAPTER 15

Growth and Development of the Eye

Normal Growth and Development

The human eye undergoes dramatic anatomical and physiologic development throughout infancy and early childhood (Table 15-1). Ophthalmologists caring for children should be familiar with the normal growth and development of the pediatric eye, because departures from the norm may indicate pathology. See also BCSC Section 2, *Fundamentals and Principles of Ophthalmology.*

Dimensions of the Eye

Most of the growth of the eye takes place in the first year of life. The change in the axial length of the eye occurs in 3 phases (Fig 15-1). The first phase (birth to age 2 years) is a

Table 15-1 Dimensions of Newborn and Adult Eyes

	Newborn	Adult
Axial length (mm)	14.5–15.5	23.0–24.0
Corneal horizontal diameter (mm)	9.5–10.5	12.0
K value (diopters)	52.00	42.00–44.00

K = keratometry.

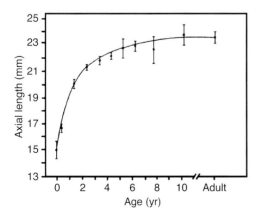

Figure 15-1 Axial length plotted with respect to age. *Dots* represent mean values for age group indicated; *bars* represent standard deviations. *(Reproduced with permission from Gordon RA, Donzis PB. Refractive development of the human eye. Arch Ophthalmol. 1985;103(6):785–789. © 1985, American Medical Association.)*

period of rapid growth. The axial length increases by approximately 4 mm in the first 6 months of life and by an additional 2 mm during the next 6 months. During the second (age 2 to 5 years) and third (age 5 to 13 years) phases, growth slows, with axial length increasing by about 1 mm per phase.

Similarly, the cornea grows rapidly during the first year of life (Fig 15-2). Keratometry values change markedly in the first year, starting at approximately 52.00 D at birth, flattening to 46.00 D by age 6 months, and reaching adult measurements of 42.00–44.00 D by age 12 months. The average horizontal diameter of the cornea is 9.5–10.5 mm in newborns and increases to 12.0 mm in adults. Mild corneal clouding may be seen in healthy newborns and is common in premature infants. It resolves as the cornea gradually thins, decreasing from an average central thickness of 691 μm at 30–32 weeks' gestation to 564 μm at birth.

The power of the pediatric lens decreases dramatically over the first several years of life—an important consideration when intraocular lens implantation is being planned for infants and young children after cataract extraction. Figure 15-3 shows the theoretical power of the pediatric lens at a given age, based on intraocular lens power calculations

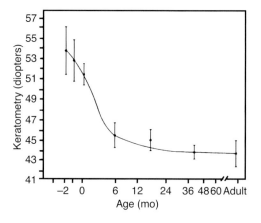

Figure 15-2 Keratometry values plotted with respect to age on a logarithmic scale. The negative number represents months of prematurity; *dots* represent the mean value for the age group indicated; and *bars,* the standard deviations. *(Reproduced with permission from Gordon RA, Donzis PB. Refractive development of the human eye. Arch Ophthalmol. 1985;103(6):785–789. © 1985, American Medical Association.)*

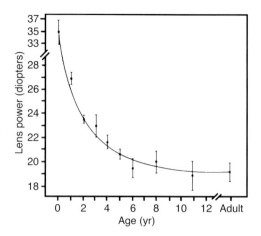

Figure 15-3 Mean values *(dots)* and standard deviations *(bars)* for calculated lens power as determined by modified SRK formula, plotted with respect to age. *(Reproduced with permission from Gordon RA, Donzis PB. Refractive development of the human eye. Arch Ophthalmol. 1985;103(6):785–789. © 1985, American Medical Association.)*

performed with the modified SRK formula, which uses pediatric keratometry and axial length values.

Kirwan C, O'Keefe M, Fitzsimon S. Central corneal thickness and corneal diameter in premature infants. *Acta Ophthalmol Scand.* 2005;83(6):751–753.

Refractive State

The refractive state of the eye changes as the eye's axial length increases and the cornea and lens flatten. In general, eyes are hyperopic at birth, become slightly more hyperopic until age 7 years, and then experience a myopic shift toward plano until the eyes reach their adult dimensions, usually by about age 16 years (Fig 15-4). Changes in refractive error vary widely, but if myopia presents before age 10 years, there is a higher risk of eventual progression to myopia of 6.00 D or more. Astigmatism is common in infants and often regresses.

The term *emmetropization* refers to the process in the developing eye in which the refractive power of the anterior segment and the axial length of the eye adjust to reach emmetropia. The reduction in astigmatism that occurs in many infant eyes and the decreasing hyperopia that occurs in eyes after age 6–8 years are examples of emmetropization.

Orbit and Ocular Adnexa

During infancy and childhood, the orbital volume increases and the shape of the orbital opening becomes less circular, resembling a horizontal oval. The lacrimal fossa becomes more superficial, and the angle formed by the axes of the 2 orbits becomes less divergent. The palpebral fissure measures approximately 18 mm horizontally and 8 mm vertically at birth and changes very little during the first year of life. However, from age 1 to 10 years, the palpebral fissure length increases rapidly, causing the round infant eye to acquire its elliptical adult shape.

Histologic studies show that the nasolacrimal duct is not fully canalized in many newborns, but most are asymptomatic.

Cornea, Iris, Pupil, and Anterior Chamber

Average central corneal thickness (CCT) decreases during the first 6–12 months of life (see the section Dimensions of the Eye). It then increases from 553 μm at age 1 year to

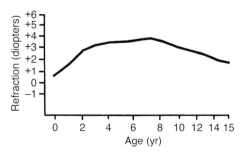

Figure 15-4 Change in mean refractive error as a function of age. *(Modified with permission from Eustis HS, Guthrie ME. Postnatal development. In: Wright KW, Strube YNJ, eds.* Pediatric Ophthalmology and Strabismus. *2nd ed. New York: Springer-Verlag; 2003:49.)*

573 μm by age 12 years and stabilizes thereafter. CCT is similar in white and Hispanic children but decreased in African American children. Most changes in iris color occur over the first 6–12 months of life, as pigment accumulates in the iris stroma and melanocytes. Compared with the adult pupil, the infant pupil is relatively small. A pupil less than 1.8 mm or greater than 5.4 mm in diameter is suggestive of an abnormality. The pupillary light reflex is normally present after 31 weeks' gestational age. At birth, the iris insertion is near the level of the scleral spur, but during the first year of life, the lens and ciliary body migrate posteriorly, resulting in formation of the angle recess.

Pediatric Eye Disease Investigator Group; Bradfield YS, Melia BM, Repka MX, et al. Central corneal thickness in children. *Arch Ophthalmol.* 2011;129(9):1132–1138.

Intraocular Pressure

Measurement of intraocular pressure (IOP) in infants can be difficult, and normal pressures vary depending on the method used to obtain them. Nevertheless, normal IOP is lower in infants than in adults, and a pressure of greater than 21 mm Hg should be considered abnormal. CCT influences the measurement of IOP, but this effect is not well understood in children. See Chapter 22 in this volume and BCSC Section 10, *Glaucoma,* for further discussion.

Extraocular Muscles

The rectus muscles of infants are smaller than those of adults; muscle insertions, on average, are 2.3–3.0 mm narrower in infants than in adults; and the tendons are thinner in infants. In newborns, the distance from the rectus muscle insertion to the limbus is roughly 2 mm less than that in adults; by age 6 months, this distance is 1 mm less; and at 20 months, it is similar to that in adults. Enlargement of the posterior segment occurs during the first 2 years of life, resulting in a separation of 4–5 mm between the superior and inferior oblique insertions and migration of the inferior oblique insertion temporally.

Extraocular muscle function continues to develop after birth. Vestibular-driven eye movements are present as early as 34 weeks' gestational age. Conjugate horizontal gaze is present at birth, but vertical gaze may not be fully functional until 6 months of age. Intermittent strabismus is present in approximately two-thirds of young infants but resolves in most by 2–3 months of age. Accommodation and fusional convergence are usually present by age 3 months.

Retina

The macula is poorly developed at birth but changes rapidly during the first 4 years of life. Most notable are changes in macular pigmentation, the annular ring, the foveal light reflex, and cone photoreceptor differentiation. Improvement in visual acuity with age is attributed to 3 processes: differentiation of cone photoreceptors, narrowing of the rod-free zone, and increase in foveal cone density (Fig 15-5). Retinal vascularization proceeds in a centrifugal manner, starting at the optic disc at 16 weeks' gestational age and reaching the temporal ora serrata by 40 weeks' gestational age.

Hendrickson A, Possin D, Lejla V, Toth CA. Histologic development of the human fovea from midgestation to maturity. *Am J Ophthalmol.* 2012;154(5):767–778.

Visual Acuity and Stereoacuity

Two major methods are used to quantitate visual acuity in preverbal infants and toddlers: *preferential looking (PL)* and *visually evoked potential (VEP)*. See Chapter 1 for a description of these methods. VEP shows that visual acuity improves from approximately 20/400 in newborns to 20/20 by age 6–7 months. However, PL studies estimate the visual acuity of a newborn to be 20/600, improving to 20/120 by age 3 months and to 20/60 by 6 months. Further, PL testing shows that visual acuity of 20/20 is not reached until age 3–5 years. The discrepancy between measurements obtained by these 2 methods may be related to the higher cortical processing required for PL compared to VEP. Stereoacuity reaches 60 seconds of arc by about age 5–6 months (see Chapter 7).

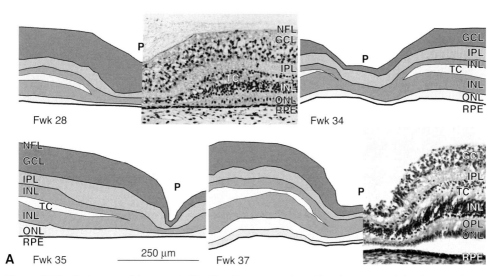

Figure 15-5 **A,** Layers of late-gestation fetal human retina. Development of the human fovea at *(top left)* Fwk 28, *(top right)* Fwk 34, *(bottom left)* Fwk 35, and *(bottom right)* Fwk 37. A transient layer of Chievitz *(TC)* is present as a gap in the INL of all eyes from this age group. The foveal pit *(P)* has thinned the GCL, IPL, and INL compared to layers surrounding the pit (the foveal slope). Scale in bottom left for all. *GCL* = ganglion cell layer; *INL* = inner nuclear layer; *IPL* = inner plexiform layer; *NFL* = nerve fiber layer; *ONL* = outer nuclear layer; *OPL* = outer plexiform layer; *RPE* = retinal pigment epithelium.

(Continued on next page)

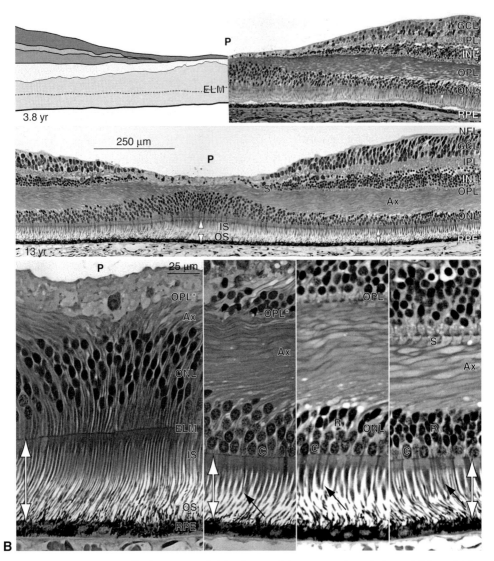

Figure 15-5 *(continued)* **B,** Layers and histology of human retina during childhood. The final maturation stages of the human fovea are shown at *(top left)* 3.8 years and *(top right)* 13 years with higher magnification of the 13 years *(middle)* foveal center, *(bottom left)* first rods at 300 μm, *(bottom middle left)* 500 μm, and *(bottom middle right)* 2 mm from the fovea. The foveal pit is wide and shallow. The foveal center is composed of long, thin cone OS; IS, and cell bodies 8–12 cones deep. The central OPL contains a thick layer of axon *(Ax)*. The foveal OPL contains only Ax *(OPL*)* out to 500 μm, where synaptic pedicles *(bottom middle left, OPL; bottom middle and far right, S)* are first encountered. Long, thin rod OS *(bottom row, black arrows)* becomes more prominent with eccentricity. Note the marked increase in cone IS diameter from the foveal center to 300 μm, with a small further increase at 2 mm. Scale in middle for top and middle rows; scale in bottom left for bottom row. *C* = cone; *ELM* = external limiting membrane; *GCL* = ganglion cell layer; *INL* = inner nuclear layer; *IPL* = inner plexiform layer; *IS* = inner segment; *OS* = outer segment; *NFL* = nerve fiber layer; *ONL* = outer nuclear layer; *OPL* = outer plexiform layer; *R* = rod; *RPE* = retinal pigment epithelium. *(Modified with permission from Hendrickson A, Possin D, Lejla V, Toth CA. Histologic development of the human fovea from mid-gestation to maturity. Am J Ophthalmol. 2012;154(5):767–778.)*

Abnormal Growth and Development

Major congenital anomalies occur in 2%–3% of live births. Causes include chromosomal anomalies, multifactorial disorders, environmental agents, and idiopathic etiologies. Regardless of etiology, from a developmental point of view, congenital anomalies may be categorized as follows (ocular examples are given in parentheses):

- *agenesis:* developmental failure (anophthalmos)
- *hypoplasia:* developmental arrest (optic nerve hypoplasia)
- *hyperplasia:* developmental excess (distichiasis)
- *dysraphia:* failure to fuse (choroidal coloboma)
- failure to divide or canalize (congenital nasolacrimal duct obstruction)
- persistence of vestigial structures (persistent fetal vasculature)

A *malformation* implies a morphologic defect present from the onset of development or from a very early stage. A disturbance to a group of cells in a single developmental field may cause multiple malformations. Multiple etiologies may result in similar field defects and patterns of malformation. A single structural defect or factor can lead to a cascade, or domino effect, of secondary anomalies called a *sequence.* The Pierre Robin group of anomalies (cleft palate, glossoptosis, micrognathia, respiratory problems) may represent a sequence caused by abnormal descent of the tongue and is seen in disorders such as Stickler and fetal alcohol syndromes. A *syndrome* is a recognizable and consistent pattern of multiple malformations known to have a specific cause, which is usually a mutation of a single gene, a chromosome alteration, or an environmental agent. An *association* represents defects known to occur together in a statistically significant number of patients. An association may represent a variety of yet-unidentified causes. Two or more minor anomalies in combination significantly increase the chance of an associated major malformation.

Jones KL, Jones MC, del Campo M. *Smith's Recognizable Patterns of Human Malformation.* 7th ed. Philadelphia: Elsevier Saunders; 2013.

CHAPTER 16

Decreased Vision in Infants and Children

When an infant has not developed good visual attention or the ability to fixate on and follow objects by 3–4 months of age, a number of causes must be considered. Ophthalmic (pregeniculate) causes of visual impairment include corneal and lenticular opacities, glaucoma, retinal anomalies or dystrophies, and optic nerve anomalies. Many of these are covered elsewhere in this volume. Other causes of reduced visual attention include delayed visual maturation and cerebral visual impairment (ie, postgeniculate visual impairment). These entities, which may be associated with other neurologic abnormalities, are discussed in this chapter.

Normal Visual Development

Visual development is a highly complex maturational process. Structural changes occur in both the eye and the central nervous system. Laboratory and clinical research has shown that normal vision develops as a result of both genetic coding and experience in a normal visual environment.

A blink reflex to bright light should be present within a few days of birth. The pupillary light reflex is usually present after 31 weeks' gestation, but it can be difficult to evaluate in the early neonatal period because the pupils are miotic in the newborn.

At about 6–8 weeks of age, the healthy full-term infant should be able to make and maintain eye contact with other humans and react with facial expressions. Infants aged 2–3 months should be interested in bright objects. By age 3–4 months, smooth pursuit asymmetry should have resolved, the eyes should be orthotropic, and fix-and-follow visual responses to a small (2–4 inches in diameter) toy should be present. Premature infants can be expected to reach these landmarks later, but there is not an exact week-for-week correlation for the attainment of these milestones.

Disconjugate eye movements, skew deviation, and *sunsetting* (tonic downward deviation of both eyes) may be noted in healthy newborns but should not persist beyond 4 months of age. Signs of poor visual development include searching eye movements, lack of response to familiar faces and objects, and nystagmus. Staring at bright lights and forceful rubbing or poking of the eyes *(oculodigital reflex)* in an otherwise visually disinterested infant are other signs of poor vision and suggest an ocular cause for the deficiency.

Evaluation of the Infant With Decreased Vision

A careful history, beginning with a review of family history, is essential. The clinician should review details of the pregnancy, including maternal infection, maternal diabetes mellitus, radiation exposure, maternal drug or alcohol use, and trauma. Perinatal problems such as prematurity, intrauterine growth retardation, fetal distress, bradycardia, meconium staining, and oxygen deprivation are important. In addition, the clinician should inquire about the presence of systemic abnormalities or delayed developmental milestones.

Comprehensive ophthalmologic examination of the infant should begin with an assessment of visual behavior. Vision in the infant is usually assessed qualitatively by clinical appraisal and observation of optokinetic nystagmus (OKN) responses, as well as quantitatively by psychophysical tests such as visually evoked potential or response (VEP or VER) and by preferential looking tests such as Teller Acuity Cards II and the Cardiff Acuity Test (see Chapter 1). Pupillary light responses, ocular alignment and motility, presence or absence of nystagmus or roving eye movements, anterior segment and fundus examinations, and cycloplegic refraction are the other important parts of the evaluation.

Pupillary responses are sluggish with anterior visual pathway disease such as retinal dystrophies and optic nerve abnormalities. Paradoxical pupils (pupillary constriction in response to darkness) are most commonly associated with retinal dystrophies, but they can also occur with optic neuropathies. Pupillary responses are normal in infants with cerebral visual impairment (see the section Retrogeniculate Visual Impairment, or Cerebral Visual Impairment). Nystagmus may be an indicator of bilateral pregeniculate visual dysfunction (see the section Pregeniculate Visual Impairment), or it may be purely a motor anomaly. The nystagmus usually starts at 2–3 months of age (see Chapter 13). Visual deficits in 1 or both eyes frequently cause abnormal ocular alignment (either esotropia or exotropia; see Chapters 8 and 9, respectively).

Classification of Visual Impairment in Infants and Children

When an infant or child presents with poor vision, the workup is predicated on localizing the visual dysfunction. It is helpful to classify disorders causing visual impairment in infants as delayed visual maturation or pregeniculate or retrogeniculate visual dysfunction (cerebral visual impairment). Although this is a useful clinical paradigm, it should be recognized that some disorders affect both the pregeniculate and retrogeniculate pathways.

Delayed Visual Maturation

Normal visual fixation and tracking usually develop in infants within the first 3 months of life. If this does not occur, the condition is referred to as *delayed visual maturation (DVM),* or *cortical inattention.* Ophthalmologic and systemic examination of infants with DVM usually reveals a cause. There are 3 subgroups of infants with DVM: otherwise healthy infants, infants with systemic/neurologic abnormalities, and infants with structural eye anomalies.

In an otherwise healthy infant with DVM, the following findings suggest a good visual and neurologic prognosis: some reaction to light, normal pupillary responses, no nystagmus, and normal ocular structures. If the visual behavior does not progress toward normal by 4–6 months of age, further investigation (neuroimaging or electrophysiologic testing) is warranted.

Azmeh R, Lueder GT. Delayed visual maturation in otherwise normal infants. *Graefes Arch Clin and Exp Ophthalmol.* 2013;251(13):941–944.

Pregeniculate Visual Impairment

Pregeniculate visual impairment denotes visual deficits resulting from pathology anterior to the lateral geniculate nucleus (the pregeniculate visual pathways). Congenital sensory nystagmus may be a clinical indicator of bilateral pregeniculate visual impairment. Strabismus is commonly seen with these disorders. Causes of pregeniculate visual impairment in infants include corneal and other anterior segment abnormalities, glaucoma, retinal disorders, and optic nerve abnormalities.

Optic nerve abnormalities are frequent causes of pregeniculate visual impairment (see also Chapter 26). The most common of these is optic nerve hypoplasia, which may be associated with central nervous system anomalies such as septo-optic dysplasia and schizencephaly. Other optic nerve disorders are optic atrophy, morning glory disc anomaly, optic disc coloboma, and staphyloma. Causes of optic nerve atrophy include hydrocephalus, brain tumors, trauma, hypoxic–ischemic injury, metabolic storage diseases, and inherited optic neuropathies such as Behr optic atrophy.

Inherited retinal disorders are also common causes of pregeniculate visual impairment and should be considered in infants with poor vision, nystagmus, and no obvious abnormality on ophthalmic examination. Inherited retinal diseases include Leber congenital amaurosis, achromatopsia, blue-cone monochromatism, and congenital stationary night blindness (see Chapter 25). Fundus examination in an infant with a retinal dystrophy is often normal because the associated retinal pigmentary changes may not appear until later. Subtle retinal vessel attenuation and optic disc pallor may be present. Electroretinography (ERG) can aid in the diagnosis of these disorders. Foveal hypoplasia can also cause pregeniculate visual impairment. It can be isolated but is more commonly associated with albinism and aniridia.

Retrogeniculate Visual Impairment, or Cerebral Visual Impairment

Cerebral visual impairment (CVI; also termed *retrogeniculate visual impairment*) is the most frequent cause of childhood visual impairment in developed countries. It denotes visual deficits resulting from pathology posterior to the lateral geniculate nucleus (the retrogeniculate visual pathways). CVI is also often referred to as *cortical visual impairment,* but the former term is preferred because subcortical visual impairment causes vision problems that are difficult to differentiate from those due to cortical visual impairment. The pathology may involve the optic radiations as well as the occipital cortex. Depending on the etiology, the visual impairment can be transient or permanent and can be an isolated finding or associated with multiple neurologic deficits.

The causes of CVI can be congenital or acquired. Prenatal and perinatal causes include periventricular leukomalacia (a prominent cause of visual impairment in premature children), intrauterine infection, hypoxia, intracranial hemorrhage, structural central nervous system abnormalities, seizures, and hydrocephalus. Acquired causes include accidental trauma, abusive head trauma, meningitis, and encephalitis.

Infants with CVI show varying degrees of visual inattentiveness. Both the family and the ophthalmologist may be uncertain as to whether the baby can see. Examination reveals normal ocular structures, normal pupillary responses, and variable levels of visual fixation, from mildly decreased to roving eye movements. Nystagmus is typically not present. Descending optic atrophy (from transsynaptic degeneration) may coexist. In preterm infants, optic disc cupping resembling that seen in glaucoma can occur as a result of transsynaptic degeneration, most commonly secondary to periventricular leukomalacia.

ERG results are normal. VEP results may be normal or subnormal. Neuroimaging studies may be normal or may reveal changes such as cerebral atrophy, porencephaly in the occipital (striate or parastriate) cortex, damage to the optic radiations, or periventricular leukomalacia. Children with normal neuroimaging studies tend to have a more favorable prognosis.

> Khetpal V, Donahue SP. Cortical visual impairment: etiology, associated findings and prognosis in a tertiary care setting. *J AAPOS*. 2007;11(3):235–239.

Pediatric Low Vision Rehabilitation

Vision rehabilitation should be recommended when a child has a visual impairment that affects his or her ability to perform visual tasks (as occurs with best-corrected visual acuity worse than 20/40 in the better-seeing eye, decreased visual field, central field loss, or reduced contrast sensitivity). At the time of diagnosis and throughout the subsequent years, the ophthalmologist plays an important role in recommending that children with low vision receive comprehensive vision rehabilitation. Early referral is essential for setting the family and child on a course to achieve optimal visual performance and to make a successful adjustment to vision loss.

Vision rehabilitation for children often involves pediatric ophthalmologists, vision rehabilitation clinicians, occupational therapists, teachers, orientation and mobility specialists, technology experts, state societies, and other professionals and organizations. An Individualized Education Plan (IEP) outlines the needs of an individual child in the school setting. The child's needs in the home and in other nonacademic settings must be considered as well. A variety of aids are available to assist patients with low vision, ranging from simple telescopes to Braille literacy. Because most children have large accommodative amplitudes that allow them to hold an object closer than normal to enlarge its image, magnifiers may not be necessary for pediatric patients with low vision. Existing and future technologies, including e-readers, audio books, and text-to-speech technology, offer continually expanding opportunities for these children.

The American Academy of Ophthalmology's Preferred Practice Pattern on vision rehabilitation (see references) outlines the rehabilitation process for preschool-aged

Table 16-1 Sources of Information on Low Vision

American Foundation for the Blind; www.afb.org

American Printing House for the Blind (APH); www.aph.org
  Large-print and braille books, tapes, talking computer software, and low vision aids

Family Support America; www.familysupportamerica.org
  Identifies parent support groups all over the country

Learning Ally; www.learningally.org
  Audiobooks for the blind and dyslexic

Lighthouse International; www.lighthouse.org

National Library Service for the Blind and Physically Handicapped (NLS), Library of Congress;
  www.loc.gov/nls
  Free library program of braille and audio materials, including books and magazines

National Organization for Albinism and Hypopigmentation (NOAH); www.albinism.org

Prevent Blindness America; www.preventblindness.org

National Toll-Free Numbers

American Council of the Blind (ACB); (800) 424-8666

New York Times Large-Print Weekly; (800) 631-2580

Reader's Digest Large Print; (800) 807-2780

---

children to young adults. The availability of rehabilitation resources varies across communities, but the following online resource, which can be searched by location, may be helpful for clinicians and families in identifying such services in their community: http://www.afb.org/directory.aspx. Other useful information can be found in the SmartSight Patient Handout (one.aao.org/smart-sight-low-vision), available on the Academy's website. See also Table 16-1, which lists resources for further information, and BCSC Section 3, *Clinical Optics,* for detailed discussion of low vision aids.

American Academy of Ophthalmology Vision Rehabilitation Committee. Preferred Practice Pattern Guidelines. *Vision Rehabilitation.* San Francisco: American Academy of Ophthalmology; 2013. Available at: www.aao.org/ppp.

Markowitz SN. Principles of modern low vision rehabilitation. *Can J Ophthalmol.* 2006;41(3): 289–312.

Eyelid Disorders

Congenital Eyelid Disorders

Congenital eyelid disorders result from abnormal differentiation of the eyelids and adnexa, developmental arrest, intrauterine environmental insults, and other unknown factors (see also BCSC Section 2, *Fundamentals and Principles of Ophthalmology,* and Section 7, *Orbit, Eyelids, and Lacrimal System*).

Eyelid malformations can be isolated, be associated with orbital malformations, or represent features of a syndrome; therefore, systematic evaluation of the eyelids, ocular adnexa, and interpupillary distance is an essential part of the clinical evaluation of a dysmorphic infant. Morphologic measurements of the eyelids and orbit can be performed with transparent rulers or calipers and compared with normal reference measures (Fig 17-1). Alternatively, indexes such as the Farkas canthal index, defined as the ratio of inner canthal distance to outer canthal distance × 10, can be used. Hypotelorism and hypertelorism are defined as having canthal indexes less than 38 and greater than 42, respectively. It is important to consider ethnic variations (see also Chapter 18).

Telecanthus

Telecanthus is a condition characterized by a greater-than-normal distance between the inner canthi. It is considered primary if the interpupillary distance is normal and secondary if the interpupillary distance is greater than normal. Telecanthus is common in many syndromes. This condition must be distinguished from hypertelorism, which is described in Chapter 18.

Dystopia Canthorum

Dystopia canthorum is characteristic of Waardenburg syndrome type 1. It is lateral displacement of both the inner canthi and the lacrimal puncta such that an imaginary vertical line connecting the upper and lower puncta crosses the cornea (Fig 17-2).

Cryptophthalmos

Cryptophthalmos, a rare condition, results from failed differentiation of eyelid structures. The skin passes uninterrupted from the forehead, over the eye, to the cheek and blends in with the cornea, which is usually malformed (Fig 17-3). Fraser syndrome is an autosomal recessive disorder that is characterized by partial syndactyly and genitourinary anomalies; it may include cryptophthalmos and other ocular malformations.

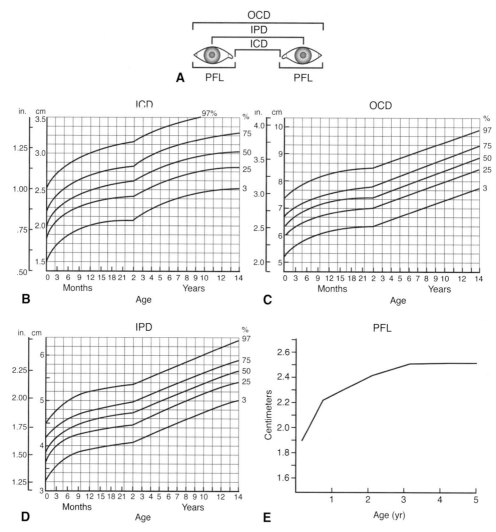

Figure 17-1 A, Schematic representation of measurements involved in the evaluation of the orbital region. *OCD* = outer canthal distance; *IPD* = interpupillary distance; *ICD* = inner canthal distance; *PFL* = palpebral fissure length. **B,** ICD measurements according to age. **C,** OCD measurements according to age. **D,** IPD measurements according to age. **E,** PFL measurements according to age. *(Modified with permission from Dollfus H, Verloes A. Dysmorphology and the orbital region: a practical clinical approach. Surv Ophthalmol. 2004;49(6):549.)*

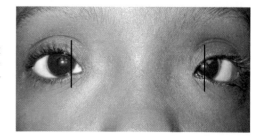

Figure 17-2 Dystopia canthorum in a patient with Waardenburg syndrome. Notice that the *vertical lines* drawn through the puncta intersect the cornea. *(Courtesy of Amy Hutchinson, MD.)*

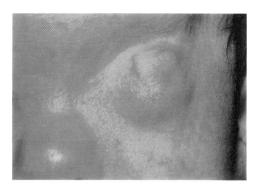

Figure 17-3 Cryptophthalmos, left eye.

Ablepharon

Ablepharon, absence or severe hypoplasia of the eyelids, is very rare. Affected patients are at high risk for exposure keratopathy. It is seen in ablepharon macrostomia syndrome.

Congenital Coloboma of the Eyelid

Congenital eyelid coloboma (eyelid clefting or notching) usually involves the upper eyelid and can range from a small notch to a defect encompassing the horizontal length of the eyelid. The eyelid may be fused to the globe (Fig 17-4). Eyelid colobomas are unrelated to other ocular colobomas and are commonly associated with Goldenhar syndrome or amniotic band syndrome. The eye of an infant with a congenital eyelid coloboma should be observed for exposure keratopathy. Surgical closure of the eyelid defect is required in most cases.

Ankyloblepharon

Fusion of part or all of the eyelid margins is known as *ankyloblepharon.* This condition may be dominantly inherited. Treatment is surgical. A variant is *ankyloblepharon filiforme adnatum,* in which the eyelid margins are connected by fine strands (Fig 17-5). This

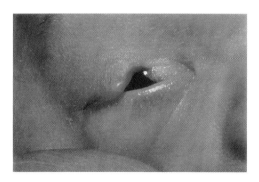

Figure 17-4 Congenital eyelid coloboma (cleft), right eye. The eyelid is fused to the globe.

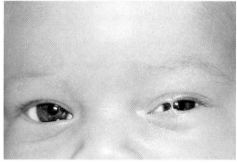

Figure 17-5 Ankyloblepharon filiforme adnatum. The eyelid margins are fused by a fine strand. The eyelids were easily separated with blunt scissors in the office, without anesthesia. *(Courtesy of Amy Hutchinson, MD.)*

variant is seen in Hay-Wells syndrome (ankyloblepharon–ectodermal dysplasia–clefting syndrome), a form of ectodermal dysplasia that includes cleft lip or palate.

Congenital Ectropion

Congenital ectropion is a disorder characterized by eversion of the eyelid margin; it usually involves the lower eyelid secondary to a vertical deficiency of the skin. Lateral tarsorrhaphy may be necessary for mild cases. More severe cases may require a skin flap or graft.

Congenital Entropion

Congenital entropion is a rare abnormality in which eyelid inversion is present at birth. It does not resolve spontaneously. Surgery should be performed when corneal integrity is threatened.

Epiblepharon

Epiblepharon is a congenital anomaly characterized by a horizontal fold of skin adjacent to either the upper or lower eyelid—most commonly, the lower eyelid—that may turn the lashes inward, against the cornea. The child's cornea often tolerates this condition surprisingly well. Unlike congenital entropion, epiblepharon often resolves spontaneously. Ocular lubricants may be beneficial. Cases that do not resolve or that cause chronic corneal irritation require surgical repair.

Congenital Tarsal Kink

In this condition, the tarsal plate of the upper eyelid is folded at birth, resulting in entropion. The cornea may be exposed and traumatized, leading to ulceration. The clinician can manage minor defects by manually unfolding the tarsus and taping the eyelid shut with a pressure dressing for 1–2 days. More severe cases require surgical incision of the tarsal plate or excision of a V-shaped wedge from the inner surface to permit unfolding.

Distichiasis

The presence of a partial or complete accessory row of eyelashes growing out of or slightly posterior to the meibomian gland orifices is known as *distichiasis* (Fig 17-6). The abnormal lashes tend to be thinner, shorter, softer, and less pigmented than normal cilia and are therefore often well tolerated. Treatment is indicated if corneal irritation is present.

Euryblepharon

In euryblepharon, the lateral aspect of the palpebral aperture is enlarged, with downward displacement of the temporal half of the lower eyelid. This condition gives the appearance of a very wide palpebral fissure or a droopy lower eyelid. Euryblepharon may be associated with Kabuki syndrome.

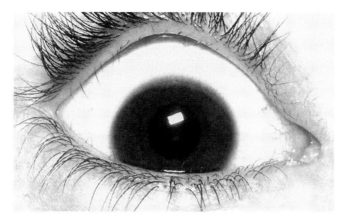

Figure 17-6 Distichiasis. An accessory row of eyelashes exits from the meibomian gland orifices. *(Reproduced with permission from Patil BB, Bell R, Brice G, Jeffery S, Desai SP. Distichiasis without lymphoedema?* Eye (Lond). *2004;18(12):1270–1272.)*

Epicanthus

Epicanthus, a crescent-shaped fold of skin running vertically between the eyelids and overlying the inner canthus, is shown in Figure 17-7. There are 4 types:

1. *epicanthus tarsalis:* fold is most prominent in the upper eyelid
2. *epicanthus inversus:* fold is most prominent in the lower eyelid
3. *epicanthus palpebralis:* fold is equally distributed between the upper and lower eyelids
4. *epicanthus supraciliaris:* fold arises from the eyebrow and terminates over the lacrimal sac

Epicanthus may be associated with blepharophimosis or ptosis, or it may be an isolated finding. Surgical correction is only occasionally required.

Palpebral Fissure Slants

In the normal eye, the eyelids are generally positioned so that the lateral canthus is approximately 1 mm higher than the medial canthus. Slight upward or downward slanting of palpebral fissures normally occurs on a familial basis or in certain ethnic groups (eg, Asians). However, certain craniofacial syndromes frequently cause palpebral fissures to have a characteristic upward or downward slant (eg, downward slant in Treacher Collins syndrome; see Chapter 18, Fig 18-9).

Blepharophimosis–Ptosis–Epicanthus Inversus Syndrome

Blepharophimosis–ptosis–epicanthus inversus syndrome (BPES) is also referred to as *congenital eyelid syndrome* or *blepharophimosis syndrome.* It consists of blepharophimosis, epicanthus inversus, telecanthus, and ptosis. BPES may occur as a sporadic or autosomal

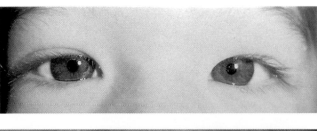

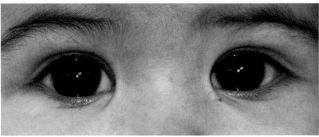

Figure 17-7 Epicanthus, bilateral. *Top,* Epicanthus tarsalis. *Bottom,* Epicanthus palpebralis. *(Top image reproduced with permission from Crouch E.* The Child's Eye: Strabismus and Amblyopia. *Slide script. San Francisco: American Academy of Ophthalmology; 1982. Bottom image courtesy of Robert W. Hered, MD.)*

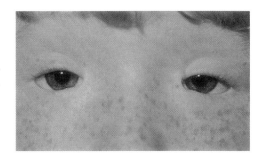

Figure 17-8 Blepharophimosis–ptosis–epicanthus inversus syndrome (BPES). Note telecanthus as well.

dominant disorder. Mutation of the *FOXL2* gene has been found to cause both BPES type II (eyelid findings only) and type I (eyelid findings and premature ovarian failure). The palpebral fissures are shortened horizontally and vertically *(blepharophimosis),* with poor levator muscle function and no eyelid fold (Fig 17-8). The horizontal palpebral fissure length, normally 25–30 mm, is only 18–22 mm in these patients. Repair of the ptosis, usually with frontalis suspension procedures, may be necessary early in life. Because the epicanthus and telecanthus may improve with age, repair of these defects is often delayed.

> Beysen D, De Paepe A, De Baere E. *FOXL2* mutations and genomic rearrangements in BPES. *Hum Mutat.* 2009;30(2):158–169.

Congenital Ptosis

Ptosis (blepharoptosis) is eyelid droop. The condition can be congenital or acquired. It is important to differentiate congenital ptosis from acquired cases with systemic associations (Table 17-1; see also BCSC Section 7, *Orbit, Eyelids, and Lacrimal System*). Congenital ptosis may be familial. Anisometropic amblyopia and strabismus are common associations.

Table 17-1 Classification of Ptosis

Pseudoptosis
Congenital ptosis
Acquired ptosis
  Myogenic ptosis
    Myasthenia gravis
    Progressive external ophthalmoplegia
  Neurogenic ptosis
    Horner syndrome
    Third nerve palsy
  Mechanical ptosis

Evaluation of ptosis requires assessment of the upper eyelid crease, the amount of ptosis, and the function of the levator muscle. In severe congenital ptosis, the eyelid crease is usually absent. The clinician can determine the amount of ptosis by measuring the palpebral fissure height and the margin–reflex distance (MRD). The MRD is the distance from the margin of the upper eyelid to the corneal light reflex when the eye is in primary gaze. The examiner can determine levator muscle function by applying finger pressure on the brow to block the frontalis muscle and then measuring the distance that the upper eyelid moves when the patient shifts from downgaze to upgaze. Tear function and corneal sensitivity should be evaluated because exposure may occur after surgical repair. If the Bell phenomenon is poor, the cornea can decompensate after ptosis repair. The clinician should also determine whether the globe is microphthalmic or whether a hypotropia is present, as either of these conditions may produce pseudoptosis.

Correction of mild or moderate ptosis can usually be delayed until the patient is several years old, although a compensatory chin-up head posture may justify earlier surgery. Marked ptosis that obstructs vision must be corrected early in infancy to prevent deprivation amblyopia. Surgical techniques include external levator muscle resection, levator aponeurosis tuck, and frontalis suspension. When levator muscle function is less than 4 mm, frontalis suspension is usually performed. Materials for suspension include autologous fascia lata, human donor fascia lata, and synthetic material such as silicone rods. Autologous fascia cannot be obtained until the patient is 3 or 4 years old. Use of synthetic material or donor fascia lata may lead to higher recurrence rates.

Marcus Gunn Jaw-Winking Syndrome

Marcus Gunn jaw-winking syndrome (co-contractive retraction with jaw–eyelid synkinesis syndrome [CCRS], type 5) results from congenital synkinesis of the jaw and levator muscles. The ptotic eyelid elevates with opening of the mouth or movement of the jaw to the contralateral side. The clinician may test an infant for this condition by having the child suck on a bottle or pacifier. Treatment may involve simple ptosis repair or a combination of disinsertion of the levator muscle and frontalis suspension. Frontalis suspension may also be performed on the normal eyelid to achieve a more symmetric appearance.

Demirci H, Frueh BR, Nelson CC. Marcus Gunn jaw-winking synkinesis: clinical features and management. *Ophthalmology.* 2010;117(7):1447–1452.

Table 17-2 Eyelid Tumor Classification

Chalazion
Hordeolum
Benign epithelial and appendage tumors: syringoma, porosyringoma, myoepithelioma, apocrine
    hidrocystoma (sudiferous cyst; originating from a blocked excretory duct of Moll glands),
    eccrine hydrocystoma (derived from eyelid eccrine sweat gland), sebaceous cyst (pilar cyst;
    retention cyst of the pilosebaceous structure), milia (cystic expansion of the pilosebaceous
    structure due to obstruction of the orifice), epidermal inclusion cyst, pilomatricoma (calcifying
    epithelioma of Malherbe; a solid or cystic mass derived from hair matrix cells), conjunctival
    inclusion cyst
Papilloma
Molluscum contagiosum
Juvenile xanthogranuloma
Cutaneous horn
Rhabdomyosarcoma

Infectious and Inflammatory Eyelid Disorders

Inflammatory masses of the eyelids are much more common than neoplasms (Table 17-2). *Chalazia* are caused by blockage of the meibomian glands, and *hordeola* arise from blocked eccrine or apocrine glands. Treatment of both includes warm compresses and management of associated blepharitis; surgical treatment is reserved for large, painful, or chronic lesions. Pyogenic granuloma is a pedunculated, fleshy pink growth of granulation tissue that develops, sometimes rapidly and exuberantly, from the conjunctiva overlying a chalazion or site of trauma. Eyelid and epibulbar lesions can develop in juvenile xanthogranuloma (see Chapter 20).

Molluscum contagiosum may present on the eyelids with characteristic lesions and secondary follicular conjunctivitis (see Chapter 21).

Neoplasms and Other Noninfectious Eyelid Lesions

Malignant tumors arising from eyelid skin or conjunctiva (eg, basal cell carcinoma, squamous cell carcinoma, melanoma) are relatively common in adults, but they are extremely rare in children. These tumors are discussed elsewhere in the BCSC (see Section 4, *Ophthalmic Pathology and Intraocular Tumors;* Section 7, *Orbit, Eyelids, and Lacrimal System;* and Section 8, *External Disease and Cornea*). Pediatric cases are likely to be associated with underlying systemic disorders that predispose the patient to malignancy, such as basal cell nevus syndrome or xeroderma pigmentosum. In rare cases, rhabdomyosarcoma may present as an eyelid or conjunctival mass.

Benign lesions of the ocular surface and surrounding skin are common, and these may be classified as originating from epithelium, melanocytes, or vascular tissue.

Capillary Malformations

Port-wine stain (PWS; also referred to as *port-wine nevus, nevus flammeus*) is a congenital vascular malformation that manifests as a flat red or pink cutaneous lesion. It may lighten

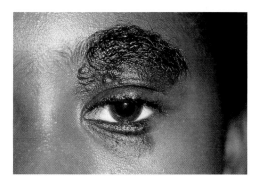

Figure 17-9 Congenital nevocellular nevus of the eyelid, present since birth. *(Courtesy of Amy Hutchinson, MD.)*

during the first year of life but then tends to become darker, thicker, and more nodular over time. PWS is associated with Sturge-Weber syndrome and Klippel-Trénaunay-Weber syndrome (see Chapter 28) and is seen in combination with ocular melanosis in phako-matosis pigmentovascularis. Glaucoma can occur in affected eyes and can be difficult to treat (see Chapter 22). Lasers can be used to decrease the skin pigmentation.

Congenital Nevocellular Nevi of the Skin

Congenital nevocellular nevi can occur on the eyelids; they may cause visual deprivation amblyopia or undergo malignant transformation (Fig 17-9). The risk of malignant trans-formation increases with the size of the lesion; large lesions (>20 cm) have a 5%–20% risk of malignant transformation. Observation is often recommended for small (<1.5 cm) and medium-sized (1.5–20.0 cm) lesions.

Other Acquired Eyelid Conditions

Trichotillomania

Trichotillomania is characterized by the pulling out of one's hair, frequently including the eyebrows and eyelashes. It may be associated with obsessive-compulsive disorder. The characteristic appearance includes madarosis, broken hairs, and regrowth of hairs of vary-ing lengths (see BCSC Section 7, *Orbit, Eyelids, and Lacrimal System*).

Excessive Blinking

Excessive blinking is common in children. Causes vary; they include anterior segment and eyelid abnormalities, psychogenic and stress-related factors, habit and motor tics, uncor-rected refractive errors, and strabismus. Isolated excessive blinking tends not to be associ-ated with vision-threatening or life-threatening disorders.

CHAPTER **18**

Orbital Disorders

Orbital anatomy is described in BCSC Section 2, *Fundamentals and Principles of Ophthalmology,* and Section 7, *Orbit, Eyelids, and Lacrimal System.* Many pediatric orbital disorders are also described in Section 7.

Abnormal Interocular Distance: Terminology and Associations

Hypertelorism, orbital Excessive distance between the medial orbital walls as a result of lateralization of the orbits. This diagnosis is made radiographically, not clinically. Hypertelorism occurs in more than 550 disorders.

Hypertelorism, ocular Excessive interpupillary distance when compared to standard nomograms; it implies orbital hypertelorism.

Hypotelorism Smaller than normal distance between the medial orbital walls, with reduced inner and outer canthal distances. The finding is associated with more than 60 syndromes. Hypotelorism can be the result of skull malformation or a failure in brain development.

Telecanthus Greater than normal distance between the medial canthi. This can be secondary to hypertelorism, or it can be a primary soft-tissue abnormality (see also Chapter 17).

Exorbitism Variously defined as prominent eyes due to shallow orbits or as an increased angle of divergence of the orbital walls.

Congenital and Developmental Disorders: Craniofacial Malformations

Craniosynostosis

Cranial sutures are present throughout the skull, which is divided into 2 parts, the *calvarium* and the *skull base,* via an imaginary line drawn from the supraorbital rims to the base of the occiput (Fig 18-1). *Craniosynostosis* is the premature closure of 1 or more cranial sutures during the embryonic period or early childhood. Bony growth of the skull occurs in osteoblastic centers located at the suture sites. Bone is laid down parallel and perpendicular to the direction of the suture. Premature suture closure prevents perpendicular growth but allows parallel growth. This growth pattern, called *Virchow's law,* results in

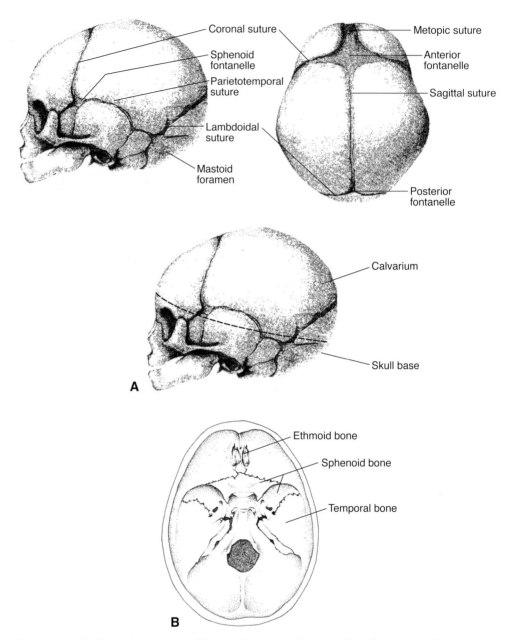

Figure 18-1 **A,** Normal sutures and fontanelles of the fetal skull. **B,** Adult cranial base, complete with sutures. *(Illustration by C. H. Wooley.)*

clinically recognizable cranial bone deformations (Fig 18-2). The following are important terms associated with craniosynostosis, in order of frequency of occurrence.

Plagiocephaly The term *plagiocephaly* literally means "oblique head." Most often plagiocephaly is deformational, the consequence of external compressive forces, occurring

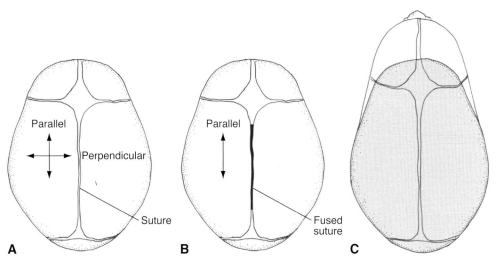

Figure 18-2　**A,** Normal sutures. Bone growth occurs at the suture, with bone laid down parallel and perpendicular to the direction of the suture. **B,** Virchow's law. Prematurely fused sutures allow bone growth only in the parallel direction; perpendicular growth is inhibited. **C,** An example of Virchow's law. Premature closure of the sagittal suture produces scaphocephaly (boatlike skull); the shaded area shows the normal skull shape. *(Illustration by C. H. Wooley.)*

prenatally or during infancy. Deformational plagiocephaly resulting from intrauterine constraint (eg, oligohydramnios) is characterized by ipsilateral occipital flattening with contralateral forehead flattening. However, this condition may also result from unilateral coronal suture synostosis. On the synostotic side, the forehead and supraorbital rim are retruded (depressed), the interpalpebral fissure is wider, and the orbit is often higher than on the nonsynostotic side. The nonsynostotic side displays a protruding or bulging forehead, a lower supraorbital rim, a narrower interpalpebral fissure, and frequently a lower orbital position (Fig 18-3).

Brachycephaly　"Short head"; specifically refers to growth in the anterior-posterior axis. Brachycephaly is frequently the result of bilateral closure of the coronal sutures. The forehead is most often wide and flat.

Scaphocephaly　"Boat head." Scaphocephaly usually results from premature closure of the sagittal suture; the skull is thus long in the anterior-posterior axis and narrow bitemporally.

Dolichocephaly　"Long head"; the skull shape is similar to that in scaphocephaly.

Kleeblattschädel　"Cloverleaf skull"; the skull shape is trilobar. Kleeblattschädel is typically the result of synostosis of the coronal, lambdoidal, and sagittal sutures.

Fusion of calvarial sutures affects cranial shape and orbital development. Fusion of the skull base sutures affects orbital development and facial development. In contrast to calvarial suture fusion, which causes varied cranial deformations, skull base suture fusion causes only *midface hypoplasia* (Fig 18-4), a constellation of abnormalities consisting of maxillary hypoplasia, beak-shaped nose, hypertelorism, shallow orbits with proptosis

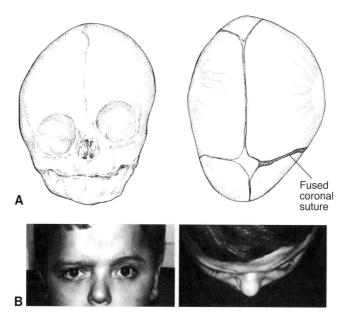

Figure 18-3 **A,** Fused coronal suture, with inhibition of perpendicular skull growth. **B,** Patient with left coronal synostosis. Note retruded left forehead, elevated brow, and wider interpalpebral fissure, with compensatory protrusion of the right forehead, lower brow, and narrowed interpalpebral fissure. *(Part A illustration by C. H. Wooley; part B courtesy of Jane Edmond, MD.)*

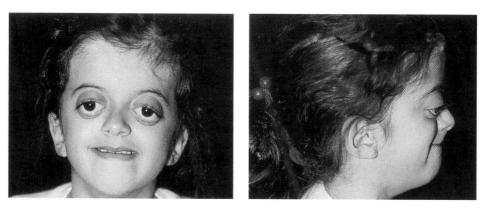

Figure 18-4 Crouzon syndrome. This patient evidences brachycephaly and "tower" skull with forehead retrusion, proptosis, inferior scleral show, and a small, beaklike nose. Also visible is the emerging midface hypoplasia. *(Reproduced with permission from Katowitz JA, ed.* Pediatric Oculoplastic Surgery. *New York: Springer; 2002:fig 31-23.)*

and lagophthalmos, high-arched palate, and a prominent-appearing jaw due to retruded maxilla.

Etiology of craniosynostosis

Early suture fusion can occur sporadically as an isolated abnormality (eg, sagittal suture synostosis and most cases of unilateral coronal suture synostosis), or it can be part of a genetic syndrome and thus associated with other abnormalities. Craniosynostosis syndromes are usually autosomal dominant conditions, often with associated limb abnormalities. Many of these syndromes have overlapping features, which makes accurate diagnosis based on clinical findings difficult. Identification of specific mutations may be diagnostic, as approximately 50% of patients with syndromic craniosynostosis are found to have mutations that result in increased calvarial cell differentiation and bone matrix formation.

Craniosynostosis syndromes

Common systemic features of the craniosynostosis syndromes include fusion of multiple calvarial sutures and skull base sutures. Syndactyly (partial fusion of the digits) and brachydactyly (short digits), ranging in severity, are hallmarks of these syndromes, with the exception of Crouzon syndrome.

Crouzon syndrome Crouzon syndrome is the most common autosomal dominant craniosynostosis syndrome. Over 30 mutations, all occurring in the *FGFR2* gene on chromosome 10, cause the Crouzon phenotype.

Calvarial bone synostosis often includes both coronal sutures, resulting in a broad, retruded forehead; brachycephaly; and tower-shaped skull. The skull base sutures are also involved, leading to varying degrees of midfacial retrusion. There is marked variability of the skull and facial features, with milder cases escaping diagnosis through multiple generations. Hypertelorism and proptosis, with inferior scleral show (lower eyelid below limbus), are the most frequent features of Crouzon syndrome (see Fig 18-4). Hydrocephalus is common, but intelligence is usually normal. Findings are usually limited to the head. The absence of hand and foot anomalies can aid the clinician in the diagnosis.

Apert syndrome Patients with Apert syndrome usually have multiple fused calvarial sutures, most often both coronal sutures, and skull base suture fusion. The skull shape and facial features of these patients resemble those of Crouzon patients, but Apert syndrome is associated with an often extreme amount of syndactyly (Fig 18-5), in which most or all digits of the hands and feet are completely fused *(mitten deformity)*. Apert syndrome is likely to be associated with internal organ malformations (cardiovascular and genitourinary) and mental deficiency. Hydrocephalus is less common in this syndrome than in Crouzon syndrome. The condition is autosomal dominant. Two mutations, both in the *FGFR2* gene on chromosome 10, account for most cases.

Pfeiffer syndrome Patients with Pfeiffer syndrome have craniofacial abnormalities resembling those of Apert patients but often have more severe craniosynostosis, resulting in a cloverleaf skull. There is a high risk of hydrocephalus. The syndactyly is much less severe, and patients have characteristic short, broad thumbs and toes. This syndrome is autosomal dominant and caused by mutations in the *FGFR1* or *FGFR2* gene.

Saethre-Chotzen syndrome The features of Saethre-Chotzen syndrome are much milder than those of other craniosynostosis syndromes; this syndrome is therefore underdiagnosed. Early suture fusion is not a constant feature but, when present, typically involves 1 coronal suture (plagiocephaly), resulting in an asymmetric face. Other common features are ptosis, low hairline, and ear abnormalities. Abnormalities of the hands and feet

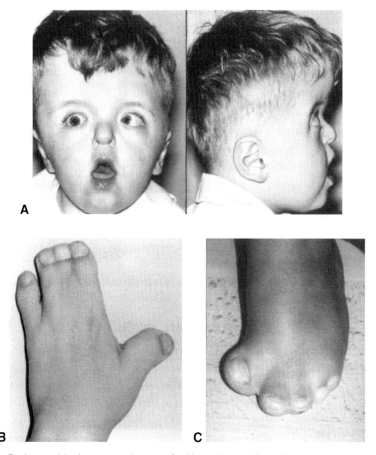

Figure 18-5 Patient with Apert syndrome. **A,** Note "tower" skull, brachycephaly, forehead and superior orbital rim retrusion, maxillary hypoplasia, beaklike nose with depression of nasal bridge, and trapezoid-shaped mouth (common in infancy in Apert syndrome). **B,** Extreme syndactyly of the digits; the thumb is spared but is broad and deviated. **C,** Syndactyly of the toes analogous to that of the hands. *(Part A reproduced with permission from Cohen MM Jr, Kreiborg S. A clinical study of the craniofacial features in Apert syndrome. Int J Oral Maxillofac Surg. 1996;25(1):45–53. Parts B and C reproduced with permission from Cohen MM Jr, Kreiborg S. Hands and feet in the Apert syndrome. Am J Med Genet. 1995;57(1):82–96.)*

include brachydactyly and mild syndactyly (Fig 18-6). Intelligence is usually normal. The condition is autosomal dominant and caused by mutations in the *TWIST* gene on chromosome 7.

Ocular complications of craniosynostosis

Proptosis Proptosis (or exorbitism) results from the reduced volume of the bony orbit. The severity of the proptosis in patients with craniosynostosis is not uniform and frequently increases with age because of the impaired growth of the bony orbit.

Corneal exposure Because the eyelids may not close completely over the proptotic globes, corneal exposure may occur secondary to inadequate blink and/or lagophthalmos, with possible development of exposure keratitis. Aggressive lubrication is necessary to prevent

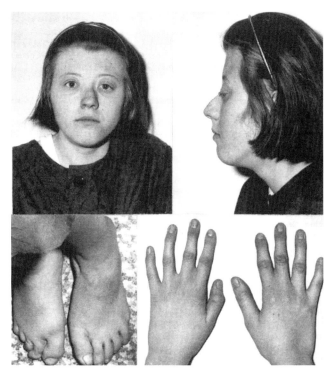

Figure 18-6   Patient with Saethre-Chotzen syndrome. Note the facial asymmetry, flat fore-head, low-set hairline, mild left ptosis, lateral deviation of the great toes, shortened toes, and partial syndactyly of fingers 2 and 3. *(Courtesy of the March of Dimes.)*

corneal drying. Tarsorrhaphy can decrease the exposure. Surgically expanding the orbital volume, thereby eliminating the proptosis, may be indicated in extreme cases.

Globe luxation   In patients with extremely shallow orbits, globe luxation may occur when the eyelids are manipulated or when there is increased pressure in the orbits, such as occurs with a Valsalva maneuver. The globe is luxated forward, the eyelids closing behind the equator of the globe. The condition is very painful and can cause corneal exposure. It may also compromise the blood supply to the globe, which is a medical emergency. Physicians and patients (or their caregivers) should quickly reposition the globe behind the eyelids. The best technique for doing this is to place a finger and thumb over the conjunctiva within the interpalpebral fissure and exert gentle but firm pressure; this technique does not damage the cornea. For recurrent luxation, the short-term solution is tarsorrhaphy; the long-term solution is orbital volume expansion.

Vision loss   Vision loss may occur in patients with craniofacial syndromes for a variety of reasons: corneal scarring from exposure, uncorrected refractive errors, and optic nerve compromise. Amblyopia is common and may be secondary to isoametropia, anisometropia, and strabismus, all of which occur more frequently in these patients. Most cases of vision loss can be prevented.

Strabismus Patients with craniosynostosis show a variety of horizontal deviations in primary position; exotropia is the most frequent. The most consistent finding, however, is a marked V pattern (see Chapter 10). This V pattern is often accompanied by a marked over-elevation in adduction, especially when 1 or both coronal sutures are synostosed, as occurs in unilateral coronal suture synostosis and Apert (Fig 18-7) and Crouzon syndromes. The apparent overaction (often pseudo-overaction) of the inferior oblique muscle on the side of the coronal suture fusion may be due to the following: orbital and globe extorsion, which converts the medial rectus muscle into an elevator when the eye is in adduction; superior oblique trochlear retrusion (because of superior orbital rim retrusion), which induces superior oblique underaction and secondary true inferior oblique overaction; anomalous extraocular muscle insertions or agenesis; or orbital pulley abnormalities (see Chapter 3).

Optic nerve abnormalities Because the synostosed cranial vault is unable to expand as the brain grows, the intracranial contents become crowded, elevating intracranial pressure (ICP). The risk of hindrance to brain growth is much greater when multiple sutures are fused. Elevated ICP can result in papilledema (discussed in Chapter 26), and chronic papilledema can lead to optic atrophy and subsequent vision loss. Optic atrophy may occur with or without antecedent papilledema. Hydrocephalus is another cause of elevated ICP and occurs in up to 40% of patients with Apert, Crouzon, and especially Pfeiffer syndromes. The severe midface retrusion that these conditions produce may cause breathing problems and sleep apnea. Idiopathic intracranial hypertension secondary to sleep apnea can also cause elevated ICP and papilledema. Because children with elevated ICP may not complain of a headache, young patients with multiple fused sutures should be examined yearly or biyearly.

Optic nerve edema and/or atrophy can also occur secondary to compression from optic nerve foramen synostosis. This is rare in patients with craniofacial syndromes but has been described.

Ocular adnexal abnormalities Common ocular adnexal abnormalities include orbital hypertelorism, telecanthus, abnormal slant of the palpebral fissures secondary to superior displacement of the medial canthi, ptosis, and nasolacrimal abnormalities such as duct obstruction and punctal anomalies. Epiphora is a common finding in patients with craniosynostosis and may be secondary to nasolacrimal duct obstruction, poor blink secondary to proptosis, obliquity of the palpebral fissures, or ocular irritation from corneal exposure.

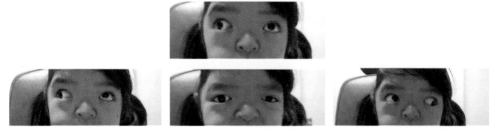

Figure 18-7 Patient with Apert syndrome. Note the good alignment in primary position with marked overelevation in adduction and exotropia in upgaze (V pattern). *(Courtesy of John Simon, MD.)*

Surgical management of craniosynostosis

Reconstructive surgery for severe craniofacial malformation is frequently extensive and involves en bloc movement of the facial structures. The status of the visual system should be documented preoperatively and monitored postoperatively, with appropriate treatment as indicated.

In many centers, a craniofacial team—composed of facial plastic surgeons, neurosurgeons, ophthalmologists, and oral surgeons—collaborates to determine the timing of the reconstructive surgery. Procedures that involve moving the orbits may significantly change the degree or type of strabismus, thereby influencing the choice of strabismus surgery. Because of this, deferring treatment of strabismus until craniofacial surgery is completed may be appropriate.

Nonsynostotic Craniofacial Conditions

Many craniofacial syndromes do not involve synostosis. A few of particular importance to the ophthalmologist are discussed in the following sections.

Anophthalmia

Anophthalmia (anophthalmos) is the absence of tissues of the eye. Anophthalmia is the most severe phenotypic expression of a spectrum of abnormalities that includes typical coloboma and microphthalmia (see Chapter 20). These conditions may be isolated, but they are frequently associated with other congenital anomalies. The genetic and environmental factors associated with these ocular abnormalities are complex and not fully defined. As with severe forms of microphthalmia, anophthalmia is associated with hypoplastic orbits and eyelids. Various techniques have been utilized for orbital expansion, and the best results are achieved with early treatment.

Branchial arch syndromes

Branchial arch syndromes are caused by disruptions in the embryonic development of the first 2 branchial arches, which are responsible for formation of the maxillary and mandibular bones, the ear, and facial musculature. The best known of these syndromes is the *oculoauriculovertebral spectrum (OAVS),* which includes hemifacial microsomia, Goldenhar syndrome, and Treacher Collins syndrome. There is no firm agreement about the nomenclature relating to this condition, but most believe that hemifacial microsomia is a forme fruste of OAVS. Patients with OAVS may have vertebral abnormalities such as hemivertebrae and vertebral hypoplasia. They may also have neurologic, cardiovascular, and genitourinary abnormalities. Most cases are sporadic, but there are rare familial cases.

Goldenhar syndrome Goldenhar syndrome is a more severe presentation of OAVS. Patients with Goldenhar syndrome have hemifacial microsoma (unilateral or bilateral), as well as characteristic ophthalmic abnormalities (Fig 18-8). Most cases are sporadic.

Epibulbar (limbal) dermoids and dermolipomas are characteristic ocular signs of Goldenhar syndrome. Dermolipomas (also termed *lipodermoids*) usually occur in the inferotemporal quadrant, covered by conjunctiva and often hidden by the lateral upper and lower eyelids. Epibulbar limbal dermoids are reported more frequently than dermolipomas and can be bilateral (approximately 25% of cases). They occasionally impinge

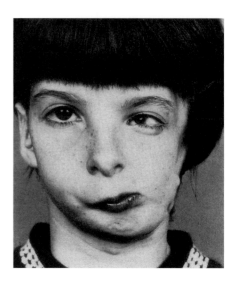

Figure 18-8 Goldenhar syndrome with hemifacial microsomia. Patient has facial asymmetry, a hypoplastic left ear (microtia), an ear tag near the right ear, epibulbar dermolipoma in the left eye, and esotropia. Patient also has Duane retraction syndrome, left eye.

on the visual axis but more commonly interfere with visual acuity by causing astigmatism and anisometropic amblyopia. Eyelid colobomas may occur. Other abnormalities include microphthalmia, cataract, and iris abnormalities. Duane retraction syndrome is more common in patients with Goldenhar syndrome than in the general population.

Treacher Collins syndrome Treacher Collins syndrome (mandibulofacial dysostosis) is due to abnormal growth and development of the first and second branchial arches, which give rise to underdevelopment and even agenesis of the zygoma and malar eminences. The cheeks and lateral orbital rims are depressed, and the palpebral fissures slant downward because of lateral canthal dystopia (Fig 18-9). Pseudocolobomas (and, uncommonly, true colobomas) are found in the outer third of the lower eyelids. Meibomian glands may be absent. The cilia of the lower eyelid may also be absent, medial to the pseudocoloboma. The ears are malformed and hearing loss is common. The mandible is typically hypoplastic, leading to micrognathia. Intelligence is normal. The syndrome is inherited in an autosomal dominant fashion and displays variable expression. Most affected patients have a mutation in the *TCOF1* gene.

Pierre Robin sequence

The Pierre Robin sequence (also *anomaly, deformity*) is characterized by respiratory problems, micrognathia, glossoptosis, and cleft palate. The sequence is a frequent finding in Stickler syndrome. Associated ocular anomalies include retinal detachment, microphthalmos, congenital glaucoma, cataracts, and high myopia.

Fetal alcohol syndrome

Fetal alcohol syndrome (FAS) is a craniofacial condition caused by in utero exposure to ethanol. It is characterized by prenatal and postnatal growth retardation, central nervous system and craniofacial abnormalities, and intellectual disability.

The classic ocular features of FAS are short palpebral fissures, telecanthus, epicanthus, ptosis, microphthalmos, and esotropia (Fig 18-10). Anterior segment dysgenesis, optic

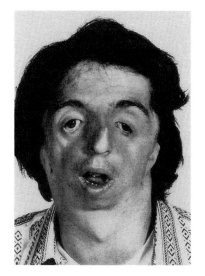

Figure 18-9 Treacher Collins syndrome (mandibulofacial dysostosis). Note downward slant of palpebral fissure, low-set abnormal ears, notch or curving of the inferotemporal eyelid margin, and maxillary and mandibular hypoplasia. *(Reproduced with permission from Peyman GA, Sanders DR, Goldberg MF. Principles and Practice of Ophthalmology. Philadelphia: Saunders; 1980:2411.)*

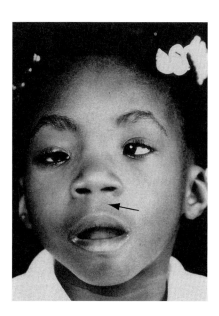

Figure 18-10 Fetal alcohol syndrome. Asymmetric ptosis; telecanthus; strabismus; long, flat philtrum *(arrow)*; anteverted nostrils. This child also had Peters anomaly, left eye, and myopia, right eye. *(Reproduced with permission from Miller MT, Israel J, Cuttone J. Fetal alcohol syndrome. J Pediatr Ophthalmol Strabismus. 1981;18(4):6–15.)*

nerve hypoplasia, and high refractive errors have been reported. Fifty percent of children with this underdiagnosed syndrome have some form of visual impairment.

Nonsynostotic disorders of bone growth

These conditions involve overgrowth of bone, thereby creating a risk of stenosis of the optic canal and resultant compressive optic neuropathy.

Infantile osteopetrosis This rare and severe form of osteopetrosis is associated with optic canal stenosis. Bone marrow transplant has been reported to reverse the stenosis. The condition is autosomal recessive.

Craniometaphyseal dysplasia Craniometaphyseal dysplasia is a rare disorder of osteoclast resorption that causes hyperostosis of the cranial bones. The typical facial appearance includes frontal and paranasal bossing. Progressive sclerosis of cranial nerve foramina can result in compressive optic neuropathy.

Infectious and Inflammatory Conditions

Preseptal and orbital cellulitis are usually more rapidly progressive and more severe in children than in adults. See also BCSC Section 7, *Orbit, Eyelids, and Lacrimal System.*

Preseptal Cellulitis

Preseptal cellulitis, a common infection in children, is an inflammatory process involving the tissues anterior to the orbital septum. Eyelid edema may extend into the eyebrow and forehead. The periorbital skin becomes taut and inflamed, and edema of the contralateral eyelids may appear. Proptosis is not a feature of preseptal cellulitis, and the globe remains noninflamed. Full ocular motility and absence of pain on eye movement help distinguish preseptal from orbital cellulitis.

Preseptal cellulitis typically develops from 1 of 3 causes. Posttraumatic cellulitis may develop following puncture, insect bite, or laceration of the eyelid skin. In these cases, organisms found on the skin, such as *Staphylococcus* or *Streptococcus* species, are most commonly responsible for the infection.

The second cause of preseptal cellulitis is severe conjunctivitis such as epidemic keratoconjunctivitis or methicillin-resistant *Staphylococcus aureus (MRSA)* conjunctivitis, or skin infection such as impetigo or herpes zoster.

The third mechanism for preseptal cellulitis is secondary to upper respiratory tract or sinus infection. *Streptococcus pneumoniae* and other streptococcal species, and *S aureus* are the most common causative organisms.

Children with nonsevere preseptal infections who are not systemically ill can be treated with oral antibiotics as outpatients. Broad-spectrum drugs effective against the most common pathogens, such as cephalosporins or ampicillin-clavulanic acid combination, are usually effective. Particularly with eyelid abscesses, clindamycin may be an appropriate choice because of the increasing prevalence of MRSA, which should also be considered in patients who do not improve with treatment. Eyelid abscesses may require urgent incision and drainage.

If the child is younger than 1 year or has signs of systemic illness such as sepsis or meningeal involvement, hospitalization—for appropriate cultures, imaging of the sinuses and orbits, and intravenous (IV) antibiotics—is appropriate. In newborns, dacryocystocele should be considered in the differential diagnosis (see Chapter 19).

Orbital Cellulitis

Orbital cellulitis is an infection of the orbit that involves the tissues posterior to the orbital septum. Orbital cellulitis is most commonly associated with ethmoid or frontal sinusitis. It can also occur following penetrating injuries of the orbit.

The etiologic agents most often responsible for orbital cellulitis vary with age. In general, children younger than 9 years have infections caused by a single aerobic pathogen. Children older than 9 years may have complex infections with multiple pathogens, both aerobic and anaerobic. *S aureus* and gram-negative bacilli are most common in the neonate. In older children and adults, *S aureus, Streptococcus pyogenes, S pneumoniae,* and various anaerobic species are common. Gram-negative organisms are found primarily in immunosuppressed patients.

Early signs and symptoms of orbital cellulitis include lethargy, fever, eyelid edema, rhinorrhea, headache, orbital pain, and tenderness on palpation. The nasal mucosa becomes hyperemic, with a purulent nasal discharge. Increased venous congestion may cause elevated intraocular pressure. Proptosis, chemosis, and limited ocular movement suggest orbital involvement.

The differential diagnosis of orbital cellulitis includes nonspecific orbital inflammation, benign orbital tumors such as lymphatic malformation and hemangioma, and malignant tumors such as rhabdomyosarcoma, leukemia, and metastases.

Paranasal sinusitis is the most common cause of bacterial orbital cellulitis (Fig 18-11). In children younger than 10 years, the ethmoid sinuses are most frequently involved. If orbital cellulitis is suspected, orbital imaging is indicated to confirm orbital involvement, to document the presence and extent of sinusitis and subperiosteal abscess (Fig 18-12), and to rule out a foreign body in a patient with a history of trauma.

It is crucial to distinguish orbital cellulitis from preseptal cellulitis because the former requires hospitalization and treatment with IV broad-spectrum antibiotics. Choice of IV

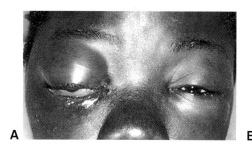 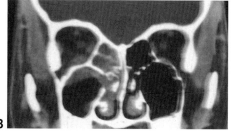

Figure 18-11 Bacterial orbital cellulitis with proptosis **(A)** secondary to sinusitis **(B).** *(Courtesy of Jane Edmond, MD.)*

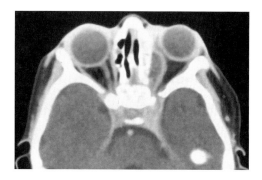

Figure 18-12 Axial computed tomography (CT) image showing a medial subperiosteal abscess of the left orbit associated with ethmoid sinusitis. *(Courtesy of Jane Edmond, MD.)*

antibiotic is based on the most likely pathogens until results from cultures are known. If associated sinusitis or subperiosteal abscess is present, pediatric otolaryngologists should be consulted. The patient should be observed closely for signs of visual compromise. Many subperiosteal abscesses in children younger than 9 years will resolve with medical management. Emergency drainage of a subperiosteal abscess is indicated for a patient of any age with *either* of the following:

- evidence of optic nerve compromise (decreasing vision, relative afferent pupillary defect) and an enlarging subperiosteal abscess
- an abscess that does not resolve within 48–72 hours of administration of antibiotics

Intraconal orbital abscesses are much less common than subperiosteal abscesses in children and require urgent surgical drainage.

Complications of orbital cellulitis include cavernous sinus thrombosis and intracranial extension (subdural or brain abscesses, meningitis, periosteal abscess), which may result in death. Cavernous sinus thrombosis can be difficult to distinguish from simple orbital cellulitis. Paralysis of eye movement in cavernous sinus thrombosis is often out of proportion to the degree of proptosis. Pain on motion and tenderness on palpation are absent. Decreased sensation along the maxillary division of cranial nerve V (trigeminal) supports the diagnosis. Bilateral involvement is virtually diagnostic of cavernous sinus thrombosis.

Other complications of orbital cellulitis include corneal exposure with secondary ulcerative keratitis, neurotrophic keratitis, secondary glaucoma, septic uveitis or retinitis, exudative retinal detachment, optic nerve edema, inflammatory neuritis, infectious neuritis, central retinal artery occlusion, and panophthalmitis.

Related conditions

Maxillary osteomyelitis is a rare condition of early infancy. Infection spreads from the nose into the tooth buds, with unilateral erythema and edema of the eyelids, cheek, and nose. Infection may spread and cause orbital cellulitis.

Fungal orbital cellulitis (mucormycosis) occurs most frequently in patients with ketoacidosis or severe immunosuppression. The infection causes thrombosing vasculitis with ischemic necrosis of involved tissue (Fig 18-13). Cranial nerves often are involved, and extension into the central nervous system is common. Smears and biopsy of the involved tissues reveal the fungal organisms. Treatment includes debridement and administration of amphotericin. *Allergic fungal sinusitis* is a less fulminant condition that frequently presents with orbital signs, including proptosis from remodeling of the bony orbit. See BCSC Section 7, *Orbit, Eyelids, and Lacrimal System*, for further discussion.

Childhood Orbital Inflammation

Several noninfectious, nontraumatic disorders cause orbital inflammation in children that may simulate infection or an orbital mass lesion; they deserve brief mention. Thyroid eye disease, the most common cause of proptosis in adults, rarely occurs in prepubescent children but occasionally affects adolescents (Fig 18-14). Bilateral orbital inflammation may occur with sarcoidosis.

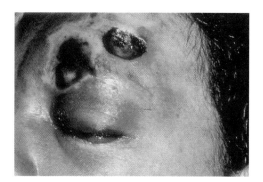

Figure 18-13 Mucormycosis, left orbit.

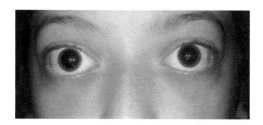

Figure 18-14 Thyroid eye disease with bilateral exophthalmos in a 15-year-old girl.

Nonspecific orbital inflammation

Nonspecific orbital inflammation (NSOI) *(orbital pseudotumor; idiopathic orbital inflammatory syndrome)* is an inflammatory cause of proptosis in childhood that differs significantly from the adult form. The typical pediatric presentation is acute and painful, more closely resembling orbital cellulitis than tumor or thyroid eye disease (Fig 18-15). NSOI is often bilateral and may be associated with systemic manifestations such as headache, nausea, vomiting, and lethargy. Uveitis is frequently present and occasionally constitutes the dominant manifestation. Imaging studies may show increased density of orbital fat, thickening of posterior sclera and the Tenon layer, or enlargement of extraocular muscles. The lacrimal gland is often involved. Sinusitis is typically not present. Treatment with a systemic corticosteroid usually provides prompt and dramatic relief, but recurrent disease is common. A slow tapering of corticosteroid dosage is usually required to prevent recurrence.

Belanger C, Zhang KS, Reddy AK, Yen MT, Yen KG. Inflammatory disorders of the orbit in childhood: a case series. *Am J Ophthalmol.* 2010;150(4):460–463.

Orbital myositis Orbital myositis describes NSOI that is confined to 1 or more extraocular muscles. The clinical presentation depends on the amount of inflammation. Diplopia, conjunctival chemosis, and orbital pain are common. Symptoms can be subacute for weeks or can progress rapidly. Vision is rarely impaired unless massive muscle enlargement is present. Imaging studies show diffusely enlarged muscles with the enlargement extending all the way to the insertion (unlike in thyroid myopathy, which mainly involves the muscle belly). Corticosteroid treatment usually produces rapid relief of symptoms; however, prolonged treatment is often necessary, and recurrence is common.

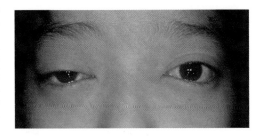

Figure 18-15 Bilateral nonspecific orbital inflammation (orbital pseudotumor) in an 11-year-old boy with a 1-week history of eye pain. Ocular rotation was markedly limited in all directions. CT confirmed proptosis and showed enlargement of all extraocular muscles. Laboratory workup was negative for thyroid disease and rheumatologic disorders. Complete resolution occurred after 1 month of corticosteroid treatment.

Neoplasms

Several of the most important pediatric malignancies show a predilection for orbital involvement. Benign adnexal masses are common and, in many cases, may threaten vision.

Differential Diagnosis

Diagnosis of space-occupying lesions in the orbit is particularly challenging because the clinical manifestations are both nonspecific and relatively limited:

- proptosis or other displacement of the globe
- swelling or discoloration of the eyelids
- palpable subcutaneous mass
- ptosis
- strabismus

The problem of differential diagnosis in childhood is compounded by the fact that many different orbital processes may cause rapid onset of symptoms. These include trauma, which may occur without a reliable history. Also, mild or moderate proptosis can be difficult to detect in an uncooperative child with associated eyelid swelling.

Nevertheless, typical presentations of the more common benign orbital and periorbital masses in infants and children (eg, hemangioma and dermoid cyst; discussed later) are sufficiently distinctive to permit confident clinical diagnosis in most cases. A malignant process should be suspected when proptosis and eyelid swelling suggestive of cellulitis are not accompanied by warmth of the overlying skin or when periorbital ecchymosis or hematoma develops in the absence of an unequivocal history of trauma. Pseudoproptosis can result when the volume of the globe exceeds the capacity of the orbit. Examples include the elongation of the eyeball from primary congenital glaucoma or high myopia.

The current widespread availability of high-quality imaging permits orbital masses to be differentiated noninvasively in many cases. Because of increasing concerns about the radiation risks associated with CT scans in children, MRI is becoming the preferred approach for orbital imaging in this patient group. CT, however, is superior at detecting disturbances of bone architecture. Ultrasonography may also provide useful diagnostic information.

Definitive diagnosis still often requires biopsy. A pediatric oncologist should be consulted when appropriate, and a metastatic workup should be considered before resorting to orbital surgery, because other, more easily accessible sites can sometimes be used as tissue sources.

Primary Malignant Neoplasms

Malignant diseases of the orbit include primary and metastatic tumors. Most primary malignant tumors of the orbit in childhood are sarcomas. Tumors of epithelial origin are extremely rare.

Rhabdomyosarcoma

The most common primary orbital malignant tumor in children is rhabdomyosarcoma, which is thought to originate from undifferentiated mesenchymal cells. The incidence of this disease (which is found in approximately 5% of pediatric orbital biopsies) exceeds that of all other sarcomas combined. The orbit is the origin of 10% of rhabdomyosarcomas; 25% of these tumors arise elsewhere in the head and neck, occasionally involving the orbit secondarily. The average age of onset is 5–7 years, but it can occur at any age. Rhabdomyosarcoma in infancy is more aggressive and carries a poorer prognosis.

Although ocular rhabdomyosarcoma usually originates in the orbit, it occasionally arises in the conjunctiva, eyelid, or anterior uveal tract. Patients generally present with proptosis (80%–100%), globe displacement (80%), blepharoptosis (30%–50%), conjunctival and eyelid swelling (60%), palpable mass (25%), and pain (10%) (Fig 18-16). Onset of symptoms and signs is usually rapid. Acute, rapidly progressive proptosis with an absence of pain should raise a high suspicion of orbital rhabdomyosarcoma. Imaging shows an irregular but well-circumscribed mass of uniform density.

A biopsy is required for confirmation of the diagnosis whenever rhabdomyosarcoma is suspected. The most common histopathologic type is embryonal, which shows few cells containing characteristic cross-striations. Second in frequency is the prognostically unfavorable alveolar pattern, showing poorly differentiated tumor cells compartmentalized by orderly connective tissue septa. Botryoid (grapelike), or well-differentiated pleomorphic tumors, are rarely found in the orbit but may originate in the conjunctiva.

Small encapsulated or otherwise well-localized rhabdomyosarcomas should be totally excised when possible. Usually, chemotherapy and radiation are used in conjunction with surgery. Exenteration of the orbit is seldom indicated.

Much of the current information on diagnosis and treatment of rhabdomyosarcoma has been obtained through the collaborative endeavors of the Intergroup Rhabdomyosarcoma Study Group (IRSG). A staging classification of rhabdomyosarcoma is employed by the IRSG. In brief, Group I is defined as localized disease that is completely resected; Group II is microscopic disease remaining after biopsy; Group III is gross disease remaining after biopsy; and Group IV is distant metastasis present at onset. This classification can help the clinician in selecting treatment and in establishing a prognosis. Primary orbital rhabdomyosarcoma has a relatively good prognosis. The 5-year

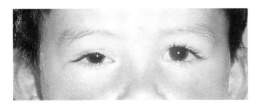

Figure 18-16 Rhabdomyosarcoma in a 4-year-old boy presenting with right upper eyelid ptosis of 3 weeks' duration and a palpable subcutaneous mass.

survival rates are 74% and 94% for patients with alveolar cell type and those with embryonal cell type, respectively.

Other sarcomas

Osteosarcoma, chondrosarcoma, and fibrosarcoma can also develop in the orbit during childhood. The risk of sarcoma is increased in children with a history of heritable retinoblastoma, particularly when external-beam radiation treatment has been given.

Metastatic Tumors

The orbit is the most common site of ocular metastasis in children, in contrast to adults, in whom the uvea is the most frequent site.

Neuroblastoma

Neuroblastoma is the most frequent source of orbital metastasis in childhood. This disorder is discussed in Chapter 28.

Ewing sarcoma

Ewing sarcoma is composed of small round cells and usually originates in the long bones of the extremities or in the axial skeleton. Among solid tumors, Ewing sarcoma is the second most frequent source of orbital metastasis. Contemporary treatment regimens involving surgery, radiation, and chemotherapy permit long-term survival in many patients with disseminated disease.

Hematopoietic, Lymphoproliferative, and Histiocytic Neoplasms

Leukemia

Leukemic infiltration of the orbit is relatively uncommon and more characteristic of acute myelogenous leukemia. Orbital involvement may be difficult to distinguish from bacterial or fungal orbital cellulitis. Orbital infiltration can cause proptosis, eyelid swelling, and ecchymosis. It may be best managed by radiation therapy. *Granulocytic sarcoma,* or *chloroma* (in reference to the greenish color of involved tissue), is a localized accumulation of myeloid leukemic cells in the orbit. This lesion may develop several months before leukemia becomes hematologically evident. Leukemia is discussed in Chapter 28.

Lymphoma

In contrast with adult disease, lymphoma in children very rarely involves the orbit. Burkitt lymphoma, endemic to East Africa and uncommon in North America, is the most likely form to involve the orbit.

Langerhans cell histiocytosis

Langerhans cell histiocytosis (*LCH;* formerly called *histiocytosis X*) is the collective term for a group of disorders, usually arising in childhood, that involve abnormal proliferation of histiocytes, often within bone. The disorders are classified as unifocal eosinophilic granuloma of the bone, multifocal eosinophilic granuloma of the bone, and diffuse soft-tissue histiocytosis.

Unifocal eosinophilic granuloma, the most localized and benign form of LCH, produces a bone lesion that involves the orbit, skull, ribs, or long bones in childhood or adolescence. Symptoms may include proptosis, ptosis, and periorbital swelling; localized pain and tenderness are relatively common. CT characteristically shows sharply demarcated osteolytic lesions without surrounding sclerosis (Fig 18-17). Treatment consists of observation of isolated asymptomatic lesions, excision or curettage, systemic or intralesional corticosteroid administration, or low-dose radiation therapy; all modalities have a high rate of success.

Multifocal eosinophilic granuloma of the bone is a disseminated and aggressive form of LCH. It usually presents between 2 and 5 years of age and may produce proptosis from involvement of the bony orbit. Diabetes insipidus is common. Chemotherapy is often required, but the prognosis is generally good.

Diffuse soft-tissue histiocytosis is the most severe form, usually affecting infants younger than 2 years. It is characterized by soft-tissue lesions of multiple viscera (liver, spleen) but rarely involves the eye.

Herwig MC, Wojno T, Zhang Q, Grossniklaus HE. Langerhans cell histiocytosis of the orbit: five clinicopathologic cases and review of the literature. *Surv Ophthalmol.* 2013;58(4):330–340.

Benign Tumors

Vascular lesions: hemangiomas

Advances in the biological characterization of vascular lesions have led to a revision of their classification. The current classification of vascular lesions establishes clear clinical, histologic, and prognostic differences between hemangiomas and vascular malformations. The older terms *capillary* and *strawberry hemangioma* should be replaced by the single term *hemangioma.* Cavernous hemangiomas, port-wine stains, and lymphangiomas all should be classified as "malformations." This nomenclature has been incorporated into the medical literature but has not been used consistently in the ophthalmic literature.

Hemangiomas are hamartomatous growths composed of proliferating capillary endothelial cells. They grow rapidly in early infancy, with a subsequent period of regression and involution. Periocular hemangiomas can be classified as follows:

- preseptal, involving the skin and preseptal orbit
- intraorbital, involving the postseptal orbit
- compound/mixed, involving the preseptal and postseptal orbit

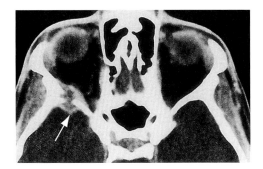

Figure 18-17 Axial CT image showing unifocal eosinophilic granuloma with partial destruction of the right posterior lateral orbital wall *(arrow)* in a 15-year-old boy, who presented with retrobulbar pain and mild edema and erythema of the right upper eyelid.

Hemangiomas occur in 1%–3% of term newborns and are more common in premature infants, in females, and after chorionic villus sampling. Most hemangiomas are clinically insignificant at birth; they can be inapparent or can appear as an erythematous macule or a telangiectasia. The natural history is one of rapid proliferation and growth over the first several months of life, rarely lasting beyond 1 year. During this phase, the lesion may ulcerate, hemorrhage, or cause amblyopia by inducing astigmatism or obstructing the visual axis. After the first year of life, the lesion usually begins to regress, although the rate and degree of involution vary.

Systemic disease associated with hemangiomas *PHACE* is an acronym for *p*osterior fossa malformations, *h*emangiomas, *a*rterial lesions, and *c*ardiac and *e*ye anomalies. The eye abnormalities include increased retinal vascularity, microphthalmia, optic nerve hypoplasia, exophthalmos, choroidal hemangiomas, strabismus, colobomas, cataracts, and glaucoma. The PHACE syndrome should be considered in any infant presenting with a large, segmental, plaquelike facial hemangioma involving 1 or more dermatomes (Fig 18-18).

Kasabach-Merritt syndrome is a thrombocytopenic coagulopathy with a high mortality rate. It is caused by sequestration of platelets within a vascular lesion.

Diffuse neonatal hemangiomatosis is a potentially lethal condition that occurs in infants, with multiple small cutaneous hemangiomas associated with visceral lesions affecting the liver, gastrointestinal tract, and brain. These hemangiomas are initially asymptomatic but can lead to cardiac failure and death within weeks. Infants with more than 3 cutaneous lesions should be evaluated for visceral lesions.

Treatment of hemangiomas The diagnosis of hemangiomas is usually clear from the clinical presentation. If not, MRI or Doppler ultrasonography may be helpful in establishing the diagnosis and delineating the posterior extent of the lesion.

Observation is indicated when hemangiomas are small and there is no risk of amblyopia from either obstruction of the visual axis or induced astigmatism.

Propranolol induces involution of most hemangiomas. Since its use was first reported in 2008, propranolol has rapidly become the treatment of choice for most cases requiring therapy. Risks of treatment with systemic β-blockers in infants include bradycardia,

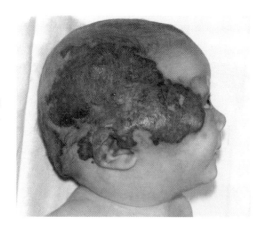

Figure 18-18 Plaque hemangioma in a child with PHACE syndrome. *(Courtesy of Ken K. Nischal, MD.)*

hypotension, hypoglycemia, and bronchospasm. Particular caution should be taken when propranolol is used in children with PHACE syndrome, because this drug may increase their risk of stroke. Timolol maleate solution applied topically has also shown efficacy in treating superficial hemangiomas.

Corticosteroids (including topical, intralesional, or systemic administration) were previously employed as the primary treatment of hemangioma but are now used infrequently because of the potential complications associated with any form of this treatment and because of the efficacy of propranolol. Interferon alfa-2a and vincristine may be used in severe cases. Pulsed-dye laser can treat superficial hemangiomas with few complications, but it has little effect on deeper components of the tumor.

Surgical excision of periocular hemangiomas is feasible for some well-localized lesions (Fig 18-19). In other cases, surgery may be used as a reconstructive tool after medical treatment.

Drolet BA, Frommelt PC, Chamlin SL, et al. Initiation and use of propranolol for infantile hemangioma: report of a consensus conference. *Pediatrics.* 2013;131(1):128–140. Epub 2012 Dec 24.

Léauté-Labrèze C, Dumas de la Roque E, Hubiche T, Boralevi F, Thambo JB, Taïeb A. Propranolol for severe hemangiomas of infancy. *N Engl J Med.* 2008;358(24):2649–2651.

Ni N, Langer P, Wagner R, Guo S. Topical timolol for periocular hemangioma: report of further study. *Arch Ophthalmol.* 2011;129(3):377–379.

Vascular lesions: malformations

Vascular malformations are developmental anomalies derived from capillary venous, arterial, or lymphatic vessels. In contrast to hemangiomas, vascular malformations remain relatively static, with growth correlating to growth of the child. The age and mode of clinical presentation vary, but in general, vascular malformations manifest later in life, although cutaneous vascular malformations such as port-wine stains are evident from birth.

Orbital lymphatic malformation Orbital lymphatic malformation (LM), also known as *lymphangioma,* may produce proptosis at birth or, more commonly, in the second or third decade of life. LM of the orbit is best managed conservatively. Exacerbations tend to

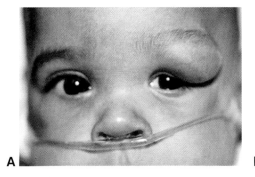
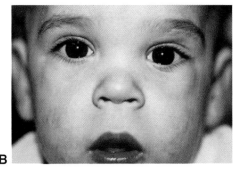

A **B**

Figure 18-19 **A,** Five-month-old boy with well-circumscribed hemangioma in left upper eyelid. Preoperative refraction was –6.00 +8.00 × 40°. **B,** Six months after the lesion was surgically excised, the induced astigmatism resolved and refraction was –0.25 +0.25 × 80°. *(Courtesy of David A. Plager, MD.)*

occur during upper respiratory tract infections and may be managed with short-course systemic corticosteroids. Rapid expansion may be seen in cases of intralesional hemorrhage (Fig 18-20). In these cases, partial resection and drainage may be required in order to manage acute orbital symptoms and compressive optic neuropathy. Because of the infiltrative character of this malformation, complete removal is usually impossible. Intralesional injection of a sclerosing agent has been used in some cases.

Orbital venous malformations Orbital venous malformations, or varices, can be divided into primary and secondary types. The primary type is confined to the orbit and has no association with arteriovenous malformations (AVMs). Secondary orbital varices occur as a result of intracranial AVM shunts that cause the orbital veins to dilate. Orbital venous malformations usually become symptomatic after years of progressive congestion and rarely manifest before the second decade of life. Treatment is reserved for highly symptomatic lesions.

Orbital arteriovenous malformations AVMs isolated to the orbit are extremely rare. Patients with congenital AVMs of the retina and midbrain, a condition known as *Wyburn-Mason syndrome* (see Chapter 28), may have orbital involvement. AVMs of the bony orbit rarely manifest in childhood but when present are characterized by pulsatile exophthalmos, chemosis, congested conjunctival vessels, and elevated intraocular pressure. AVMs may be treated by embolization, surgical resection, or both.

Other vascular tumors

Other orbital tumors composed of vascular elements are rare in childhood. *Hemangiopericytoma* is a benign tumor of pericytes that manifests as slowly progressive proptosis of the globe and has the potential for malignant transformation. Port-wine stains are discussed in Chapter 17.

Tumors of bony origin

During the early years of life, a variety of uncommon benign orbital tumors of bony origin can present with gradually increasing proptosis. *Fibrous dysplasia* and *juvenile ossifying fibroma* are similar disorders in which normal bone is replaced by fibro-osseous tissue. In both conditions, orbital CT shows varying degrees of lucency and sclerosis.

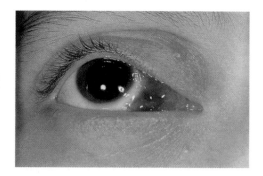

Figure 18-20 Lymphatic malformation with hemorrhage involving the right orbit, upper eyelid, and conjunctiva in a 15-year-old girl.

Fibrous dysplasia has a slow progression that ceases when skeletal maturation is complete. The most serious complication is vision loss caused by optic nerve compression, which may occur acutely. Periodic assessment of vision, pupil function, and optic disc appearance is indicated. Surgical treatment is indicated for functional deterioration or disfigurement.

Juvenile ossifying fibroma is distinguished histologically by the presence of osteoblasts. It tends to be more locally invasive than fibrous dysplasia; some authorities recommend early excision.

Brown tumor of bone is an osteoclastic giant cell reaction resulting from hyperparathyroidism. *Aneurysmal bone cyst* is a degenerative process in which normal bone is replaced by cystic cavities containing fibrous tissue, inflammatory cells, and blood, producing a characteristic radiographic appearance.

Tumors of connective tissue origin

Benign orbital tumors originating from connective tissue are rare in childhood. *Juvenile fibromatosis* may present as a mass in the inferoanterior portion of the orbit. These tumors, sometimes called *myofibromas* or *desmoid tumors,* are composed of relatively mature fibroblasts. They tend to recur locally after excision and can be difficult to control, but they do not metastasize.

Tumors of neural origin

Optic pathway glioma is the most important orbital tumor of neural origin in childhood. Optic pathway gliomas are usually low-grade astrocytomas, but the rate of growth with or without therapeutic intervention is unpredictable. Management of these tumors is thus controversial and depends largely on their location. Approximately 30% of optic pathway gliomas are associated with neurofibromatosis type 1. *Plexiform neurofibroma* nearly always occurs in the context of neurofibromatosis and frequently involves the eyelid and orbit. These tumors are discussed in Chapter 28. Orbital *meningioma* and *schwannoma* (neurilemoma, neurinoma) are rare before adulthood.

Ectopic Tissue Masses

The term *choristoma* is applied to growths consisting of normal cells and tissues appearing at an abnormal location. The growths may result from abnormal sequestration of germ layer tissue during embryonic development or from faulty differentiation of pluripotential cells. Masses composed of such ectopic tissue growing in the orbit can also be a consequence of herniation of tissue from adjacent structures.

Cystic Lesions

Dermoid and epidermoid cysts

Dermoid cysts are the most common space-occupying orbital lesions of childhood. They are benign developmental choristomas that arise from primitive dermal and epidermal elements sequestered in fetal suture lines at the time of closure. The tissue forms a cyst lined with keratinized epithelium and dermal appendages, including hair follicles, sweat glands, and sebaceous glands. Cysts containing squamous epithelium without dermal appendages are called *epidermoid cysts.*

Orbital dermoid cysts in childhood most commonly arise in the superotemporal and superonasal quadrants (Fig 18-21) but sometimes extend into the bony suture line. Clinically, they present as painless, smooth masses that are mobile and unattached to overlying skin. Episodes of inflammation may occur with small ruptures of the cyst wall and consequent extrusion of cyst contents. Most patients have no visual symptoms. Clinical examination is often sufficient for diagnosis. In some cases, imaging is indicated to identify and delineate the extent of the cyst. Imaging reveals a well-circumscribed lesion with a low-density lumen and often bony remodeling (Fig 18-22).

Management of dermoid cysts is surgical. Early excision can eliminate the risk of traumatic rupture and subsequent inflammation. An infrabrow or eyelid crease incision is used, and the cyst is carefully dissected. If possible, rupture of the cyst at the time of surgery is avoided to limit lipogranulomatous inflammation and scarring. If the cyst is entered, the intraluminal material should be thoroughly removed. Sutural cysts often cannot be removed intact because of their extension into or through bone. To limit the possibility of recurrence, the surgeon must attempt removal of all remaining cyst lining.

Microphthalmia with cyst

Also known as *colobomatous cyst,* microphthalmia with cyst is composed of tissues that originate from the eye wall of a malformed globe with posterior segment coloboma. Most fundus colobomas show some degree of scleral ectasia. In extreme cases, a bulging

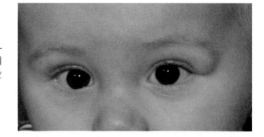

Figure 18-21 Eight-month-old boy with periorbital dermoid cyst, left eye, with typical superotemporal location. *(Courtesy of Robert W. Hered, MD.)*

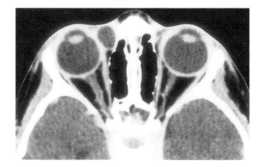

Figure 18-22 Axial CT image showing a dermoid cyst of the superonasal anterior orbit, right eye, in a 6-year-old boy.

globular appendage grows to become as large as or larger than the globe itself, which is invariably microphthalmic, sometimes to a marked degree.

Microphthalmia with cyst may occur either as an isolated congenital defect or in association with a variety of intracranial or systemic anomalies. Frequently, the fellow eye shows evidence of coloboma as well. The usual location of the cyst is inferior or posterior to the globe, with which the cyst is always in contact. The cyst communicates with the vitreous cavity, sometimes through a channel so small it is undetectable even with high-resolution imaging.

Whether posteriorly located cysts cause proptosis depends on the size of the globe and the cyst. Inferiorly located cysts present as a bulging of the lower eyelid or a bluish subconjunctival mass (Fig 18-23). If fundus examination does not make the diagnosis obvious, orbital imaging may reveal a cystic lesion that is attached to the globe and has the uniform internal density of vitreous. The goal of treatment is to promote normal growth of the orbit. A variety of methods are used, including aspiration of the cyst, surgical excision of the cyst, and use of orbital expanders and conformers.

Mucocele

Mucoceles are cystic lesions that originate from obstructed paranasal sinus drainage. They may expand over time, potentially causing destruction of bone and eroding into the orbit or intracranial space. These lesions most commonly arise from the frontal or anterior ethmoid sinuses, resulting in inferior or medial displacement of the globe. The differential diagnosis includes encephalocele with skull base deformity. Treatment involves reestablishing normal sinus drainage and removing the cyst wall.

Encephalocele and meningocele

Encephaloceles and meningoceles in the orbital region may result from a congenital bony defect that permits herniation of intracranial tissue, or they may develop after trauma that disrupts the bone and dura mater of the anterior cranial fossa. An intraorbital location leads to proptosis or downward displacement of the globe. Anterior presentation takes the

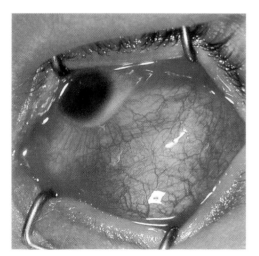

Figure 18-23 Microphthalmia with cyst (colobomatous cyst), left eye.

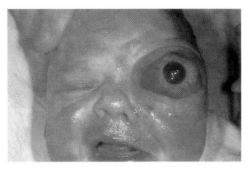

Figure 18-24 Congenital cystic teratoma originating in the left orbit of a 1-day-old girl.

form of a subcutaneous mass that can be misdiagnosed as a dacryocystocele. However, encephaloceles and meningoceles are typically located above the medial canthal tendon; dacryocystoceles are typically located below it (see Chapter 19). Pulsation of the globe or the mass from the transmission of intracranial pulse pressure is characteristic. Neuroimaging readily confirms the diagnosis.

Teratoma

Choristomatous tumors that contain multiple tissues derived from all 3 germinal layers (ectoderm, mesoderm, and endoderm) are referred to as *teratomas*. Most teratomas are partially cystic, with varying fluid content. Orbital teratomas account for a very small fraction of both orbital tumors and teratomas in general. The clinical presentation of orbital teratomas is particularly dramatic, with massive proptosis evident at birth (Fig 18-24). In contrast with teratomas in other locations, which tend to show malignant growth, most orbital lesions are benign. Surgical excision, facilitated by prior aspiration of fluid, can often be accomplished without sacrificing the globe. Permanent optic nerve damage from stretching and compression usually results in poor vision in the involved eye.

Ectopic Lacrimal Gland

These are rare choristomatous lesions that may present with proptosis in childhood. Cystic enlargement and chronic inflammation sometimes aggravate the condition.

CHAPTER 19

Lacrimal Drainage System Abnormalities

Disorders of the lacrimal system, particularly nasolacrimal duct obstruction (NLDO), are among the most common problems encountered in pediatric ophthalmology. Symptoms of NLDO, most of which resolve spontaneously, develop in approximately 5% of infants. The pertinent anatomical features of the lacrimal drainage system and their development are discussed in BCSC Section 2, *Fundamentals and Principles of Ophthalmology,* and Section 7, *Orbit, Eyelids, and Lacrimal System.*

One point about the evaluation of children with suspected lacrimal drainage system abnormalities deserves emphasis. While lacrimal obstruction occurs most often in patients aged 0–12 months, the presence of excessive tearing in such patients should always prompt the clinician to consider primary congenital (infantile) glaucoma. Tearing in an infant can be an important sign of this condition. Other signs and symptoms of glaucoma are photophobia, corneal clouding with or without enlargement, and breaks in Descemet membrane (see Chapter 22).

Congenital and Developmental Anomalies

Atresia of the Lacrimal Puncta or Canaliculi

Atresia of the lacrimal puncta or canaliculi refers to failure of canalization during development of the upper lacrimal system structures. Patients usually present with overflow of clear tears; there is no infection because bacteria cannot reach the lacrimal sac to produce one. If a patient with atresia of either the upper or lower canaliculus has symptoms that include mucopurulent discharge, this usually indicates concomitant obstruction of the distal NLD, with reflux of discharge through the normal canaliculus.

There are 2 main causes of upper lacrimal system obstruction. One is a thin membrane that obstructs the lacrimal puncta. The puncta otherwise appear normal. Simple puncture of the membrane with a punctal dilator eliminates this obstruction. For concomitant obstruction of the distal NLD, probing of the distal system is necessary. The second cause of upper lacrimal system obstruction is atresia of the puncta and canaliculi. In these patients, no puncta can be seen (Fig 19-1). If only 1 of the canaliculi is atretic and

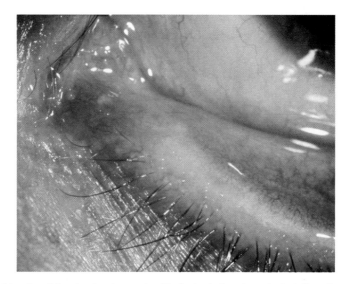

Figure 19-1 Atresia of the lacrimal puncta. No indentation is noted at the site of the normal punctal opening. *(Reproduced with permission from Lueder GT. Neonatal lacrimal system anomalies. Semin Ophthalmol. 1997;12(2):109.)*

there is mucopurulent discharge, probing of the distal duct through the patent canaliculus may be curative. If both the upper and lower canaliculi are absent, an incision through the eyelid margin at the expected location of the canaliculi may reveal structures that can be cannulated. However, many patients ultimately require conjunctivodacryocystorhinostomy, which is usually deferred until they are older. Conjunctivodacryocystorhinostomy is discussed in BCSC Section 7, *Orbit, Eyelids, and Lacrimal System.*

Congenital Lacrimal Fistula

A congenital lacrimal fistula is an epithelium-lined tract extending from the common canaliculus or lacrimal sac to the overlying skin surface. It usually presents as a small dimple medial to the eyelids, which may be difficult to detect in the absence of symptoms (Fig 19-2). If patients are asymptomatic, no treatment is necessary. Discharge from the fistula is often associated with distal NLDO and may cease after probing of the distal obstruction. If discharge persists despite a patent lacrimal duct, surgical excision of the fistula between the skin and normal lacrimal structures is required.

Dacryocystocele

Congenital dacryocystocele *(dacryocele, mucocele, amniotocele)* is present in approximately 3% of infants with NLDO. It develops when a distal blockage causes distention of the lacrimal sac. Kinking of the common canaliculus does not allow retrograde discharge of accumulated secretions, thereby preventing decompression of the lacrimal sac. Most patients with dacryocystoceles have associated cysts of the distal NLD, which may be seen beneath the inferior turbinate. Involvement is bilateral in 20%–30% of cases.

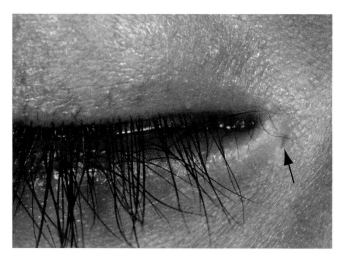

Figure 19-2 Lacrimal fistula. *(Reproduced with permission from Lueder GT. Neonatal lacrimal system anomalies. Semin Ophthalmol. 1997;12(2):109.)*

Clinical features

Dacryocystocele presents at birth or within the first few days of life as a bluish swelling just below and nasal to the medial canthus. The differential diagnosis includes hemangioma, dermoid cyst, and encephalocele. Hemangiomas are not typically present at birth. They have a vascular appearance and are generally less firm than dacryocystoceles. Dermoid cysts and encephaloceles present most often above the medial canthal tendon. The diagnosis is clinically apparent when a newborn has a nasal mass beneath the medial canthus that is associated with symptoms of NLDO (discussed later in the chapter). Imaging is usually not required in this case.

Dacryocystoceles are prone to infection, which differs in severity from the low-grade, chronic dacryocystitis commonly seen in older infants with typical NLDO. When dacryocystoceles are infected, acute dacryocystitis usually develops. The skin over the distended lacrimal sac becomes erythematous (Fig 19-3), and pressure on the sac may produce reflux of frank purulent material.

Infants who have large intranasal cysts may present with respiratory symptoms, because infants are obligate nasal breathers. Symptoms range from difficulty during feeding (due to obstruction of the mouth) to frank respiratory distress.

Management

Early treatment of dacryocystoceles is advised to prevent complications related to the infection associated with these lesions, which is more severe than that seen in typical NLDO. Infants are relatively immunocompromised and are therefore at risk for local or systemic spread of infection should dacryocystoceles become infected.

Dacryocystoceles associated with acute respiratory distress require immediate treatment, including nasal endoscopy to remove the intranasal cysts. Noninfected dacryocystoceles sometimes resolve with decompression by careful digital massage or by bedside

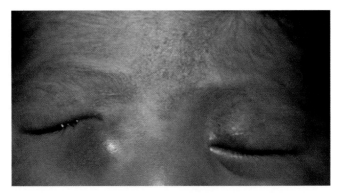

Figure 19-3 Infected congenital dacryocystocele, right eye, in a newborn. Note typical location and erythema overlying the distended lacrimal sac. *(Courtesy of Edward L. Raab, MD.)*

NLD probing. If the lesions do not resolve within the first 1–2 weeks of life or if they become acutely infected at any time, surgical treatment is indicated. Nasolacrimal probing alone may be curative, but in approximately 25% of patients, symptoms persist after probing. Nasolacrimal probing in conjunction with endoscopy and cyst removal is effective in more than 95% of infants. Systemic antibiotics should be used perioperatively if acute dacryocystitis is present. Because approximately 20%–30% of patients have bilateral nasal cysts, sometimes without visible dacryocystoceles, bilateral endoscopy is recommended. Surgical treatment of an infected dacryocystocele via a skin incision should be avoided because of the risk of creating a persistent fistulous tract.

Lueder GT. The association of neonatal dacryocystoceles and infantile dacryocystitis with nasolacrimal duct cysts (an American Ophthalmological Society thesis). *Trans Am Ophthalmol Soc.* 2012;110:74–93.

Nasolacrimal Duct Obstruction

Nasolacrimal duct obstruction is by far the most common lacrimal system disorder encountered in pediatric ophthalmology, occurring in approximately 5% of full-term newborns. Usually, a thin mucosal membrane at the lower end of the NLD, at the valve of Hasner, is the cause (see Fig 19-7A).

Clinical Features

Infants who have typical NLDO usually present within the first month of life with epiphora, recurrent periocular crusting, or both (Fig 19-4). Symptoms are usually chronic and intermittent, and bilateral involvement is common. Digital pressure over the lacrimal sac usually results in retrograde discharge of mucoid or mucopurulent material. Culture of the discharge typically reveals the presence of multiple strains of bacteria, but this information is ordinarily not necessary for clinical management.

The differential diagnosis of NLDO includes infantile glaucoma, conjunctivitis, epiblepharon with corneal irritation due to misdirected eyelashes, and various corneal disorders. The presence of epiphora is the primary reason that these entities may be mistaken

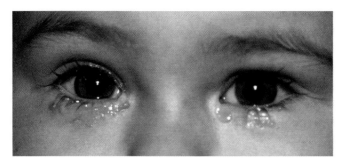

Figure 19-4 Bilateral nasolacrimal duct obstruction. Note epiphora and periocular crusting without evidence of inflammation. *(Reproduced with permission from Lueder GT. Pediatric Practice Ophthalmology. New York: McGraw-Hill Professional; 2011:55.)*

for NLDO, but the associated findings (eg, enlarged corneas and Haab striae in glaucoma, conjunctival injection in conjunctivitis, visible eyelid abnormalities in epiblepharon, and corneal surface abnormalities in corneal disorders) make the diagnosis of NLDO relatively easy to establish.

An important clinical characteristic of NLDO is that infants with this disorder typically do not appear bothered by it. In addition, the cornea and conjunctiva are usually otherwise normal. The presence of photophobia, visible conjunctival changes, or corneal surface abnormalities should prompt the examiner to look for diseases other than NLDO.

Some studies have shown an association between NLDO and anisometropia, which may cause amblyopia. Because of this, and because of the need to rule out the disorders noted previously, children with NLDO who present to an ophthalmologist should undergo a full ophthalmic examination, including refraction.

Nonsurgical Management

There is a high rate of spontaneous resolution of NLDO, with approximately 90% of patients improving within the first 9–12 months of life. For this reason, conservative treatment is recommended initially for these patients. Because most pediatricians are familiar with NLDO and its early treatment, patients with this condition who present to an ophthalmologist are usually older and have symptoms that have persisted beyond the normal time frame for resolution.

Conservative treatment includes lacrimal massage and use of topical antibiotics. Massage serves 2 purposes: it empties the sac, thereby reducing the opportunity for bacterial growth, and it applies hydrostatic pressure to the obstruction, which may open the duct and resolve the condition. Massage is performed by pressing over the lacrimal sac, at the medial canthus, a few times per day. This is the only location where application of external pressure on the lacrimal sac can be effective. Passing the finger along the nares, which is often mistakenly recommended by primary care providers, is not effective because the lacrimal duct is covered by bone at this site.

Topical antibiotics are often recommended if patients have significant periocular discharge. There are 3 important points with regard to topical antibiotic use in this disorder.

First, the antibiotics do not cure the obstruction. They may temporarily improve the associated infection, but they do not cause the distal lacrimal membrane to resolve. Second, the infection in NLDO is due to stasis of fluid within the lacrimal sac. Therefore almost any bacteria, including normal flora, may cause infection. Most broad-spectrum antibiotics are effective in reducing the associated symptoms, so culturing the mucoid or mucopurulent material is usually not necessary. Third, antibiotic use for a few days often produces improvement, and prolonged use may not be necessary. Parents may be instructed to administer the antibiotics as needed when the amount of discharge increases.

Surgical Management

Nasolacrimal probing is one of the most common procedures performed by pediatric ophthalmologists. It is used to treat infants with NLDO whose symptoms do not resolve with age and conservative treatment. There are 2 common approaches to the surgical management of this disorder. Some ophthalmologists recommend probing at age 3–6 months in an awake infant in the office, whereas others prefer to delay treatment until age 9–12 months, at which time surgery is performed in the operating room. The advantages of early in-office probing are that it avoids general anesthesia and resolves symptoms earlier. The disadvantages are that a painful procedure is performed on an awake infant and that surgery is performed on many infants who would spontaneously improve without surgery (approximately 75%). The advantages of later surgery in the operating room are that fewer infants require treatment and that surgery is performed in a more controlled environment, in which additional procedures can be performed concurrently. Either of these approaches is acceptable.

Surgical procedures for NLDO are also discussed in BCSC Section 7, *Orbit, Eyelids, and Lacrimal System.*

Pediatric Eye Disease Investigator Group. A randomized trial comparing the cost-effectiveness of 2 approaches for treating unilateral nasolacrimal duct obstruction. *Arch Ophthalmol.* 2012; 130(12):1525–1533.

Probing

When nasolacrimal probing is to be performed in the operating room, placement of an oxymetazoline-soaked pledget beneath the inferior turbinate before surgery may decrease intraoperative bleeding. The initial step in nasolacrimal probing is dilation of the puncta and proximal canaliculi. Punctal membranes and atretic canaliculi are sometimes not recognized until surgery. Their management is discussed earlier in this chapter. Because the lacrimal system cannot be visualized beyond the puncta, knowledge of the anatomy and normal course of the system's structures is essential for passing lacrimal probes properly. The probes are initially inserted in the puncta, perpendicular to the eyelid. Within 1–2 mm of the eyelid margin, the canaliculi turn approximately 90°; the probes are therefore turned almost immediately and passed along the course of the canaliculi until the nasal bone is encountered on the medial side of the lacrimal sac. The probes are held flat on the patient's face and rotated until they are almost vertical; they are then passed gently into the distal duct (Fig 19-5A). Most surgeons feel a slight popping sensation as the probe passes through the membrane causing the obstruction.

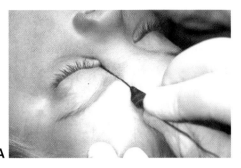 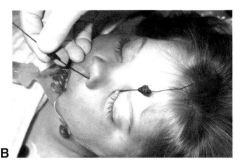

Figure 19-5 Probing for lacrimal obstruction. **A,** The probe is advanced through the lacrimal sac and nasolacrimal duct, in this instance via the lower canaliculus. **B,** A second probe introduced into the nares is used to verify the position of the probe tip. *(Courtesy of Edward L. Raab, MD.)*

A wide variety of techniques are used for probing in NLDO. Most surgeons begin with a size 0 or 1 Bowman probe, and some pass successively larger probes to enlarge the distal duct. Irrigation may be performed following probing in order to verify that the system is patent. Introducing a second metal probe into the nares and making direct contact with the previously placed lacrimal probe verifies the position of the latter (Fig 19-5B). Alternatively, direct inspection with a nasal speculum and headlamp or with a nasal endoscope can determine the precise position of the probe. Infracture of the inferior turbinate may be employed to widen the area where the fluid drains beneath the inferior turbinate. The surgeon accomplishes this by placing a small periosteal elevator beneath the turbinate or by grasping it with a hemostat and then rotating the instrument.

Postoperatively, minor bleeding from the nose or into the tears commonly occurs and usually requires no treatment. Optional postoperative medications include antibiotic drops, corticosteroid drops, or both instilled 1–4 times daily for 1–2 weeks. Phenylephrine or oxymetazoline nasal spray may be used to control nasal bleeding or congestion. Because transient bacteremia can occur after probing, systemic antibiotic prophylaxis should be considered for patients with cardiac disease.

Resolution of signs after probing may not occur until 1 week or more postoperatively. Recurrence after unsuccessful probing is usually evident within 1–2 months. The success rate of properly performed initial probing for congenital NLDO exceeds 80% in infants younger than 15 months.

Significant complications of probing are rare. In some patients, mild epiphora occurs occasionally, particularly outdoors in cold weather or in conjunction with an upper respiratory tract infection. This epiphora is probably attributable to a patent but narrow lacrimal drainage channel. Usually no additional treatment is required.

Patients with persistent symptoms following initial probing

A variety of treatment options are available for patients whose symptoms persist following initial probing. A second probing can be used in such patients, with or without infracture of the inferior turbinate.

Some surgeons employ balloon catheter dilation, intubation, or nasal endoscopy (discussed in the following subsections) during the first surgery for NLDO, but most reserve their use for patients who require a second procedure.

Balloon catheter dilation Balloon catheter dilation (BCD) is performed by passing a catheter into the distal NLD and inflating a balloon at the site of obstruction (Fig 19-6). This procedure is particularly useful for patients with diffuse, rather than localized, obstruction of the distal duct.

Intubation Intubation of the lacrimal system is usually recommended when 1 or more probings or BCD has failed. Several methods of intubation are available. Bicanalicular intubation is performed by passing stents through the upper and lower canaliculi and recovering them in the nares. Most surgeons secure the stents in the nares by using a bolster or by suturing the stents to the nasal mucosa. Monocanalicular stents are placed by passing them through either the upper or lower canaliculus or sometimes by passing separate stents through both canaliculi.

Complications associated with stents include elongation of the lacrimal puncta, dislodging and protrusion of the stents, and corneal abrasions. In some cases, the stent can be repositioned, but early removal may be necessary.

Stents are usually left in place for 2–6 months, but shorter periods can be successful. The technique used for stent removal depends on the age of the patient, the measure employed to secure the stent, and the position of the stent (in place or partially dislodged).

Nasal endoscopy Anatomical abnormalities of the distal NLD account for some of the failures of initial probing. These abnormalities include cysts similar to those seen in infants with dacryocystoceles and flaccid mucosal membranes obstructing the distal duct. In addition, false passages may be recognized endoscopically, in which case the probe may be re-placed so that it is in the proper position. Removal of abnormal structures is performed under endoscopic guidance. Endoscopy may be performed by the ophthalmologist alone or in conjunction with an otolaryngologist.

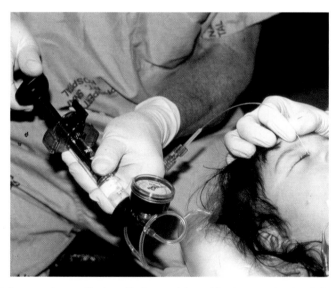

Figure 19-6 Balloon catheter dilation. Probe positioned in the nasolacrimal duct. The surgeon inflates the balloon. *(Courtesy of Edward L. Raab, MD.)*

Older children with lacrimal obstruction

Previous studies suggested that children who present with NLDO after 18–24 months of age may be less likely to show improvement following NLD probing. However, many of these studies did not account for anatomical variations of the distal NLD. Some older children with NLDO have the same membranous obstruction of the distal duct that is present in younger children with NLDO (Fig 19-7A). This obstruction is identified by a distinct

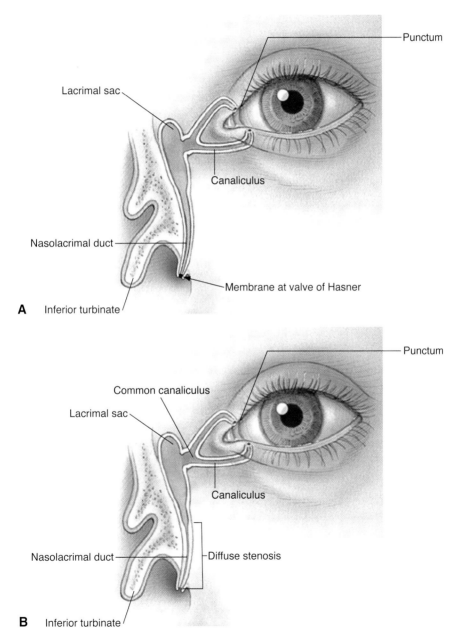

Figure 19-7   A, Typical location of membrane causing nasolacrimal duct obstruction *(arrow).* **B,** Diffuse stenosis of distal nasolacrimal duct. *(Adapted from an illustration by Christine Gralapp.)*

popping sensation as the probe is passed into the distal duct. Probing in older patients with this finding has a success rate similar to that in younger children. Diffuse stenosis of the distal duct (Fig 19-7B) is another anatomical abnormality that may be found in patients with NLDO. It is identified by palpation of a tight passage occurring throughout the distal duct. Because probing is less likely to be successful when diffuse stenosis is present, BCD or stent placement (discussed earlier) should be considered in patients with this finding.

Dacryocystorhinostomy

Dacryocystorhinostomy involves creation of a new opening between the lacrimal sac and the nasal cavity. It is a final option when the procedures described in the preceding sections are unsuccessful and NLDO persists or recurs. The decision of when to perform this procedure is affected by the severity of the signs and symptoms of obstruction.

See BCSC Section 7, *Orbit, Eyelids, and Lacrimal System,* for further discussion of this procedure.

CHAPTER 20

Diseases of the Cornea, Anterior Segment, and Iris

This chapter discusses diseases of the cornea, anterior segment, and iris whose onset is during infancy and childhood. Familiarity with the embryology of the eye will help the reader better understand the developmental anomalies covered in this chapter (see BCSC Section 2, *Fundamentals and Principles of Ophthalmology*). Many of the disorders in this chapter are also discussed in BCSC Section 8, *External Disease and Cornea*.

Congenital and Developmental Anomalies of the Cornea

Abnormalities of Corneal Size and Shape

Abnormalities of corneal size and shape in childhood include isolated megalocornea, microcornea, keratoglobus, and keratoconus.

Megalocornea

Megalocornea is a nonprogressive enlargement of the cornea in which the diameter is 13 mm or greater. Megalocornea is a rare, usually bilateral, congenital condition. Inheritance is usually X-linked but may be autosomal recessive or dominant; 90% of affected patients are male. At birth, X-linked megalocornea is associated with iris transillumination and a deep anterior chamber. Late changes include corneal mosaic degeneration (shagreen), arcus juvenilis, presenile cataracts, and glaucoma. Treatment includes lubrication if patients have exposure keratopathy.

Microcornea

Microcornea is a clear cornea of normal thickness with a diameter less than 9 mm in the newborn and less than 10 mm after 2 years of age (Fig 20-1). Isolated microcornea is very rare. In *microphthalmos,* the entire eye is small and malformed, whereas in *nanophthalmos,* the eye is small but normal.

Microcornea may be autosomal dominant or recessive. It usually accompanies other abnormalities of the eye, including cataracts, colobomas, high hyperopia, cornea plana, and persistent fetal vasculature. It may be seen in oculodentodigital syndrome, Warburg micro syndrome, and Ehlers-Danlos syndrome.

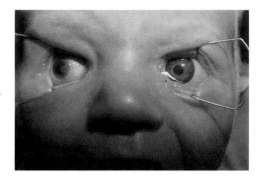

Figure 20-1 Microcornea, right eye.

Keratoglobus

Keratoglobus is a very rare autosomal recessive, bilateral noninflammatory condition present at birth. It may occur in Ehlers-Danlos syndrome type VI. The corneal curvature is steep, with thinning of the cornea in the periphery and a very deep anterior chamber. Spontaneous breaks in Descemet membrane may produce acute corneal edema, and the cornea is easily ruptured by minor blunt trauma. Patients with keratoglobus should routinely wear protective lenses. Scleral contact lenses may be helpful.

Keratoconus

In keratoconus, the central or paracentral cornea bulges and progressively thins such that the cornea takes on the shape of a cone. Keratoconus may present and progress during the adolescent years. It can occur with Down syndrome, atopic diseases, and chronic eye rubbing. Keratoconus may be familial. Unlike in keratoglobus, iron lines, stress lines (Vogt striae), and apical scarring are often seen. Tears in Descemet membrane can cause acute corneal edema (hydrops) in patients with keratoconus.

Abnormalities of Peripheral Corneal Transparency

Posterior embryotoxon

Posterior embryotoxon, also called a *prominent Schwalbe line,* is a thickening and anterior displacement of the Schwalbe line. This anomaly is visible at the slit lamp; it looks like an irregular white line just concentric with and anterior to the limbus (Fig 20-2). Through the gonioscope, the condition looks like a continuous or broken ridge protruding into the anterior chamber. Pigmented spots may be seen on the internal surface of the ridge. This anomaly is most often associated with Axenfeld-Rieger syndrome but is also found in arteriohepatic dysplasia (Alagille syndrome) and velocardiofacial syndrome (22q11 deletion syndrome); it may be an isolated finding in 15% of normal patients.

Cornea plana

Cornea plana is a rare, bilateral, often autosomal recessive condition that features flat corneas, peripheral scleralization of the cornea, and a shallow anterior chamber. Patients are often hyperopic, and glaucoma may develop secondary to angle closure due to the shallow anterior chamber. Refractive correction and glaucoma management are the mainstays of treatment.

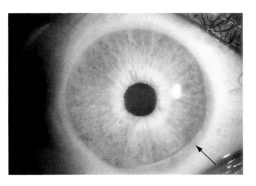

Figure 20-2 Posterior embryotoxon *(arrow)* in Axenfeld-Rieger syndrome.

Epibulbar dermoid

An epibulbar (limbal) dermoid is a choristoma composed of fibrofatty tissue covered by keratinized epithelium. It is present from birth, and little if any postnatal growth occurs. Dermoids may contain hair follicles, sebaceous glands, or sweat glands. They can be up to 10 mm in diameter and usually straddle the limbus. They may extend into the corneal stroma and adjacent sclera but seldom occupy the full thickness of either cornea or sclera. Most epibulbar dermoids are on the inferior temporal limbus. Many produce a lipoid infiltration of the corneal stroma at their leading edge. They are sometimes continuous with subconjunctival dermolipomas that involve the lateral quadrant of the eye.

Epibulbar dermoids can produce anisometropic astigmatism with secondary amblyopia. Large epibulbar dermoids can cover the visual axis. Removal of epibulbar dermoids may be indicated if they cause ocular irritation or amblyopia. Surgical excision may result in scarring and astigmatism, which can also lead to amblyopia. Although excision will not eliminate the preexisting astigmatism, surgery may be useful for treating very elevated lesions (Fig 20-3). Tumor removal involves excising the episcleral portion flush with the plane of surrounding tissue. In general, the surgeon need not remove underlying clear corneal tissue, mobilize surrounding tissue, or apply a patch graft over the resulting surface defect; however, because some lesions extend into the anterior chamber, tissue should be available in the event that a patch graft is required. Cornea and conjunctiva heal within a few days to several weeks, generally with some scarring and imperfect corneal transparency; nevertheless, the appearance can be improved considerably.

Epibulbar dermoids are often seen with Goldenhar syndrome (oculoauriculovertebral spectrum; see also Chapter 18). These patients may have a variety of other anomalies, including ear deformities (Fig 20-4), maxillary or mandibular hypoplasia, vertebral deformities, eyelid colobomas, and Duane retraction syndrome.

Dermolipoma

A conjunctival lesion, the dermolipoma is usually located near the temporal fornix and is composed of adipose tissue and dense connective tissue. The overlying conjunctival epithelium is normal, and hair follicles are absent. Dermolipomas may be extensive, sometimes involving orbital tissue, the lacrimal gland, and extraocular muscle. Like limbal dermoids, conjunctival dermolipomas are frequently associated with Goldenhar syndrome (see also Chapter 18).

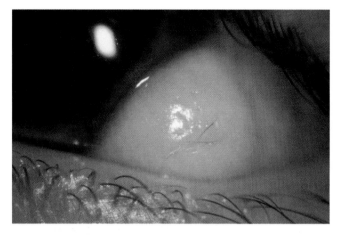

Figure 20-3 Epibulbar dermoid with hair growing in the center. *(Courtesy of Ken K. Nischal, MD.)*

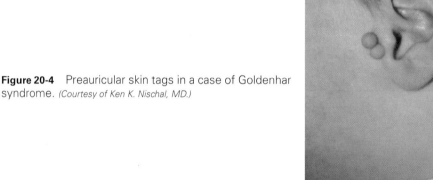

Figure 20-4 Preauricular skin tags in a case of Goldenhar syndrome. *(Courtesy of Ken K. Nischal, MD.)*

Dermolipomas rarely require excision. If surgery is undertaken, the surgeon should attempt to remove only the portion of the lesion visible within the palpebral fissure, disturbing conjunctiva and the Tenon layer as little as possible to minimize scarring. Cicatrization may occur even with a conservative operative approach.

Abnormalities of Central and Diffuse Corneal Transparency

The mnemonic *STUMPED* is helpful for remembering the differential diagnosis for congenital corneal opacities (Table 20-1): *s*clerocornea, *t*ears in Descemet membrane (usually due to forceps trauma or congenital glaucoma), *u*lcers (infection; see Chapter 28), *m*etabolic (eg, mucopolysaccharidosis), *P*eters anomaly, *e*dema (eg, congenital hereditary endothelial

Table 20-1 Differential Diagnosis of Infantile Corneal Opacities

Entity	Location and Description of Opacity	Other Signs	Method of Diagnosis
Sclerocornea (total corneal opacification)	Peripheral opacity, clearest centrally; unilateral or bilateral; often vascularized	Flat cornea	Inspection; anterior segment imaging
Forceps injury	Central opacity; unilateral	Breaks in Descemet membrane	History
Posterior corneal defect	Central opacity; unilateral or bilateral	Iris adherence to cornea; posterior keratoconus	Inspection
Infection	Central or diffuse; unilateral or bilateral	Dendrites, infiltrate, ulceration	Culture, PCR, serologic tests
Mucopolysaccharidosis, mucolipidosis	Diffuse opacity; bilateral	Smooth epithelium	Biochemical testing
Congenital hereditary stromal dystrophy (CHSD)	Diffuse opacity; bilateral	Stromal opacities; normal thickness; normal epithelium	Examination of family members for autosomal dominance
Congenital hereditary endothelial dystrophy (CHED)	Diffuse opacity; bilateral	Thickened cornea	Inspection
Infantile glaucoma	Diffuse opacity; unilateral or bilateral	Enlarged cornea; breaks in Descemet membrane	Tonometry for elevated intraocular pressure
Dermoid	Inferotemporal opacity; unilateral; elevated; surface hair; keratinized; usually limbal	Associated with Goldenhar syndrome	Inspection

dystrophy [CHED], posterior polymorphous dystrophy, congenital hereditary stromal dystrophy [CHSD], glaucoma), and dermoid. An alternative classification of corneal opacities is based on whether they are primary or secondary (Table 20-2).

Primary causes

Congenital hereditary endothelial dystrophy CHED is an uncommon corneal dystrophy. The cornea is diffusely and uniformly edematous because of a defect of the corneal endothelium and Descemet membrane. The edema involves both the stroma and the epithelium. The appearance of the cornea is similar to that in congenital glaucoma but without increased corneal diameter and elevated intraocular pressure. The hallmark of CHED is increased corneal thickness. CHED type I is the same entity as posterior polymorphous dystrophy (PPMD); both are autosomal dominant on the same locus at pericentromeric chromosome 20 and present in the first or second decade of life without nystagmus.

Table 20-2 Primary and Secondary Corneal Opacities: An Alternative Classification

Primary
Corneal dystrophies (eg, CHED, PPMD, CHSD)
Corneal dermoid

Secondary
Posterior corneal depression
Kerato-irido-lenticular dysgenesis (KILD)
Iridocorneal adhesions only (Peters anomaly type 1)
Failure of lens to separate from cornea (Peters anomaly type 2)
Lens separation but failure to form thereafter (sclerocornea)
Failure of lens to form (sclerocornea)
Congenital or infantile glaucoma
Traumatic breaks in Descemet membrane
Infection
Metabolic causes

CHED = congenital hereditary endothelial dystrophy; CHSD = congenital hereditary stromal dystrophy; PPMD = posterior polymorphous dystrophy.

Adapted with permission from Nischal KK. A new approach to the classification of neonatal corneal opacities. *Curr Opin Ophthalmol.* 2012;23(5):344–354.

CHED type II presents at birth with nystagmus and is autosomal recessive. Deafness and CHED are seen in Harboyan syndrome.

Posterior polymorphous dystrophy PPMD presents at birth only rarely; it usually presents later. See BCSC Section 8, *External Disease and Cornea.*

Congenital hereditary stromal dystrophy CHSD is a very rare congenital stationary opacification of the cornea transmitted in an autosomal dominant manner. A flaky or feathery clouding of the stroma, which is of normal thickness, is covered by a smooth, normal epithelium. These features are in contrast with those of CHED, which exhibits a thickened stroma and epithelial edema.

> Weiss JS, Møller HU, Lisch W, et al. The IC3D classification of the corneal dystrophies. *Cornea.* 2008;27(Suppl 2):S1–S83.

Secondary causes

Posterior corneal depression Posterior corneal depression (central posterior keratoconus), a discrete posterior corneal indentation, produces an abnormal red reflex during examination with a retinoscope or direct ophthalmoscope. A highly convex posterior corneal surface is visible with slit-lamp examination. Pigment deposits sometimes appear on the border of the posterior defect. The anterior curvature of the cornea is normal. This defect usually causes irregular astigmatism and can result in amblyopia. If refractive correction is not successful, Descemet stripping endothelial keratoplasty (DSEK) can be considered.

Peters anomaly Peters anomaly, also known as *iridocorneal* or *keratolenticular adhesions,* is a posterior corneal defect with an overlying stromal opacity, often accompanied by adherent iris strands (Peters anomaly type 1; Fig 20-5A). The size and density of the opacity

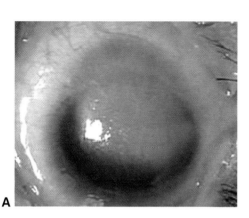
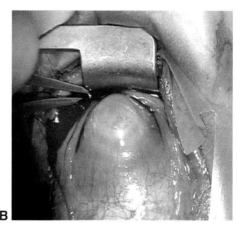

Figure 20-5 **A,** Corneal opacity secondary to iridocorneal adhesion (Peters anomaly type 1). **B,** Corneal opacity secondary to keratolenticular adhesion (Peters anomaly type 2). *(Courtesy of Ken K. Nischal, MD.)*

can range from a mild to dense central leukoma. The strands from the iris to the borders of this defect vary in number and density. In severe cases, the central leukoma may be vascularized and protrude above the level of the cornea. The stromal opacity may decrease with time. Lysis of adherent iris strands has been reported to improve corneal clarity. A more severe variety includes adherence of the lens to the cornea at the site of the central defect (Peters anomaly type 2; Fig 20-5B).

Peters anomaly can be caused by many different diseases, including genetic conditions (eg, Axenfeld-Rieger syndrome) and nongenetic conditions (eg, congenital rubella). Unilateral cases are usually isolated. Bilateral cases are often associated with systemic disorders and warrant a complete genetic workup. A syndrome called *microphthalmia with linear skin defects (MLS)* includes microphthalmos, reddish linear skin lesions, and life-threatening cardiac arrhythmias. Peters-plus syndrome is bilateral Peters anomaly associated with congenital brain defects, heart defects, and craniofacial anomalies.

Bhandari R, Ferri S, Whittaker B, Liu M, Lazzaro DR. Peters anomaly: review of the literature. *Cornea.* 2011;30(8):939–944.

Mataftsi A, Islam L, Kelberman D, Sowden JC, Nischal KK. Chromosome abnormalities and the genetics of congenital corneal opacification. *Mol Vis.* 2011;17:1624–1640.

Sclerocornea Sclerocornea (total corneal opacification) is a congenital disorder in which the cornea is opaque and resembles the sclera, making the limbus indistinct (Fig 20-6). The central cornea is clearer than the periphery in nearly all cases, in contradistinction to Peters anomaly, in which the periphery is generally clearer. Severe cases show no increased corneal curvature and no apparent scleral sulcus. Sclerocornea is often associated with other ocular or systemic abnormalities. Anterior segment imaging is important for detecting other abnormalities and guiding treatment.

Congenital or infantile glaucoma Glaucoma in an infant can cause the cornea to become edematous, cloudy, and enlarged (see Chapter 22).

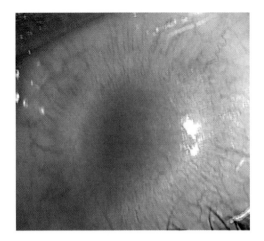

Figure 20-6 Sclerocornea with cornea plana. *(Courtesy of Ken K. Nischal, MD.)*

Traumatic breaks in Descemet membrane Injuries to Descemet membrane may be caused by forceps trauma to the eye during delivery. These are usually vertical and linear, whereas the Haab striae seen in congenital glaucoma are curvilinear. Rupture of Descemet membrane leads to stromal and sometimes epithelial edema. Other signs of trauma are frequently apparent on the child's head. In most cases, the stromal and epithelial edema regresses, but the edges of the broken Descemet membrane persist and can be seen as ridges protruding slightly from the posterior corneal surface. Amblyopia may result from the corneal opacity. Anisometropic astigmatism induced by the trauma can cause severe amblyopia even if the corneal haze resolves quickly. Follow-up examinations are indicated, as optical correction and patching may be required. Trauma from amniocentesis is a rare cause of unilateral corneal opacification in a newborn.

Corneal ulcers Corneal ulcers that are present at or develop around birth are rare and may be caused by herpes simplex keratitis or other infection (bacterial) (see Chapter 28).

Treatment of Corneal Opacities

The treatment of congenital corneal opacities is difficult but can be rewarding as long as the clinician understands that the goals include both corneal graft clarity and improvement in visual function. If bilateral dense opacities are present, early keratoplasty should be considered for 1 eye so that deprivation amblyopia can be minimized. If the opacity is unilateral, the decision is more difficult. Keratoplasty should be undertaken only if the family and the ophthalmologists are prepared for the significant commitment of time and effort needed to deal with corneal graft rejection, which often occurs in children, as well as with amblyopia. The team should include ophthalmologists skilled in pediatric corneal surgery, pediatric glaucoma, and amblyopia. Contact lens expertise is important for infants with small eyes and large refractive errors. Repeated examinations under anesthesia are often required.

In addition to penetrating keratoplasty, treatment options include optical iridectomy, deep anterior lamellar keratoplasty (DALK; used for stromal disease with healthy endothelium), DSEK (used to replace diseased endothelium or Descemet membrane), and keratoprostheses.

Ashar JN, Ramappa M, Vaddavalli PK. Paired-eye comparison of Descemet's stripping endothelial keratoplasty and penetrating keratoplasty in children with congenital hereditary endothelial dystrophy. *Br J Ophthalmol.* 2013;97(10):1247–1249. Epub 2013 Apr 23.

Harding SA, Nischal KK, Upponi-Patil A, Fowler DJ. Indications and outcomes of deep anterior lamellar keratoplasty in children. *Ophthalmology.* 2010;117(11):2191–2195.

Congenital and Developmental Anomalies of the Globe

Microphthalmos

Microphthalmos refers to a small, disorganized globe, often with an associated cystic outpouching of the posteroinferior sclera. It may be isolated or syndromic. Mutations of the *CHX10, MAF, PAX6, PAX2, RAX, SHH, SIX3,* and *SOX2* genes have been reported in microphthalmos.

Anophthalmos

True anophthalmos (absence of any ocular globe tissue) is very rare and often extreme. Usually, severe microphthalmos is present, giving a clinical picture of anophthalmos. The genes involved in anophthalmos are the same as those involved in microphthalmos.

Nanophthalmos

Nanophthalmos refers to a small but normal eye. The patient has a high degree of hyperopia (+7–+10 D) due to the short eye. There is a high lens-to-eye ratio, leading to a shallow anterior chamber and angle-closure glaucoma.

Congenital and Developmental Anomalies of the Iris and Pupil

Abnormalities of the Iris

Persistent pupillary membranes

Persistent pupillary membranes (Fig 20-7) are the most common developmental abnormality of the iris. They are present in approximately 95% of newborns, and remnants are common in older children and adults. Persistent pupillary membranes are rarely of any visual significance. However, if especially prominent, they can adhere to the anterior lens capsule, causing a small anterior polar cataract. They may also be associated with other anterior segment abnormalities.

Ramappa M, Murthy SI, Chaurasia S, et al. Lens-preserving excision of congenital hyperplastic pupillary membranes with clinicopathological correlation. *J AAPOS.* 2012;16(2): 201–203.

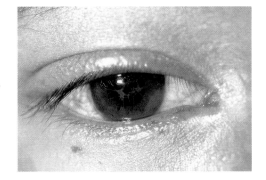

Figure 20-7 Persistent pupillary membranes. Uncorrected visual acuity is 20/40.

Iris hypoplasia

When the iris stroma is underdeveloped, it is termed *iris hypoplasia.* When the posterior pigment epithelium is underdeveloped, it results in iris transillumination (discussed later). When the condition involves both structures, it may be focal (iris coloboma) or diffuse (aniridia).

Axenfeld-Rieger syndrome Axenfeld-Rieger syndrome is the commonest cause of iris (stromal) hypoplasia. This syndrome represents a spectrum of developmental disorders characterized by posterior embryotoxon, with attached iris strands, iris hypoplasia, and a 50% lifetime risk of glaucoma (Figs 20-8, 20-9, 20-10). The conditions—previously called *Axenfeld anomaly, Rieger anomaly* or *syndrome, iridogoniodysgenesis anomaly* or *syndrome, iris hypoplasia,* and *familial glaucoma iridogoniodysplasia*—all overlap genotypically and phenotypically and are now considered a single entity known as *Axenfeld-Rieger syndrome.* With the identification of several causative genes and loci for these disorders, it is now known that the same ocular appearance can be caused by different genes, and very different ocular presentations can be caused by the same mutated gene. In the latter circumstances, the different ocular presentations previously would have been classified as distinct conditions—Peters anomaly, Rieger anomaly, or primary glaucoma, for example.

Axenfeld-Rieger syndrome may include a smooth, cryptless iris surface and a high iris insertion, sometimes accompanied by iris transillumination. Iris hypoplasia can range from mild stromal thinning to marked atrophy with hole formation, corectopia, and ectropion uveae. The severity of the iris hypoplasia may be so great as to mimic aniridia. Posterior embryotoxon, megalocornea (secondary to glaucoma), or microcornea may occur. Associated nonocular abnormalities include abnormal teeth, redundant periumbilical skin, hypospadias, and anomalies in the region of the pituitary gland.

Autosomal dominant inheritance is most common. Mutations in the *PITX2* gene on band 4q25 have been identified. This is a paired homeobox gene that regulates expansion of other genes during embryonic development. Patients with mutations of *PITX2* have been reported to have phenotypes of aniridia, Peters anomaly, and Axenfeld-Rieger syndrome. The nonocular findings are more consistent and should be sought with any of these ocular phenotypes. Mutations in the forkhead transcription factor gene *FOXC1* (formerly called *FKHL7*) also cause Axenfeld-Rieger syndrome, generating features such as

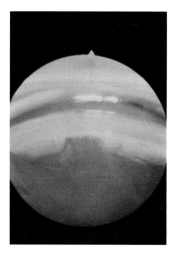

Figure 20-8 Gonioscopic view in Axenfeld-Rieger syndrome.

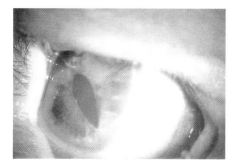 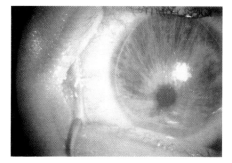

Figure 20-9 Axenfeld-Rieger syndrome, bilateral.

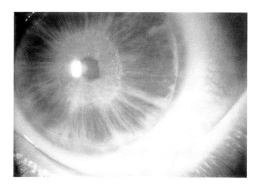

Figure 20-10 Axenfeld-Rieger syndrome. Note variation compared with Figures 20-2 and 20-9. *(Courtesy of Jane D. Kivlin, MD.)*

autosomal dominant iris hypoplasia, glaucoma, Axenfeld-Rieger syndrome, posterior embryotoxon, Peters anomaly, and primary congenital glaucoma. *FOXC1* is also expressed in the heart, and some patients have cardiac valve abnormalities.

Iris transillumination In albinism, diffuse iris transillumination results from the absence of pigment in the posterior epithelial layers. Iris hypoplasia can also lead to iris transillumination, especially as part of Axenfeld-Rieger syndrome or iridocorneal endo-thelial (ICE) syndrome. In addition, iris transillumination may occur in Marfan syn-drome, ectopia lentis et pupillae, X-linked megalocornea, and microcoria. Patchy areas of transillumination can also be seen after trauma, surgery, or uveitis. Scattered iris transil-lumination defects may be a normal variant in individuals with very lightly pigmented irides.

Coloboma of the iris Iris colobomas are classified as *typical* if they occur in the inferona-sal quadrant and can thus be explained by failure of the embryonic fissure to close in the fifth week of gestation. With a typical iris coloboma, the pupil is shaped like a lightbulb, keyhole, or inverted teardrop (Fig 20-11). Typical colobomas may also involve the lens, ciliary body, choroid, retina, and optic nerve. These colobomas are part of a continuum that extends to microphthalmos and anophthalmos. Isolated colobomatous microphthalmos is inherited as an autosomal dominant trait in approximately 20% of cases. Parents of an affected child may have small, previously undetected chorioretinal or iris defects in an inferonasal location, so careful examination of family members is indicated.

Atypical iris colobomas occur in areas other than the inferonasal quadrant and are not usually associated with posterior uveal colobomas. These colobomas probably result from fibrovascular remnants of the anterior hyaloid system and pupillary membrane.

Aniridia Aniridia is a panocular, bilateral disorder. The term *aniridia* is a misnomer, be-cause at least a rudimentary iris is always present. The degree of iris formation ranges from almost total absence to only mild hypoplasia, the latter of which can be confused with Axenfeld-Rieger syndrome. The typical presentation is an infant with nystagmus who appears to have absent irides or dilated, unresponsive pupils. Photophobia may be present. Examination findings commonly include small anterior polar cataracts, at times with attached strands of persistent pupillary membranes (Fig 20-12). Foveal hypoplasia is usually present, with visual acuity less than 20/100. Glaucoma and optic nerve hypoplasia are common. Corneal opacification often develops later in childhood and may lead to progressive deterioration of visual acuity. The corneal abnormality is due to a stem cell deficiency and therefore keratolimbal allograft stem cell transplantation may be a more effective treatment than corneal transplantation.

A defect in the *PAX6* gene on band 11p13 is the cause of aniridia, which can be spo-radic or familial. The familial form is autosomal dominant with complete penetrance but

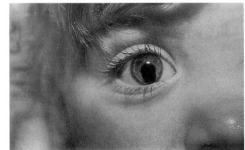

Figure 20-11 Typical iris coloboma, right eye.

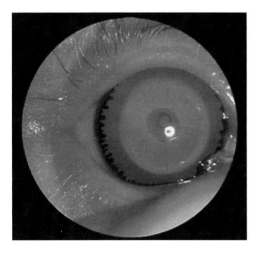

Figure 20-12 Aniridia in an infant. Both the ciliary processes and the edge of the lens are visible. Also present are persistent pupillary membrane fibers and a small central anterior polar cataract.

variable expressivity. There are reports of autosomal dominant pedigrees in which patients have severe glaucoma but normal maculae and good central vision. Two-thirds of all aniridic children have affected parents. The *PAX6* gene is the master control gene for eye morphogenesis. This gene is involved in the complex interactions between the optic cup, surface ectoderm, and neural crest during formation of the iris and other ocular structures. Many mutations of the *PAX6* gene have been reported. It is likely that they cause aniridia by reducing the amount of functional PAX6 protein.

Sporadic aniridia is associated with Wilms tumor (nephroblastoma) in as many as one-third of cases. When associated with aniridia, Wilms tumor is diagnosed before patients reach age 5 in 80% of cases. The combination of aniridia and Wilms tumor represents a contiguous gene syndrome in which the adjacent *PAX6* and Wilms tumor *(WT1)* genes are both deleted. Some deletions create the WAGR complex of *W*ilms tumor, *a*niridia, *g*enitourinary malformations, and mental *r*etardation. All children with sporadic aniridia should undergo chromosomal deletion analysis to exclude the possibility of Wilms tumor formation. Positive results require consultation with an oncologist along with repeated abdominal ultrasonographic examinations. Because Wilms tumor has been reported in patients with familial aniridia, these patients should also undergo chromosomal analysis.

Congenital iris ectropion

Ectropion of the posterior pigment epithelium onto the anterior surface of the iris is called *ectropion uveae* in much of the literature. This term is a misnomer, however, because the iris posterior epithelium is derived from neural ectoderm and is not considered part of the uvea. Iris ectropion can occur as an acquired tractional abnormality, often associated with rubeosis iridis, or as a congenital nonprogressive abnormality. The combination of unilateral congenital iris ectropion, a glassy-smooth cryptless iris surface, a high iris insertion, dysgenesis of the drainage angle, and glaucoma has been called *congenital iris ectropion syndrome*. Congenital iris ectropion may occur in patients with neurofibromatosis, facial hemihypertrophy, and Prader-Willi syndrome.

Abnormalities in the Size, Shape, or Location of the Pupil

Dyscoria

Dyscoria is an abnormality of the shape of the pupil. The term is usually reserved for congenital malformations, which include iris colobomas and sectoral hypoplasia. Slitlike pupils have been described in Axenfeld-Rieger syndrome (see Fig 20-9), in ectopia lentis et pupillae, and, in rare cases, as an isolated condition with normal vision. Acquired inflammatory conditions can lead to posterior synechiae, which can also produce a misshapen pupil.

Congenital miosis

Congenital miosis, or *microcoria,* may represent an absence or malformation of the dilator pupillae muscle. Congenital miosis can also occur secondary to contracture of fibrous material on the pupil margin due to remnants of the tunica vasculosa lentis or neural crest cell anomalies. The condition may be unilateral or bilateral and sporadic or hereditary. Severe cases require surgical pupilloplasty.

The pupil rarely exceeds 2 mm in diameter, is often eccentric, and reacts poorly to mydriatic drops. Some patients with eccentric microcoria also have lens subluxation; this combination is thus part of the spectrum of ectopia lentis et pupillae. Congenital miosis may be associated with microcornea, cataract, megalocornea, iris atrophy, iris transillumination, myopia, glaucoma, congenital rubella syndrome, hereditary ataxia, and Lowe syndrome.

Congenital mydriasis

Pupils that are dilated and fixed at birth but accompanied by normal-appearing irides have been reported; this has been called *familial iridoplegia* and *congenital bilateral mydriasis.* Iris sphincter trauma, pharmacologic mydriasis, and acquired neurologic disease affecting the parasympathetic innervation to the pupil are differential diagnoses. Many cases of congenital mydriasis fall within the aniridia spectrum, especially if the central iris structures from the collarette to the pupillary sphincter are absent. Congenital heart defects may be associated in patients with *ACTA2* mutations.

Milewicz DM, Østergaard JR, Ala-Kokko LM, et al. De novo *ACTA2* mutation causes a novel syndrome of multisystemic smooth muscle dysfunction. *Am J Med Genet A.* 2010;152A(10): 2437–2443.

Corectopia

Corectopia refers to displacement of the pupil. Normally, the pupil is situated approximately 0.5 mm inferonasally from the center of the iris. Minor deviations up to 1.0 mm are usually cosmetically insignificant and are not considered abnormal. Sector iris hypoplasia or other colobomatous lesions can lead to corectopia, and isolated noncolobomatous, autosomal dominant corectopia has been reported. More commonly, however, corectopia is associated with lens subluxation, and this combination is called *ectopia lentis et pupillae.* This autosomal recessive condition is almost always bilateral, with the pupils and lenses displaced in opposite directions. The pupils may be very small and misshapen. They often dilate poorly. Iris transillumination may occur, and microspherophakia has been reported.

Progressive corectopia can be associated with Axenfeld-Rieger or ICE syndrome. Vision may be good, even with eccentric pupils.

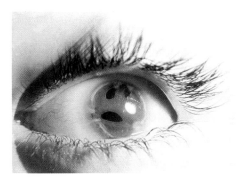

Figure 20-13 Pseudopolycoria that is secondary to Axenfeld-Rieger syndrome. *(Courtesy of John W. Simon, MD.)*

Polycoria and pseudopolycoria

True polycoria, which by definition must include a sphincter mechanism in each pupil, is very rare. The majority of accessory iris openings can be classified as *pseudopolycoria*. These iris holes may be congenital or may develop in response to progressive corectopia and iris hypoplasia in Axenfeld-Rieger (Fig 20-13) or ICE syndrome. Pseudopolycoria can also result from trauma, surgery, or persistent pupillary membranes.

Acquired Corneal Conditions

Keratitis

Keratitis may be epithelial, stromal, peripheral, or, in rare cases, endothelial.

Infectious causes

Congenital syphilis Interstitial keratitis may occur in the first decade of life secondary to congenital syphilis. The keratitis presents as a rapidly progressive corneal edema followed by abnormal vascularization in the deep stroma adjacent to Descemet membrane. Intense vascularization may give the cornea a salmon-pink color—hence the term *salmon patch*. Blood flow through these vessels gradually ceases over several weeks to several months, leaving empty "ghost" vessels in the corneal stroma. Immune-mediated uveitis, arthritis, and hearing loss may also develop and recur even after treatment of syphilis. Immunosuppression may be necessary to diminish sequelae. See also Chapter 28.

Herpes simplex infection Eye involvement in congenital HSV infection can include conjunctivitis, keratitis, retinochoroiditis, and cataracts. Congenital HSV infection is discussed in Chapter 28.

Adenovirus Punctate epithelial keratitis is most often seen after adenoviral infection and is due to subepithelial immune complex deposition.

Noninfectious causes

Punctate epithelial erosions are most commonly seen in patients with lagophthalmos or dry eye disease. Peripheral (marginal) keratitis is usually associated with blepharokeratoconjunctivitis secondary to meibomian gland disease.

Thygeson superficial punctate keratitis The etiology of this condition is unclear, but it is thought to be immune mediated. It can occur in children and presents with tearing, photophobia, and reduced vision. It is bilateral but often asymmetric. Characteristic features include slightly elevated gray corneal epithelial lesions that do not stain. It is treated with mild steroids (eg, fluorometholone 0.1%) or topical cyclosporine 0.05%.

Cogan syndrome Cogan syndrome is a rare vasculitis that presents with ocular, audiovestibular, and systemic features. Interstitial keratitis, uveitis, conjunctivitis, episcleritis, or a combination of these features may be seen.

Systemic Diseases Affecting the Cornea or Iris

Metabolic Disorders Affecting the Cornea or Iris

See the section Inborn Errors of Metabolism in Chapter 28 for additional discussion of some of the disorders covered here.

Mucopolysaccharidosis

Corneal haze may be present in early life in 3 lysosomal disorders: by age 6 months in mucopolysaccharidosis I H *(Hurler syndrome);* by age 12–24 months in mucopolysaccharidosis I S *(Scheie syndrome);* and as early as age 6 weeks in mucopolysaccharidosis IV *(Morquio syndrome).* Treatment options for significant opacities include penetrating keratoplasty and DALK.

Cystinosis

Cystinosis is a rare metabolic disease characterized by elevated levels of cystine within the cell. Cystine crystals are deposited in various places throughout the body. The major presenting symptoms of the infantile form of cystinosis are failure to thrive, rickets, and progressive renal failure, collectively resulting in Fanconi syndrome. The ocular findings of cystinosis are pathognomonic. Iridescent elongated corneal crystals appear at approximately age 1 year, first in the peripheral part of the cornea and the anterior part of the stroma (Fig 20-14). Severe photophobia can make slit-lamp examination difficult. These crystals are also present in the uvea and on the surface of the iris. As survival has

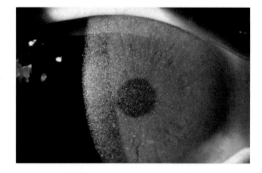

Figure 20-14 Cystinosis with corneal involvement. *(Courtesy of Gregg T. Lueder, MD.)*

improved, reports of angle-closure glaucoma secondary to crystal deposition in the ciliary body have increased. Oral cysteamine has been shown to alleviate the systemic problems but not the corneal crystal deposition. Topical cysteamine can reduce crystal deposition in the cornea. However, the medication may be difficult to obtain and has an unpleasant odor, and treatment is complicated by the need for frequent application.

Tyrosinemia

Children with tyrosinemia often present with photophobia, pseudodendritic ulcers on the cornea, and ulceration on the palms and soles. Systemic problems include liver and kidney dysfunction.

Hepatolenticular degeneration

Hepatolenticular degeneration *(Wilson disease),* an autosomal recessive inborn error of metabolism, results in excess copper deposition in the liver, kidneys, and basal ganglia of the brain, leading to cirrhosis, renal tubular damage, and a Parkinson-like disorder of motor function. The characteristic copper-colored Kayser-Fleischer ring is limited to Descemet membrane and can be several millimeters in width. It may resolve with treatment. Because this ring can develop fairly late, laboratory tests for serum copper and ceruloplasmin are better than an eye examination for early diagnosis.

Fabry disease

Fabry disease is a rare X-linked lysosomal storage disease due to α-galactosidase deficiency. Vortex keratopathy (verticillata) can be seen in affected males and in female carriers.

Schnyder crystalline dystrophy

Schnyder crystalline dystrophy is caused by mutations in the *UBIAD1* gene and is thought to be a local disorder of corneal lipid metabolism.

Other Systemic Diseases Affecting the Cornea or Iris

Familial dysautonomia

Familial dysautonomia *(Riley-Day syndrome),* a complex autosomal recessive condition, occurs largely in children of Eastern European Jewish (Ashkenazi) descent. It is characterized by autonomic dysfunction, relative insensitivity to pain, temperature instability, and absence of the fungiform papillae of the tongue. Exposure keratitis and corneal ulcers with secondary opacification are frequent problems because of abnormal lacrimation and decreased corneal sensitivity. Failure to respond with a wheal and flare to intradermal injection of 1:1000 histamine solution is characteristic of this condition. Treatment includes artificial tears and tarsorrhaphy. Most cases of familial dysautonomia are caused by a mutation in the *IKBKAP* gene.

Waardenburg syndrome

Waardenburg syndrome is a rare neurocristopathy characterized by Hirschsprung disease, deafness, and depigmentation of hair (a white forelock), skin, and iris.

Tumors of the Cornea, Iris, and Anterior Segment

Cornea

Tumors of the cornea are extremely rare in children, but squamous cell carcinomas have been reported in cases of xeroderma pigmentosum.

Iris

Nodules

Lisch nodules Lisch nodules occur in patients with neurofibromatosis (see Chapter 28).

Juvenile xanthogranuloma Juvenile xanthogranuloma is a nonneoplastic histiocytic pro-liferation that develops in infants younger than 2 years. It is characterized by the presence of Touton giant cells. Skin involvement—consisting of 1 or more small, round, orange or tan papules—is typically but not always present. Iris lesions are relatively rare and virtu-ally always unilateral. The fleshy yellow-brown masses may be small and localized or may diffusely infiltrate the entire iris, resulting in heterochromia. Spontaneous bleeding with hyphema is a characteristic clinical presentation. Secondary glaucoma may cause acute pain, photophobia, and vision loss. Those at greatest risk for ocular involvement are chil-dren with multiple skin lesions.

Juvenile xanthogranuloma is a self-limited condition that usually regresses spontane-ously by age 5 years, but to avoid complications, treatment is indicated for ocular involve-ment. Topical corticosteroids and pharmacologic agents to lower intraocular pressure, given as necessary, are generally sufficient to control the problem. Surgical excision or radiation should be considered if intractable glaucoma is present.

Iris mammillations Iris mammillations may be unilateral or bilateral. They appear as nu-merous tiny, diffuse, pigmented nodules on the surface of the iris (Fig 20-15). They are more common in darkly pigmented eyes and are usually the same color as the iris. These nodules may be bilateral, autosomal dominant, and isolated, or they may be associated with oculodermal melanocytosis or phakomatosis pigmentovascularis type IIb (nevus flammeus with persistent, aberrant mongolian spots). Iris mammillations have also been reported in cases of ciliary body tumor and choroidal melanoma. They must be differ-entiated from Lisch nodules; mammillations are usually dark brown, smooth, uniformly distributed, and equal in size or slightly larger near the pupil. The incidence of iris mam-millations is higher among patients with neurofibromatosis 1.

Brushfield spots Focal areas of iris stromal hyperplasia surrounded by relative hypo-plasia occur in up to 90% of patients with Down syndrome; in such patients, these areas are known as *Brushfield spots*. They are hypopigmented. Similar lesions, known as *Wolf-flin nodules,* occur in up to 24% of healthy individuals. Neither condition is visually significant.

Cysts

Primary iris cysts These cysts may originate from the iris pigment epithelium or the iris stroma.

CYSTS OF IRIS PIGMENT EPITHELIUM Spontaneous cysts of the iris pigment epithelium result from a separation of the 2 layers of epithelium anywhere between the pupil and ciliary body (Fig 20-16). These cysts tend to be stable and rarely cause ocular complications. They are usually not diagnosed until the teenaged years.

CENTRAL CYSTS Pigment epithelial cysts at the pupillary border are sometimes hereditary. They are usually diagnosed in infancy. They may enlarge slowly but generally remain asymptomatic and rarely require treatment. Rupture of these cysts can result in iris flocculi. Cholinesterase-inhibiting eyedrops such as echothiophate may produce similar pupillary cysts, especially in young phakic eyes. Discontinuation of the drug or concomitant administration of phenylephrine generally results in improvement.

CYSTS OF IRIS STROMA Primary iris stromal cysts are often diagnosed in infancy. They are most likely caused by sequestration of epithelium during embryologic development. The epithelium-lined stromal cysts usually contain goblet cells, and they may enlarge, causing obstruction of the visual axis, glaucoma, corneal decompensation, or iritis from cyst leakage. Numerous treatments have been described, including cyst aspiration and photocoagulation or photodisruption, but the sudden release of cystic contents may result in transient iritis and glaucoma. Because of these potential complications and frequent cyst recurrence, surgical excision may be the preferred treatment method. Iris stromal cysts account for approximately 16% of childhood iris cysts. The visual prognosis is guarded.

Secondary iris cysts Secondary iris cysts have been reported in childhood after trauma; they are also associated with tumors and iris nevi.

Ciliary Body

Medulloepithelioma

A medulloepithelioma *(diktyoma)* originates from the nonpigmented epithelium of the ciliary body and most often presents as an iris mass during the first decade of life. Secondary

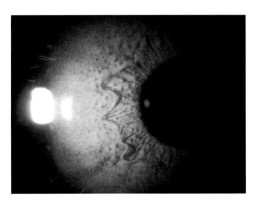

Figure 20-15 Iris mammillations. Nodules are diffuse and are the same color as the iris (Lisch nodules, by contrast, are lighter or darker than the surrounding iris). *(Courtesy of Arlene Drack, MD.)*

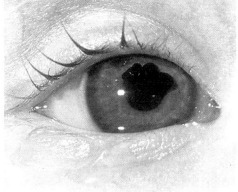

Figure 20-16 Cysts of the pigmented epithelium of the iris at the pupillary border (flocculi).

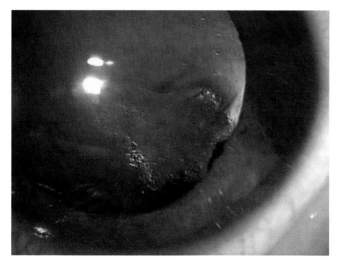

Figure 20-17 Sectoral cataract adjacent to medulloepithelioma. *(Courtesy of Ken K. Nischal, MD.)*

glaucoma, hyphema, and ectopia lentis et pupillae or sectoral cataract (Fig 20-17) are less frequent initial manifestations. This rare lesion shows a spectrum of clinical and pathologic characteristics, ranging from benign to malignant. Although distant metastasis is rare, local invasion can lead to death. Teratoid elements are often present. Enucleation is usually required and is curative in most cases.

Miscellaneous Clinical Signs

Pediatric Iris Heterochromia

The differential diagnosis of pediatric iris heterochromia is extensive. Causes can be classified based on whether the condition is congenital or acquired and whether the affected eye is hypopigmented or hyperpigmented (Fig 20-18; Table 20-3). Trauma, chronic iridocyclitis, intraocular surgery, and use of topical prostaglandin analogues are important causes of acquired hyperpigmented heterochromia. Whether congenital or acquired, hypopigmented heterochromia that is associated with a more miotic pupil and ptosis on the ipsilateral side should prompt a workup for Horner syndrome (see the discussion later in this chapter).

Anisocoria

Inequality in the diameters of the 2 pupils is called *anisocoria*. For a detailed discussion of anisocoria and the following conditions, see BCSC Section 5, *Neuro-Ophthalmology*.

Physiologic anisocoria

Physiologic anisocoria is a common cause of a difference in size between the 2 pupils. This difference is usually less than 1 mm and can vary from day to day in an individual. The inequality does not change significantly when the patient is in dim light or bright light.

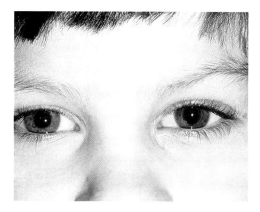

Figure 20-18 Iris heterochromia. The left iris has become darker since development of a traumatic cataract. *(Courtesy of John W. Simon, MD.)*

Table 20-3 Causes of Pediatric Iris Heterochromia

Hypochromic heterochromia
Horner syndrome (congenital or early in life)
Incontinentia pigmenti (Bloch-Sulzberger syndrome; rare)
Fuchs heterochromia
Waardenburg syndrome
Nonpigmented tumors
Hypomelanosis of Ito
Hyperchromic heterochromia
Oculodermal melanocytosis (associated with glaucoma in nonwhite adults)
Pigmented tumors
Siderosis
Iris ectropion syndrome
Extensive rubeosis
Port-wine stain

Modified with permission from Roy FH. *Ocular Differential Diagnosis*. 3rd ed. Philadelphia: Lea & Febiger; 1984.

Tonic pupil

Features of a tonic pupil include anisocoria that is greater in bright light and a pupil that is sluggishly and segmentally responsive to light and more responsive to near effort. Greater than normal constriction in response to dilute pilocarpine is diagnostic. Possible etiologic causes in children include varicella-zoster virus and Adie syndrome with absence of deep tendon reflexes.

Horner syndrome

A lesion at any location along the oculosympathetic pathway may lead to Horner syndrome. Affected patients have anisocoria that is greater in dim light and ptosis secondary to paralysis of the Müller muscle. Congenital cases may be associated with iris heterochromia in which the affected iris is lighter in color. However, the heterochromia may not be present in infants because the normal pupil needs time to acquire pigment.

The diagnosis of Horner syndrome can be confirmed with the use of topical cocaine or apraclonidine drops. Apraclonidine reverses the anisocoria, causing dilation of the affected (smaller) pupil and having no effect on the normal pupil. This agent should be used with caution in young children, as it may cause excessive sedation due to its central nervous system effects. Additional pharmacologic testing may not be necessary in the presence of typical clinical findings.

Horner syndrome in children may be idiopathic or due to trauma, surgery, or the presence of neuroblastoma affecting the sympathetic chain in the chest. For children with acquired Horner syndrome but no history of trauma or surgery that could explain the anisocoria, evaluation should include imaging studies of the brain, neck, and chest. The value of measuring catecholamine excretion has been questioned because some patients with catecholamine measurements that are not abnormal have been found to have neuroblastomas.

CHAPTER 21

External Diseases of the Eye

This chapter focuses on external diseases of the eye that are seen in the pediatric population. Many of the topics covered in this chapter are also discussed in BCSC Section 8, *External Disease and Cornea.*

Infectious Conjunctivitis

Bacterial and viral infections are the most common causes of infectious conjunctivitis in children in developed countries. Patients with infectious conjunctivitis commonly present with burning, stinging, foreign-body sensation, ocular discharge, and matting of the eyelids. Symptoms and signs may present unilaterally or bilaterally. The character of the discharge, which can provide some diagnostic help, may be serous, mucopurulent, or purulent. Purulent discharge suggests a polymorphonuclear response to a bacterial infection; mucopurulent discharge suggests a viral or chlamydial infection; and a serous or watery discharge suggests a viral or allergic reaction. Membrane or pseudomembrane formation may be seen in severe viral or bacterial conjunctivitis, Stevens-Johnson syndrome, ligneous conjunctivitis, and chemical burns. Table 21-1 lists common causes of conjunctival injection, or *red eye,* in infants and children.

Table 21-1 Common Causes of Conjunctival Injection in Children

Infectious conjunctivitis
  Bacterial infection
    Chlamydial infection
  Viral infection
Blepharitis
Allergic conjunctivitis
Trauma
Foreign body
Drug, toxic, or chemical reaction
Nasolacrimal duct obstruction
Iritis
Episcleritis or scleritis

Ophthalmia Neonatorum

Ophthalmia neonatorum refers to conjunctivitis occurring in the first month of life. This condition can be caused by bacterial, viral, and chemical agents. Widespread effective prophylaxis has diminished its occurrence to very low levels in industrialized countries, but ophthalmia neonatorum remains a significant cause of ocular infection, blindness, and even death in medically underserved areas around the world.

Epidemiology and etiology

Worldwide, the incidence of ophthalmia neonatorum is greater in areas with high rates of sexually transmitted disease and poor health care. The prevalence ranges from 0.1% in highly developed countries with effective prenatal and perinatal care to 10% in areas such as East Africa. Because a mother may have multiple sexually transmitted diseases, infants with one type of ophthalmia neonatorum should be screened for other such diseases. Public health authorities should be contacted to initiate evaluation and treatment of other maternal contacts in cases of sexually transmitted diseases.

The causative organism usually infects the infant through direct contact during passage through the birth canal. Infection can ascend to the uterus, especially if there is prolonged rupture of membranes, so even infants delivered by cesarean section can be infected.

Neisseria gonorrhoeae

Ophthalmia neonatorum caused by *Neisseria gonorrhoeae* typically presents in the first 3–4 days of life. Patients may present with mild conjunctival hyperemia and discharge. In severe cases, there is marked chemosis, copious discharge, and potentially rapid corneal ulceration and perforation of the eye (Fig 21-1). Systemic infection can cause sepsis, meningitis, and arthritis.

Gram stain of the conjunctival exudate showing gram-negative intracellular diplococci allows for a presumptive diagnosis of *N gonorrhoeae* infection; treatment should be started immediately. Ophthalmia neonatorum from *Neisseria meningitidis* has also been reported. Definitive diagnosis is based on culture of the conjunctival discharge. Treatment of gonococcal ophthalmia neonatorum includes systemic ceftriaxone and topical irrigation with saline. Topical antibiotics may be indicated if there is corneal involvement.

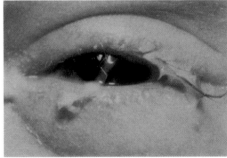

Figure 21-1 *Neisseria gonorrhoeae* conjunctivitis.

Chlamydia trachomatis

Chlamydia trachomatis is an obligate intracellular bacterium that causes neonatal inclusion conjunctivitis. Onset of conjunctivitis usually occurs around 1 week of age, although onset may be earlier, especially in cases with premature rupture of membranes. Eye infection is characterized by minimal to moderate discharge, mild swelling of the eyelids, and hyperemia with a papillary reaction of the conjunctiva. Severe cases may be accompanied by more copious discharge and pseudomembrane formation. Chlamydial infection in infants differs from that in adults in several ways: in infants, there is no follicular response, membrane formation may occur, and there is greater mucopurulent discharge.

Chlamydial infections can be diagnosed by culture of conjunctival scrapings, polymerase chain reaction, direct fluorescent antibody tests, and enzyme immunoassays. Systemic treatment of neonatal chlamydial disease is indicated because of the risk of pneumonia and otitis media. The treatment of choice is oral erythromycin, 50 mg/kg per day in 4 divided doses for 14 days.

Herpes simplex virus

Infection with herpes simplex virus (HSV) is usually secondary to HSV type 2 and typically presents later than infection with *N gonorrhoeae* or *C trachomatis,* frequently in the second week of life. See the discussion of congenital HSV infection in Chapter 28.

Chemical conjunctivitis

Chemical conjunctivitis refers to a mild, self-limited irritation and redness of the conjunctiva occurring in the first 24 hours after instillation of silver nitrate, a preparation used for prophylaxis against ophthalmia neonatorum. This condition improves spontaneously by the second day of life.

Prophylaxis for ophthalmia neonatorum

In 1880, Credé introduced the concept of widespread prophylaxis for gonorrheal ophthalmia neonatorum with 2% silver nitrate. Silver nitrate prophylaxis significantly reduced the incidence of gonorrheal conjunctivitis and is still used in some parts of the world. Silver nitrate is not effective against *C trachomatis* and thus has been supplanted by agents that act against both *N gonorrhoeae* and *C trachomatis,* such as erythromycin and tetracycline ointments.

A clinical trial for ophthalmia neonatorum conducted in Kenya showed that povidone-iodine drops are more effective and less toxic than erythromycin or silver nitrate ointment. Povidone-iodine is particularly useful in developing countries because of its low cost and ease of application.

Bacterial Conjunctivitis

The most common causes of bacterial conjunctivitis in school-aged children are *Streptococcus pneumoniae, Haemophilus* species, *Staphylococcus aureus,* and *Moraxella.* The incidence of infection from *Haemophilus* has decreased because of widespread immunization.

More severe forms of bacterial conjunctivitis accompanied by copious discharge suggest infection with more virulent organisms, including *N gonorrhoeae* and *N meningitidis*.

Diagnosis is by clinical presentation. Culture to identify the offending agent is usually not necessary in mild cases but should be done in severe cases. If untreated, symptoms are self-limited but may last up to 2 weeks. A broad-spectrum topical ophthalmic drop or ointment should shorten the course to a few days. Topical medications that are usually effective include polymyxin combinations, aminoglycosides, erythromycin, bacitracin, fluoroquinolones, and azithromycin. The fluoroquinolones are considerably more expensive than other medications and may give rise to drug-resistant organisms. Patients with *N meningitidis* conjunctivitis, and others exposed to these patients, require systemic treatment because of the high risk of meningitis.

Parinaud oculoglandular syndrome

Parinaud oculoglandular syndrome (POS) manifests as unilateral granulomatous conjunctivitis associated with preauricular and submandibular adenopathy that can be very marked (Fig 21-2). *Bartonella henselae*, a pleomorphic gram-negative bacillus that is endemic in cats and causes cat-scratch disease, is the most common cause of POS. Other causative organisms include *Mycobacterium tuberculosis*, *Mycobacterium leprae*, *Francisella tularensis*, *Yersinia pseudotuberculosis*, *Treponema pallidum*, and *C trachomatis*. Cat-scratch disease is usually associated with a scratch from a kitten, but a cat bite or even touching the eye with a hand that has been licked by an infected kitten can cause the disease.

Serologic testing is an effective means of diagnosing POS. Presence of antibodies to *B henselae*, detected by indirect fluorescent antibody testing or enzyme immunoassay, can confirm a diagnosis of cat-scratch disease. Treatment can be supportive in mild cases of cat-scratch disease because the disease is self-limited. In more severe cases systemic treatment, usually with azithromycin, may be indicated. Appropriate systemic antibiotics are used to treat the other organisms that cause POS.

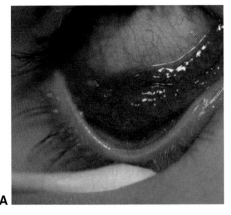 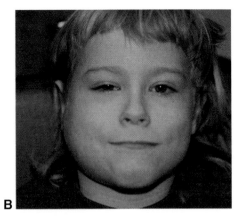

A   **B**

Figure 21-2 Parinaud oculoglandular syndrome. **A,** Marked follicular reaction in lower fornix. **B,** Massive enlargement of submandibular lymph node on affected right side. *(Courtesy of David A. Plager, MD.)*

Chlamydial infections

Two different diseases can be caused by *C trachomatis* in children and adolescents: trachoma and adult inclusion conjunctivitis.

Trachoma Trachoma is the most common cause of preventable blindness in the world. This disease is uncommon in Europe and the United States, except in areas of the southern United States and on Native American reservations. It is caused by poor hygiene and inadequate sanitation and is spread from eye to eye or by flies or fomites. Clinical manifestations include acute purulent conjunctivitis, a follicular reaction, papillary hypertrophy, vascularization of the cornea, and progressive cicatricial changes of the cornea and conjunctiva. Diagnosis is made by Giemsa stain, cell culture, or polymerase chain reaction. Treatment includes both topical and systemic erythromycin. Tetracycline can be used in children 8 years of age and older.

Adult inclusion conjunctivitis Adult inclusion conjunctivitis is a sexually transmitted disease that can be found in sexually active teenagers in association with chlamydial urethritis or cervicitis. Patients present with follicular conjunctivitis, scant mucopurulent discharge, and preauricular adenopathy. There is no membrane formation. This condition can be diagnosed by culture of conjunctival scrapings, polymerase chain reaction, direct fluorescent antibody tests, and enzyme immunoassays. If untreated, inclusion conjunctivitis resolves spontaneously in 6–18 months. The recommended treatment is oral tetracycline, doxycycline, or azithromycin. The clinician should consider whether the patient has been sexually abused, especially if adult inclusion conjunctivitis is found in a young child.

Viral Conjunctivitis

Adenovirus

Viral conjunctivitis is most often caused by adenovirus, a DNA virus that can cause a range of human diseases, including upper respiratory tract infection and gastroenteritis. The following adenovirus diseases are listed with their associated serotypes: epidemic keratoconjunctivitis (serotypes 8, 19, and 37), pharyngoconjunctival fever (serotypes 3 and 7), acute hemorrhagic conjunctivitis (serotypes 11 and 21), and acute follicular conjunctivitis (serotypes 1, 2, 3, 4, 7, and 10).

Epidemic keratoconjunctivitis Epidemic keratoconjunctivitis (EKC) is a highly contagious conjunctivitis that tends to occur in epidemic outbreaks. This infection is an acute bilateral follicular conjunctivitis that is usually unilateral at onset and associated with preauricular adenopathy. Initial symptoms are foreign-body sensation and periorbital pain. A diffuse superficial keratitis is followed by focal epithelial lesions that stain. After 11–15 days, subepithelial opacities begin to form under the focal epithelial infiltrates. The epithelial component fades by day 30, but the subepithelial opacities may remain for up to 2 years. In severe infections, particularly in infants, a conjunctival membrane forms and marked swelling of the eyelids occurs; these signs must be differentiated from those of orbital or preseptal cellulitis. In severe cases, complications include persistent subepithelial opacities and conjunctival scar formation.

Because EKC is easily transmitted, medical personnel who become infected should be excluded from patient contact for up to 2 weeks, and isolation areas should be designated for examination of patients known or suspected to have adenoviral infections.

Diagnosis is usually based on clinical presentation but can be confirmed in the office by a rapid immunodetection assay. The organism can be recovered from the eyes and throat for 2 weeks after onset, demonstrating that patients are infectious during this period. Treatment is supportive in most cases. Artificial tears and cold compresses can provide symptomatic relief. Topical steroids may be used judiciously to decrease symptoms in severe cases and in cases of decreased vision secondary to subepithelial opacities; however, such agents may prolong the time to full recovery. Steroid use in adenovirus infection is seldom indicated in children.

Pharyngoconjunctival fever Pharyngoconjunctival fever presents with conjunctival hyperemia, subconjunctival hemorrhage, conjunctival edema, epiphora, and eyelid swelling, accompanied by sore throat and fever. Within a few days, a follicular conjunctival reaction and preauricular adenopathy develop. Symptoms may last for 2 weeks or more. Treatment is supportive because no topical or systemic treatment alters the course of the disease.

Herpes simplex virus

Conjunctivitis caused by HSV type 1 is covered in BCSC Section 8, *External Disease and Cornea*. Neonatal HSV infection is discussed in Chapter 28.

Varicella-zoster virus

Varicella-zoster virus (VZV) is a herpesvirus that can cause varicella and herpes zoster.

Varicella Varicella (chickenpox) is a contagious viral exanthem of childhood caused by primary infection with VZV. It presents with fever and vesicular eruptions of the skin and mucous membranes. Varicella vaccine is very effective in preventing severe disease, but immunized children exposed to VZV may develop mild symptoms. Clinical manifestations of primary VZV infection include fever and characteristic skin lesions. Except for eyelid vesicles and follicular conjunctivitis, ocular involvement is uncommon. Treatment of conjunctival disease is usually not necessary. Intravenous or oral acyclovir may be considered in the treatment of immunocompromised children with varicella.

Herpes zoster Reactivation of latent VZV from dorsal root and cranial nerve ganglia results in herpes zoster. Vesicular lesions may erupt on the periorbital skin in a dermatome configuration, with subsequent ocular involvement (Fig 21-3). Keratitis and anterior uveitis are most likely if the nasociliary branch of cranial nerve V is affected. Oral acyclovir is indicated in healthy children to shorten the course of the illness and decrease the risk of bacterial superinfection. Intravenous antiviral agents (famciclovir, valacyclovir, acyclovir) are indicated in immunocompromised patients or patients with severe disseminated disease. Antiviral medications should be started within 72 hours of onset of symptoms.

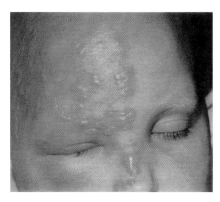

Figure 21-3 Herpes zoster.

Epstein-Barr virus

Epstein-Barr virus is a herpesvirus that can cause infectious mononucleosis. This disease usually occurs between ages 15 and 30 years and is benign and self-limited. Findings include fever, widespread adenopathy, pharyngitis, hepatic involvement, and the presence of atypical lymphocytes in the circulating blood. Conjunctivitis is the most common ocular finding. Nummular keratitis may also be seen. Diagnosis is confirmed with detection of immunoglobulin M (IgM) antibodies to viral capsid antigens or with a positive heterophile antibody test. Ocular treatment is cool compresses to the eyes.

Molluscum contagiosum

Molluscum contagiosum is caused by a DNA poxvirus and usually presents as numerous umbilicated skin lesions (Fig 21-4A). Lesions on or near the eyelid margin can release viral particles onto the conjunctival surface, resulting in a follicular conjunctivitis (Fig 21-4B). Most lesions do not require treatment because they tend to resolve spontaneously; however, resolution can take months or years. Lesions causing conjunctivitis can be treated by

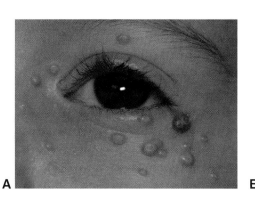
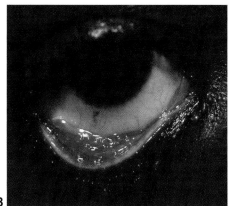

A **B**

Figure 21-4 Molluscum contagiosum. **A,** Eyelid lesions. **B,** Secondary follicular conjunctivitis.
(Part A courtesy of Edward L. Raab, MD; part B courtesy of Gregg T. Lueder, MD.)

incising each lesion and debriding the central core. For young children, such treatment usually requires general anesthesia.

Inflammatory Disease

Blepharitis

Though less common in children than in adults, blepharitis is a common cause of chronic conjunctivitis in children. The signs and symptoms in children are similar to those in adults and include ocular irritation, morning crusting, eyelid margin erythema, and meibomian gland obstruction. Intermittent blurred vision may be present because of tear-film instability. Inferior keratitis may develop in more severe cases. Recurrent chalazia in children may indicate underlying blepharitis. Acne rosacea in children may present with chronic blepharitis and facial telangiectasias, papules, and pustules. *Demodex* (human mites that inhabit the hair follicles) may play a role in the pathogenesis of blepharitis.

Initial treatment of blepharitis includes warm compresses, eyelid scrubs with baby shampoo, and topical antibiotic ointment. Severe cases may benefit from either oral erythromycin or tetracycline. Erythromycin is most commonly used in young children to avoid the potential dental staining associated with use of tetracycline. Judicious use of topical steroids may be indicated in patients with corneal disease. Dietary supplementation with flaxseed oil (omega-3 fatty acid) may benefit some patients.

> Jones SM, Weinstein JM, Cumberland P, et al. Visual outcome and corneal changes in children with chronic blepharokeratoconjunctivitis. *Ophthalmology.* 2007;114(12):2271–2280.

Ocular Allergy

Allergies are thought to affect approximately 20% of the US population, and more than 50% of patients who seek treatment present with ocular symptoms. Allergic ocular disease is a common problem in children and is often associated with asthma, allergic rhinitis, and atopic dermatitis. Marked itching and bilateral conjunctival inflammation of a chronic, recurrent, and possibly seasonal nature are hallmarks of external ocular disease of allergic origin. Other signs and symptoms may be nonspecific and include tearing, stinging, burning, and photophobia.

Three specific types of ocular allergy are discussed in this section: seasonal allergic conjunctivitis, vernal keratoconjunctivitis (VKC), and atopic keratoconjunctivitis (AKC). All have some element of a type I hypersensitivity reaction caused by the interaction between an allergen and specific immunoglobulin E (IgE) antibodies on the surface of mast cells in the conjunctiva. This interaction initiates a cascade of biochemical events involved in mediation of the allergic response. Among the mediators released is histamine, which causes much of the itching, vasodilation, and edema that are characteristic of the ocular allergic response.

Seasonal allergic conjunctivitis

Seasonal allergic conjunctivitis is a common clinical entity that affects approximately 40 million people in the United States, including many children. It occurs in the spring and fall and is triggered by environmental contact with specific airborne allergens such as pollens from grasses, flowers, weeds, and trees. Patients typically present with red, watery eyes; boggy-appearing conjunctiva; and ocular itching. Blue-gray to purple discoloration of the lower eyelids, termed *allergic shiners,* can occur secondary to venous stasis from nasal congestion. Perennial allergic conjunctivitis is similar to seasonal allergic conjunctivitis and is a type I hypersensitivity reaction that occurs after contact with ubiquitous household allergens, such as dust mites and dander from domestic pets. This condition is diagnosed based on clinical presentation. Conjunctival scrapings reveal eosinophils, a finding that is almost diagnostic of an allergic response.

Treatment of all ocular allergy disorders is fundamentally similar to that of other allergy-related disorders. The most effective treatment is to remove the offending allergens from the patient's environment. Unfortunately, attempts at removal may not be adequate to alleviate the patient's symptoms. Medical treatment can be systemic or topical. Although oral antihistamines may be less effective at relieving specific ocular symptoms, they are often better tolerated in children, because many have an aversion to eyedrops.

Topical medications include mast-cell stabilizers, H_1-receptor blockers, vasoconstrictors, corticosteroids, nonsteroidal anti-inflammatory agents, or combinations of these drugs (Table 21-2). Mast-cell stabilizers are often effective, but they must be used

Table 21-2 Topical Drops for Treatment of Allergic Eye Disorders

Over-the-counter antihistamines/vasoconstrictors
Naphazoline/antazoline (Vasocon-A)
Naphazoline/pheniramine (Naphcon-A, Opcon-A, Visine-A)

Mast-cell stabilizers
Cromolyn sodium 4%/2% (Crolom, Opticrom)
Lodoxamide tromethamine 0.1% (Alomide)
Nedocromil sodium 2% (Alocril)
Pemirolast potassium 0.1% (Alamast)

H_1-receptor antagonist
Emedastine difumarate 0.05% (Emadine)

Drops with both mast-cell stabilizer and H_1-blocker
Alcaftadine 0.25% (Lastacaft)
Azelastine hydrochloride 0.05% (Optivar)
Bepotastine besilate 1.5% (Bepreve)
Epinastine hydrochloride 0.05% (Elestat) [also H_2 blocker]
Ketotifen fumarate 0.025% (Alaway, Zaditor)
Olopatadine hydrochloride 0.1% (Patanol)
Olopatadine hydrochloride 0.2% (Pataday)

Corticosteroids
Fluorometholone 0.1%/0.25% (FML, Fluor-Op/FML Forte)
Loteprednol etabonate 0.5%/0.2% (Lotemax, Alrex)
Medrysone 1% (HMS)
Prednisolone acetate 1%/0.12% (Pred Forte, Econopred Plus/Pred Mild)
Rimexolone 1% (Vexol)

Nonsteroidal anti-inflammatory drug
Ketorolac tromethamine 0.5% (Acular)

Anti-inflammatory drug
Cyclosporine 0.05% (Restasis)

for a few days before an effect is seen. Nonsteroidal anti-inflammatory drops should be used with caution because associated corneal perforation has been reported. Topical steroid drops used in pulsed doses can effectively reduce severe allergic ocular symptoms, but patients must be closely monitored for adverse effects, including glaucoma and cataracts.

Vernal keratoconjunctivitis

VKC is caused by type I and type IV hypersensitivity reactions. This condition most commonly affects males in the first 2 decades of life and, like seasonal allergic conjunctivitis, usually occurs in the spring and fall. It occurs in 2 forms: palpebral and limbal (or bulbar). Both types present with severe itching. The limbal form is more common in patients of African or Asian decent and is more prevalent in hotter climates.

Clinically, the palpebral form of VKC preferentially affects the tarsal conjunctiva of the upper eyelid (Fig 21-5). In the early stages, the eye may be diffusely injected, with little discharge. There may be no progression beyond this stage. However, papillae may multiply, covering the tarsal area with a mosaic of flat papules. A thick, ropy, whitish discharge may develop.

The limbal form of VKC presents early with thickening and opacification of the conjunctiva at the limbus, usually most marked at the upper margin of the cornea. The discrete limbal nodules that appear are gray, jelly-like, elevated lumps with vascular cores. A whitish center may appear in the raised lesion filled with eosinophils and epithelioid cells. This complex is called a *Horner-Trantas dot*. Limbal nodules may increase in number and become confluent. They persist as long as the seasonal exacerbation of the disease lasts.

The cornea may become involved with punctate epithelial erosions, especially superiorly. Corneal involvement may progress to a large confluent area of epithelial defect, typically in the upper half of the cornea, called a *shield ulcer*. The ulcer is sterile and clinically resembles an ovoid corneal abrasion.

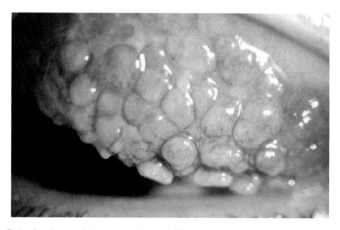

Figure 21-5 Palpebral vernal keratoconjunctivitis, upper eyelid. *(Courtesy of Ken K. Nischal, MD.)*

Treatment of VKC is usually less effective than that of seasonal allergic conjunctivitis. Eyedrops combining a mast-cell stabilizer and an H_1-receptor blocker may be used initially. Severe cases may require topical steroids or topical cyclosporine. Supratarsal injection of corticosteroids may be used in patients with refractory palpebral VKC.

Atopic keratoconjunctivitis

AKC is a nonseasonal disorder that occurs in patients with atopic disease. It is relatively rare in children. See BCSC Section 8, *External Disease and Cornea,* for further discussion.

Ligneous Conjunctivitis

Ligneous conjunctivitis is a rare bilateral chronic disorder characterized by firm, "woody," yellowish, fibrinous pseudomembranes on the palpebral conjunctiva. It is thought to be secondary to severe deficiency in type I plasminogen. No single treatment is consistently effective. Surgical removal, amniotic membrane transplantation, fresh frozen plasma, and heparin have been used.

Miscellaneous Conjunctival Disorders

Papillomas

Papillomas are benign epithelial proliferations that usually appear as sessile masses at the limbus or as pedunculated lesions of the caruncle, fornix, or palpebral conjunctiva. They may be transparent, pale yellow, or salmon colored. They are sometimes speckled with red dots. Papillomas in children usually result from viral infection. They often resolve spontaneously. Surgical excision is indicated if there is persistent associated conjunctivitis or keratitis or if new lesions continue to appear. Recurrence following surgical excision is possible. Oral cimetidine can induce papilloma regression.

Conjunctival Epithelial Inclusion Cysts

Conjunctival inclusion cysts are clear, fluid-filled cysts on the conjunctiva. These cysts are often seen in patients who had ocular surgery or trauma. Excision is indicated if the cysts cause irritation.

Conjunctival Nevi

Conjunctival nevi are relatively common in childhood. The lesions may be flat or elevated. Histologically, most of these nevi are compound (nevus cells found in both epithelium and substantia propria); others are junctional (nevus cells confined to the interface between epithelium and substantia propria). Nevi are typically brown, but approximately one-third are nonpigmented and have a pinkish appearance. The lesions are occasionally noted at birth; more commonly, they develop during later childhood or adolescence (Fig 21-6). Removal may be indicated if significant growth occurs, although transformation to malignant melanoma is extremely rare in childhood.

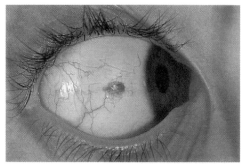

Figure 21-6 Pigmented nevus of the bulbar conjunctiva, right eye, recently developed in a 4-year-old girl.

Ocular Melanocytosis

Ocular melanocytosis *(melanosis oculi)* is a congenital abnormality characterized by unilateral patchy but extensive slate-gray or bluish discoloration of the sclera (Fig 21-7). Intraocular pigmentation is also increased, which is associated with a higher incidence of glaucoma and risk of malignant melanoma. Some patients, particularly persons of Asian ancestry, may have associated involvement of eyelid and adjacent skin with dermal hyperpigmentation that produces brown, bluish, or black discoloration without thickening *(oculodermal melanocytosis, nevus of Ota)*. Small patches of slate-gray scleral pigmentation, typically bilateral and without clinical significance, are common in black and Asian children. Melanosis of skin and sclera is occasionally associated with Sturge-Weber syndrome and Klippel-Trénaunay-Weber syndrome.

Stevens-Johnson Syndrome and Toxic Epidermal Necrolysis

Stevens-Johnson syndrome (SJS) and toxic epidermal necrolysis (TEN) are rare, life-threatening conditions that represent different intensities of an acute inflammatory systemic disease affecting skin and mucous membranes. In the pediatric population, the male to female ratio is 2:1. The mortality rate in the pediatric population, at 1%, is much lower than that of adults, although the morbidity is 45% and the recurrence rate is 18%. The most common etiologies of SJS and TEN in children are medications (usually anticonvulsants and sulfonamides) and infections (usually Mycoplasma species or herpes simplex virus). The pathogenesis of SJS and TEN is unknown.

Systemic manifestations range from mild to severe. A prodrome of fever, malaise, and upper respiratory tract infection is followed by bullous mucosal and skin lesions. These lesions rupture, ulcerate, and become covered by gray-white membranes and a hemorrhagic crust.

Ocular involvement, which occurs in as many as 50% of patients, varies from mild mucopurulent conjunctivitis to severe perforating corneal ulcers. Ocular involvement in SJS and TEN begins with edema, erythema, and crusting of the eyelids. The palpebral conjunctiva becomes hyperemic, and distinct vesicles or bullae may occur. In many instances, epithelial defects or ulcers involving the tarsus and fornices develop. In severe cases, membranous or pseudomembranous conjunctivitis may occur (Fig 21-8) and lead to symblepharon formation. Superinfection, most commonly with *Staphylococcus* species, may develop.

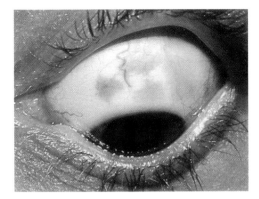

Figure 21-7 Congenital ocular melanocytosis.

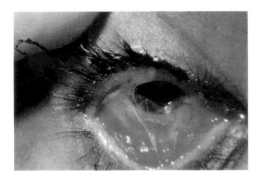

Figure 21-8 Stevens-Johnson syndrome. Early, severe involvement of conjunctiva, right eye.

Late ocular complications, possibly accompanied by a decrease in vision, occur in approximately 27% of pediatric patients. These complications include anomalies of eyelid position (ectropion and entropion), dry eye disease, trichiasis, chronic conjunctivitis, corneal defects, corneal vascularization, and symblepharon.

SJS and TEN are diagnosed based on clinical presentation and skin biopsy. Initial management includes treatment of any underlying infection and discontinuation of any inciting drug. Systemic therapy with corticosteroids or intravenous immunoglobulin is controversial. A full discussion of systemic treatment is beyond the scope of this book. A dermatologist and a specialist in pediatric infectious diseases should be consulted.

Early intervention is important in preventing the late ocular complications of SJS and TEN. Ocular lubrication with artificial tears and ointments (preferably preservative free) should be applied frequently. Associated microbial infections should be treated. Sweeping of the fornices to lyse adhesions may be performed, although some ophthalmologists believe that doing so may stimulate inflammation and cause further scarring. In severe cases, a symblepharon ring may be useful in cooperative patients. In patients with significant ocular disease, amniotic membrane grafting should be considered early to decrease the risk of late ocular complications.

Gregory DG. Treatment of acute Stevens-Johnson syndrome and toxic epidermal necrolysis using amniotic membranes. *Ophthalmology.* 2011;118(5):908–914.

CHAPTER 22

Pediatric Glaucomas

Pediatric glaucomas are a heterogeneous group of diseases that may result from an isolated congenital abnormality of the aqueous outflow pathways (primary glaucoma) or from abnormalities affecting other regions of the eye (secondary glaucoma). A variety of systemic abnormalities are associated with pediatric glaucoma. Primary congenital glaucoma (PCG) is the most common type of childhood glaucoma. BCSC Section 10, *Glaucoma*, also discusses the topics covered in this chapter.

Genetics

Although PCG usually occurs sporadically, it may be inherited as an autosomal recessive trait. When no other family history of PCG exists, the chance of an affected parent having an affected child is approximately 2%. Four chromosomal loci for PCG have been identified: *GLC3A* on band 2p21, *GLC3B* on 1p36, *GLC3C* on 14q24.3, and *GLC3D* on 14q24.3. Two genes, *LTBP2* (at the *GLC3D* locus) and *CYP1B1* (at the *GLC3A* locus), have been shown to cause PCG. Populations in which consanguinity is common have higher incidences of PCG, especially those in which the carrier rate of the *CYP1B1* gene is high. Individuals who carry the *CYP1B1* gene but who are nonpenetrant for PCG remain at higher risk for adult-onset glaucoma.

Juvenile open-angle glaucoma (JOAG) is inherited as an autosomal dominant trait and has been linked to the *GLC1A* myocilin gene *(MYOC),* which is also responsible for some adult open-angle glaucomas.

The genetic causes of many conditions associated with secondary childhood glaucoma have been identified; they are discussed in the chapters associated with their primary conditions.

Suri F, Yazdani S, Narooie-Nejhad M, et al. Variable expressivity and high penetrance of *CYP1B1* mutations associated with primary congenital glaucoma. *Ophthalmology.* 2009; 116(11):2101–2109.

Classification

Several classifications for pediatric glaucomas have been proposed; they are based on ocular anatomy, age of onset, associated systemic disorders, and inheritance. Most classifications distinguish between primary and secondary glaucomas. The World Glaucoma Association recently approved a new classification system (Table 22-1).

Table 22-1 Classification of Childhood Glaucoma

Primary childhood glaucoma
  Primary congenital glaucoma (PCG)
    Neonatal or newborn onset (age 0–1 month)
    Infantile onset (age 1–24 months)
    Late-onset or late-recognized (age ≥24 months)
  Juvenile open-angle glaucoma (JOAG)
Secondary childhood glaucoma
  Glaucoma associated with nonacquired ocular anomalies
  Glaucoma associated with nonacquired systemic disease or syndrome
  Glaucoma associated with acquired condition
  Glaucoma following cataract surgery

Data from Beck A, Chang TCP, Freedman S. Definition, classification, differential diagnosis. In: Weinreb RN, Grajewski AL, Papadopoulos M, Grigg J, Freedman S, eds. *Childhood Glaucoma.* Amsterdam: Kugler Publications; 2013:3–15.

Papadopoulos M, Cable N, Rahi J, Khaw PT; BIG Eye Study Investigators. The British Infantile and Childhood Glaucoma (BIG) Eye Study. *Invest Ophthalmol Vis Sci.* 2007;48(9):4100–4106.

Yeung HH, Walton DS. Clinical classification of childhood glaucomas. *Arch Ophthalmol.* 2010; 128(6):680–684.

Primary Childhood Glaucoma

Primary Congenital Glaucoma

PCG is also called *congenital* or *infantile glaucoma.* The incidence of PCG varies in different populations, ranging from 1 in 2500 to 1 in 68,000. PCG results in blindness in 2%–15% of cases. Visual acuity remains worse than 20/50 in at least 50% of cases. PCG is bilateral in about two-thirds of patients and occurs more frequently in males (who account for 65% of cases) than in females.

Although diagnosis is made at birth in only 25% of affected infants, disease onset occurs within the first year of life in more than 80% of cases. Neonatal-onset and late-recognized PCG are associated with guarded prognoses.

Pathophysiology

The basic pathologic defect is increased resistance to aqueous outflow due to abnormal development of anterior chamber angle tissue, which is derived from neural crest cells. The anomaly occurs late in embryologic development.

Clinical manifestations and diagnosis

PCG usually presents in the neonatal or infantile period. Epiphora, photophobia, and blepharospasm constitute the classic clinical triad of PCG. Eye redness may be present. Other signs include clouding and enlargement of the cornea (Fig 22-1).

Corneal edema results from elevated intraocular pressure (IOP) and may be gradual or sudden in onset. Corneal edema is often the presenting sign in infants younger than 3 months and is responsible for the clinical triad. Microcystic edema initially involves

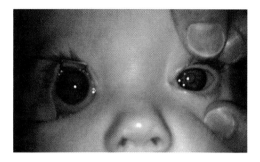

Figure 22-1 Primary congenital glaucoma, right eye. The cornea is enlarged. *(Courtesy of Gregg T. Lueder, MD.)*

the corneal epithelium but later extends to the stroma, often accompanied by 1 or more curvilinear breaks in Descemet membrane *(Haab striae)*. Although edema may resolve with IOP reduction, the split in Descemet membrane persists as paired curved lines. Significant corneal scarring and persistent opacification may require penetrating keratoplasty.

Corneal enlargement occurs with gradual stretching of the cornea as a result of elevated IOP. In newborns, the normal horizontal corneal diameter is 9.5–10.5 mm; a diameter greater than 11.5 mm suggests glaucoma. By age 1 year, the normal corneal diameter is 10.0–11.5 mm; a diameter greater than 12.5 mm suggests abnormality. Glaucoma should be suspected in any child with a corneal diameter greater than 13.0 mm.

The signs and symptoms of PCG can occur in infants with other forms of glaucoma as well. Nonglaucomatous conditions may also cause some of the signs and symptoms seen in PCG (Table 22-2).

Diagnostic examination A full ophthalmic examination of every child suspected of having glaucoma is imperative, despite the challenges. Both office examination and examination under general anesthesia are usually required. Although it is helpful in following disease progression in older children, visual field testing is rarely reliable in children younger than 6–8 years. Vision is usually poorer in the affected eye in unilateral cases and may be poor in both eyes when glaucoma is bilateral. Fixation and following behavior and the presence of nystagmus should be noted. Refraction measurement, when possible, often reveals myopia and astigmatism from eye enlargement and corneal irregularity.

CORNEAL INSPECTION The cornea should be examined for size, clarity, and Haab striae. A difference in corneal diameter of the eyes as small as 0.5 mm may be significant. Haab striae are best seen against the red reflex after pupil dilation (Fig 22-2).

TONOMETRY If the child is struggling during measurement of IOP, pressure readings may be falsely elevated. IOP is unpredictably altered (usually lowered) when systemic sedatives or anesthetics are administered. A useful technique is to have a parent bottle-feed the hungry infant at the time of pressure measurement. The Tono-Pen (Reichert Ophthalmic Instruments, Depew, NY), Icare (Icare Finland Oy, Helsinki, Finland), and Perkins (Haag-Streit USA, Mason, OH) tonometers are most commonly used for infants and young children. Goldmann applanation readings are preferred when a child is old enough to cooperate.

Table 22-2 Differential Diagnosis of Signs in Primary Congenital Glaucoma

Conditions sharing signs of epiphora and red eye
Conjunctivitis
Congenital nasolacrimal duct obstruction
Corneal epithelial defect/abrasion
Keratitis
Ocular inflammation (uveitis, trauma, foreign body)

Conditions sharing sign of corneal edema or opacification
Corneal dystrophy: congenital hereditary endothelial dystrophy, posterior polymorphous
    dystrophy
Obstetric birth trauma with Descemet tears
Storage disease: mucopolysaccharidoses, cystinosis, sphingolipidosis
Congenital anomalies: sclerocornea, Peters anomaly, choristomas
Keratitis: maternal rubella, herpes, phlyctenules
Keratomalacia (vitamin A deficiency)
Skin disorders affecting the cornea: congenital ichthyosis, congenital dyskeratosis
Idiopathic (diagnosis of exclusion only)

Conditions sharing sign of corneal enlargement
Axial myopia
Megalocornea

Conditions sharing sign of optic nerve cupping (real or apparent)
Physiologic optic nerve cupping
Cupping associated with prematurity, periventricular leukomalacia
Optic nerve coloboma
Optic atrophy
Optic nerve hypoplasia
Optic nerve malformation

Adapted with permission from Buckley EG. Primary congenital open-angle glaucoma. In: Kahook M, Schuman J, eds. *Chandler and Grant's Glaucoma.* 5th ed. Thorofare, NJ: Slack Incorporated; 2013.

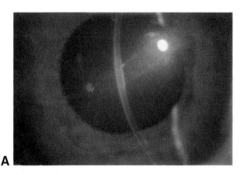 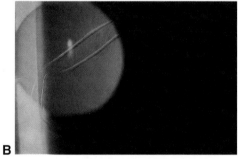

Figure 22-2 **A,** Breaks in Descemet membrane (Haab striae), right eye. **B,** Retroillumination, same eye.

The normal mean IOP in infants and young children is lower than in adults: between 10 and 12 mm Hg in newborns and approximately 14 mm Hg by age 7–8 years. In PCG, IOP commonly ranges between 30 and 40 mm Hg, and it is usually greater than 20 mm Hg even under anesthesia. Asymmetric IOP readings in a quiet or anesthetized child should raise suspicion of glaucoma.

MEASUREMENT OF CENTRAL CORNEAL THICKNESS Portable ultrasonic pachymeters may be used to measure central corneal thickness (CCT), which is typically higher in infants with glaucoma. The CCT affects the IOP measurement, but current evidence is inadequate to quantify these effects. See also Chapter 15.

> Freedman SF. Central corneal thickness in children—does it help or hinder our evaluation of eyes at risk for glaucoma? *J AAPOS.* 2008;12(1):1–2.

ANTERIOR SEGMENT EXAMINATION A portable slit lamp allows detailed inspection of the anterior segment. An abnormally deep anterior chamber and hypoplasia of the peripheral iris stroma are common findings in PCG.

Gonioscopy provides important information regarding the mechanism of glaucoma. It is best performed with the use of a goniolens and a portable slit lamp or loupes. The anterior chamber angle of a normal infant's eye (Fig 22-3A) differs from that of an adult in the following ways:

- The trabecular meshwork is more lightly pigmented.
- The Schwalbe line is often less distinct.
- The uveal meshwork is translucent, so the junction between the scleral spur and the ciliary body band is often not well seen.

In PCG, the iris often shows an insertion more anterior than that in a normal infant, and the translucence of the uveal meshwork is altered, making the ciliary body band, trabecular meshwork, and scleral spur indistinct. The scalloped border of the iris pigment epithelium is often unusually prominent, especially when peripheral iris stromal hypoplasia is present (Fig 22-3B).

OPTIC NERVE EXAMINATION The optic nerve, when visible, usually shows increased cupping in PCG. Generalized enlargement of the optic cup in very young patients with glaucoma

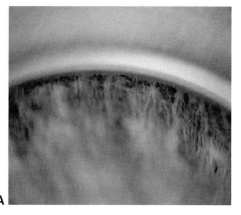 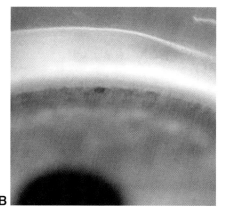

Figure 22-3 **A,** The anterior chamber angle of a normal infant's eye, as seen by direct gonioscopy with a Koeppe lens. **B,** Typical appearance of the anterior chamber angle of an infant with congenital glaucoma. *(Courtesy of Ken K. Nischal, MD.)*

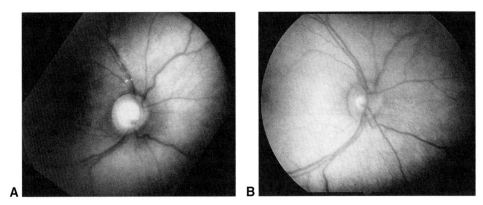

Figure 22-4 Optic nerve changes after treatment of congenital glaucoma. **A,** Preoperative enlarged optic disc cup. **B,** Reduction in disc cupping after intraocular pressure is reduced by goniotomy. *(Courtesy of Sharon Freedman, MD.)*

has been attributed to stretching of the optic canal and backward bowing of the lamina cribrosa (Fig 22-4). In most cases of PCG, the cup–disc ratio exceeds 0.3; in contrast, most normal newborn eyes have a cup–disc ratio of less than 0.3. Cup–disc asymmetry greater than 0.2 between the 2 eyes is also suggestive of glaucoma. In young children, optic nerve cupping may reverse after IOP is lowered. Whenever possible, optic disc photographs should be taken for comparison during later examinations.

MEASUREMENT OF AXIAL LENGTH Serial measurement of axial length is useful for monitoring disease progression in infant eyes. Excessive growth in an eye, especially compared with the fellow eye, may indicate inadequate IOP control.

OPTICAL COHERENCE TOMOGRAPHY Newer methods of optic nerve and retinal nerve fiber analysis such as optical coherence tomography (OCT) are being evaluated for efficacy in monitoring childhood glaucoma.

Natural history

Untreated PCG almost always progresses to blindness. The cornea irreversibly opacifies and may vascularize. It may continue to enlarge through the first 2–3 years of life, reaching a diameter of up to 17 mm. As the entire eye enlarges, pseudoproptosis and an "ox eye" appearance *(buphthalmos)* may result. Scleral thinning and myopic fundus changes may occur, and spontaneous lens dislocation can result. Optic nerve damage progresses, leading to complete blindness.

Juvenile Open-Angle Glaucoma

JOAG is an autosomal dominant condition that presents after 4 years of age. Unlike in late-recognized PCG, the cornea is not enlarged, Haab striae are not present, and the anterior chamber angle usually appears normal. Management is similar to that of adult primary open-angle glaucoma, but the condition frequently requires surgery.

Secondary Childhood Glaucoma

All other types of glaucoma are considered secondary—they are caused by other congenital or acquired ocular anomalies or are associated with systemic disease. Some common secondary glaucomas are discussed in the following sections.

Glaucoma Associated With Nonacquired Ocular Anomalies

Anterior segment abnormalities

Aniridia Aniridia is a bilateral condition characterized by complete or nearly complete absence of the iris. Glaucoma develops frequently in this disorder. Aniridia is discussed in Chapter 20.

Anterior segment developmental anomalies Glaucoma occurs in more than 50% of patients with Axenfeld-Rieger syndrome. Peters anomaly, sclerocornea, microcornea, and congenital iris ectropion are also associated with childhood glaucoma. See also Chapter 20.

Posterior segment abnormalities

Glaucoma may be associated with persistent fetal vasculature (PFV), retinopathy of prematurity (ROP), familial exudative vitreoretinopathy (FEVR), or retinal, iris, or ciliary body tumors.

Glaucoma Associated With Nonacquired Systemic Disease or Syndrome

Sturge-Weber syndrome

Sturge-Weber syndrome (SWS) is a phakomatosis that includes a port-wine stain (*nevus flammeus*) of the face, intracranial calcifications, and glaucoma. See Chapter 28 for a discussion of glaucoma associated with SWS.

Neurofibromatosis

Glaucoma associated with neurofibromatosis 1 (NF1) can be bilateral or unilateral (see Chapter 28).

Lowe syndrome

Lowe syndrome (oculocerebrorenal syndrome) is an X-linked disorder that presents with glaucoma and bilateral disciform cataracts (see Chapter 28).

Lens-associated disorders

Secondary mechanical glaucoma occurs in Marfan syndrome, homocystinuria, Weill-Marchesani syndrome, and microspherophakia (see Chapter 23).

Secondary Glaucoma Associated With an Acquired Condition

In children, as in adults, glaucoma may also develop secondary to corticosteroid use, uveitis, infection, or ocular trauma. Topiramate causes acute, usually bilateral angle-closure glaucoma secondary to ciliary effusion. Forward displacement of the iris–lens diaphragm causes acute high myopia followed by elevated IOP. Peripheral iridectomy is not effective as treatment, but timely cessation of the medication is.

Glaucoma Following Cataract Surgery

Aphakic glaucoma is a common cause of secondary glaucoma in childhood. The incidence of open-angle aphakic glaucoma after congenital cataract surgery varies from 15% to 50% or higher. Aphakic glaucoma often develops years after cataract surgery, but it can occur within weeks to months of surgery and remains a lifelong risk. Consequently, patients who have undergone cataract surgery in childhood require regular ophthalmic examination.

The mechanism that results in aphakic glaucoma is unclear. The anterior chamber angle usually appears open on gonioscopy; the outflow channels are compromised by some combination of abnormal development of the anterior chamber angle and perhaps susceptibility of the infant eye to surgically induced inflammation, loss of lens support, retained lens epithelial cells, or vitreous factors. The children at highest risk for glaucoma development following cataract surgery are those who have surgery during infancy, and the risk appears to be even higher in patients with microcornea or persistent fetal vasculature. Surgery before 6 weeks of age may be an independent risk factor. Contradicting earlier reports, recent studies have not confirmed a lower incidence of glaucoma in pseudophakic compared with aphakic eyes.

Acute or subacute angle closure with iris bombé is a rare form of aphakic glaucoma. Although it usually occurs soon after surgery, onset can be delayed by a year or more. The diagnosis should be apparent with a slit lamp, but examination at the slit lamp may be difficult in young children. Treatment consists of anterior vitrectomy to relieve the pupillary block, often with surgical iridectomy and goniosynechialysis.

Beck AD, Freedman SF, Lynn MJ, Bothun E, Neely DE, Lambert SR; Infant Aphakia Treatment Study Group. Glaucoma-related adverse events in the Infant Aphakia Treatment Study: 1-year results. *Arch Ophthalmol.* 2012;130(3):300–305.

Chak M, Rahi JS; British Congenital Cataract Interest Group. Incidence of and factors associated with glaucoma after surgery for congenital cataract: findings from the British Congenital Cataract Study. *Ophthalmology.* 2008;115(6):1013–1018.

Treatment

The primary treatment for most childhood glaucoma is surgery. PCG is usually effectively treated with angle surgery (goniotomy or trabeculotomy). Although angle surgery may be used in some secondary pediatric glaucomas—most notably Axenfeld-Rieger syndrome, SWS, and aniridia—the outcome is often less successful. The treatment of most secondary childhood glaucomas is similar to that of open-angle or secondary glaucomas in adults. Medical treatment often has value prior to surgery and may have long-term benefit, particularly in JOAG and some secondary childhood glaucomas.

Surgical Therapy

Surgical intervention is the treatment of choice for PCG. Angle surgery is the preferred initial procedure. In a *goniotomy,* an incision is made, under direct gonioscopic visualization, across the trabecular meshwork (Fig 22-5). In a *trabeculotomy,* an external approach is used to identify and cannulate the Schlemm canal, then connect it with the anterior chamber through incision of the trabecular meshwork (Fig 22-6). A modification of this technique uses a 6-0 polypropylene monofilament suture or illuminated microcatheter to cannulate and open the Schlemm canal for its entire 360° circumference in one surgery. If the cornea is clear, either a goniotomy or a trabeculotomy can be performed at the surgeon's

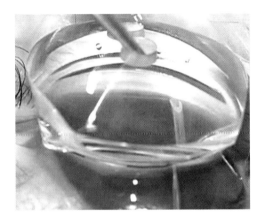

Figure 22-5 Goniotomy needle with its tip in the trabecular meshwork. The trabecular meshwork to the left of the needle has been incised. *(Courtesy of Ken K. Nischal, MD.)*

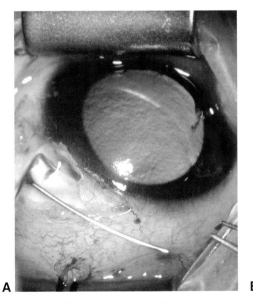
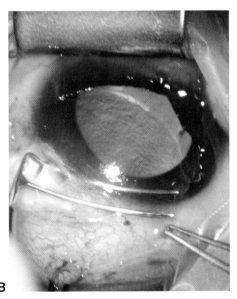

A   **B**

Figure 22-6 Trabeculotomy. **A,** The trabeculotome has entered the Schlemm canal. **B,** The trabeculotome has been rotated into the anterior chamber. *(Courtesy of Steven Archer, MD.)*

discretion. Preoperative glaucoma medications or stripping of edematous epithelium from the cornea can temporarily clear the cornea. If the view through the cornea is compromised, trabeculotomy or combined trabeculotomy-trabeculectomy can be performed.

In approximately 80% of infants with PCG presenting from 3 months to 1 year of age, IOP is controlled with 1 or 2 angle surgeries. If the first procedure is not sufficient, at least 1 additional angle surgery is usually performed before a different procedure is used.

For children in whom angle surgery is not successful or is not indicated (as is the case in many secondary glaucomas) and medical therapy is inadequate, additional surgical options include trabeculectomy with or without antifibrotic therapy (eg, mitomycin C [MMC]), glaucoma implant procedures, and cycloablative procedures.

Trabeculectomy with the use of MMC is successful in approximately 50% of children. Reported success rates vary considerably by surgical technique and type of glaucoma and decrease as the length of follow-up increases. Patients younger than 1 year and those who are aphakic are more prone to treatment failure. Although the success rate of trabeculectomy improves with the use of antifibrotics such as MMC, the long-term risk of bleb leaks and endophthalmitis also increases. Long-term risk is reduced by using a fornix-based rather than a limbus-based trabeculectomy flap. The reported success rate of glaucoma implant surgery with Molteno (Molteno Ophthalmic, Dunedin, New Zealand), Baerveldt (Abbott Medical Optics, Abbott Park, IL), and Ahmed (New World Medical, Rancho Cucamonga, CA) devices varies between 54% and 85%. Although most of these children must remain on adjunct topical medical therapy to control IOP after surgery, their blebs are thicker and are less prone to leaking and infection than those of patients undergoing MMC-augmented trabeculectomy. Potential complications include shunt failure, tube erosion and migration, tube–cornea touch, cataract, restrictive strabismus, and endophthalmitis.

Laser cycloablation and cyclocryotherapy are generally reserved for resistant cases or those not amenable to other surgical procedures. These techniques decrease ciliary body production of aqueous humor. *Cyclocryotherapy* (freezing the ciliary processes through the sclera) may be successful, but the complication rate is high. Repeated applications are often necessary, and the risk of phthisis and blindness is significant (approximately 10%). *Transscleral laser cycloablation* with the Nd:YAG or diode laser has a lower risk of complications. The short-term success rate is about 50%. Patients usually require more than one treatment.

Endoscopic cyclophotocoagulation (ECP) has been used in children with glaucomas that are difficult to treat. In ECP, a microendoscope applies laser energy to the ciliary processes under direct observation (Fig 22-7). Success rates of up to 50% have been reported. Although this is an intraocular procedure, the complication rate may be lower than that of external cyclodestructive procedures. Use of the microendoscope is advantageous in eyes with abnormal anterior segment anatomy. Some studies have shown encouraging results for patients with aphakic glaucoma.

O'Malley Schotthoefer E, Yanovitch TL, Freedman SF. Aqueous drainage device surgery in refractory pediatric glaucomas: I. Long-term outcomes. *J AAPOS*. 2008;12(1):33–39.

Wells AP, Cordeiro MF, Bunce C, Khaw PT. Cystic bleb formation and related complications in limbus- versus fornix-based conjunctival flaps in pediatric and young adult trabeculectomy with mitomycin C. *Ophthalmology*. 2003;110(11):2192–2197.

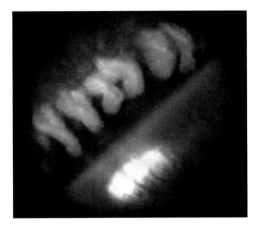

Figure 22-7 Endoscopic view of ciliary processes during endoscopic cyclophotocoagulation. The white structure at the bottom right of the photo is the lens. *(Courtesy of Endo Optiks, Little Silver, NJ.)*

Medical Therapy

Generally, medical therapy for childhood glaucoma has lower success rates and greater risks than that for adult glaucomas. Medical therapy, however, serves several important roles in preoperative, postoperative, and long-term management, particularly in childhood glaucoma other than PCG.

Because of the greater dosage per body weight and the limited number of controlled clinical trials in children, medical therapy for pediatric glaucoma carries unique risks (Table 22-3). Although punctal occlusion may be used to reduce systemic absorption of topical medications, it may be impractical in many young children. Limiting the frequency of eyedrop administration in young children may enhance adherence.

Topical medications

Topical β-blocker therapy may reduce IOP by 20%–30%. The major risks of this therapy are respiratory distress caused by apnea or bronchospasm and bradycardia, which occur mostly in small infants and in children with a history of bronchospasm. Betaxolol is a cardioselective β_1-adrenergic antagonist, but its pressure-lowering effect is less than that of nonselective agents.

Topical carbonic anhydrase inhibitors (CAIs) are effective in children, but they produce a smaller reduction in IOP (<15%) than do β-blockers. Corneal edema is a risk of topical CAIs; they should be used with caution in children with coexisting corneal disease.

A combined β-adrenergic antagonist–CAI (dorzolamide/timolol) is available for children who require dual therapy.

Prostaglandin analogues are effective in many pediatric patients. Their low systemic risk and once-daily dosage are advantageous.

Miotics are rarely used in children; perioperative pilocarpine, however, may facilitate angle surgery. Pilocarpine and echothiophate may be effective for patients with aphakic glaucoma.

The α_2-adrenergic agonist apraclonidine may be useful for short-term IOP reduction, but it has a high incidence of tachyphylaxis and allergy in young children. The α_2-adrenergic agonist brimonidine effectively reduces IOP in some cases of pediatric glaucoma. Both

Table 22-3 Systemic and Ocular Risks of Glaucoma Medications in Children

Drugs	Risks	Precautions
β-Adrenergic antagonists		
Betaxolol hydrochloride, carteolol, levobunolol, metipranolol, timolol hemihydrate, timolol maleate	Hypotension, bradycardia, bronchospasm, apnea Hallucinations Masking of hypoglycemia in diabetic children	Avoid in premature or small infants Use with caution in infants, children with asthma, cardiac disease Select lower concentrations Use punctal occlusion Consider cardioselective β-blocker to reduce risk of bronchospasm
Prostaglandin analogues		
Bimatoprost, latanoprost, tafluprost, travoprost	May exacerbate uveitis Risk of retinal detachment in Sturge-Weber syndrome Low systemic risk. Possible sleep disturbance or exacerbation of asthma	Avoid in uveitis Use caution following intraocular surgery
α₂-Adrenergic agonists		
Apraclonidine, brimonidine	Apraclonidine: tachyphylaxis, allergy Apraclonidine and brimonidine: hypotension, bradycardia, hypothermia, central nervous system depression, coma Risks are greater for brimonidine	Brimonidine contraindicated in children <2 years of age Caution in children <10 years of age or <20 kg Use low dosage Avoid with cardiovascular disease, hepatic or renal impairment
Topical carbonic anhydrase inhibitors		
Brinzolamide, dorzolamide	Metabolic acidosis (rare) Stevens-Johnson syndrome Corneal edema	Contraindicated in infants with renal insufficiency Contraindicated in sulfonamide hypersensitivity Monitor infant feeding and weight gain Caution in corneal disease
Oral carbonic anhydrase inhibitors		
Acetazolamide, methazolamide	Metabolic acidosis Stevens-Johnson syndrome Aplastic anemia (reported in adults) Headaches, nausea, dizziness, paresthesias Growth suppression, failure to thrive, weight loss Bed-wetting	Contraindicated in renal insufficiency, hypokalemia, hyponatremia Contraindicated in sulfonamide hypersensitivity Monitor for metabolic acidosis Monitor infant feeding and weight gain
Parasympathomimetic agents (miotics)		
Echothiophate, pilocarpine	Pilocarpine: bronchospasm, hypertension, vomiting, diarrhea, dizziness, weakness, headache Echothiophate: diarrhea, urinary incontinence, cardiac arrhythmia, weakness, headache, fatigue, iris cysts Risk of pupillary block Paradoxical rise in intraocular pressure	Avoid in uveitis Caution in cardiac disease, asthma, urinary tract obstruction Limit dosage and use lower concentrations Echothiophate: avoid succinylcholine

medications can produce somnolence and respiratory depression in infants and small children. Brimonidine is contraindicated in children younger than 2 years.

Oral medications

CAIs may be used effectively in children, particularly to delay the need for surgery or to clear the cornea before goniotomy. The usefulness of oral CAIs may be limited because of their systemic adverse effects.

Coppens G, Stalmans I, Zeyen T, Casteels I. The safety and efficacy of glaucoma medication in the pediatric population. *J Pediatr Ophthalmol Strabismus.* 2009;46(1):12–18.

Prognosis and Follow-Up

If PCG presents at birth, the prognosis for IOP control and visual preservation is poor; at least half of these patients become legally blind. If the corneal diameter is greater than 14 mm at diagnosis, the visual prognosis is similarly poor. Up to 90% of cases in the "favorable prognostic group" (onset at 3–12 months of age) can be controlled with angle surgery and medications. The remaining 10%, and many of the remaining cases of primary and secondary glaucomas, often present a lifelong challenge.

Vision loss in childhood glaucoma is multifactorial. It may result from corneal scarring and opacification, optic nerve damage, myopic astigmatism, and associated anisometropic and strabismic amblyopia. Myopia results from axial enlargement of the eye in the setting of high IOP; astigmatism may result from unequal expansion of the anterior segment or corneal scarring. Careful treatment of refractive errors and amblyopia is needed to optimize outcomes.

All cases of childhood glaucoma, as well as suspected but unconfirmed glaucoma, require diligent follow-up. After any surgical intervention or change in medical therapy, control of IOP should be assessed within a few weeks. Examination under sedation or anesthesia is often necessary for accurate assessment. The IOP should be considered not as an isolated finding but rather in conjunction with other measurements obtained from the examination, including refractive error (measured serially), corneal diameter, axial length, and cup–disc ratio. If the IOP is less than 20 mm Hg under anesthesia but clinical evidence shows persistent corneal edema or enlargement, progressive optic nerve cupping, or myopic progression, further intervention should be pursued despite the IOP reading. In contrast, an IOP of about 20 mm Hg in a young child who shows evidence of clinical improvement may be followed carefully.

Long-term follow-up of children with glaucoma is important. Relapse can occur years later, with elevated IOP and subsequent vision loss. Parents, and patients themselves as they become older, should be educated about the need for lifelong monitoring and management.

Walton DS, Katsavounidou G. Newborn primary congenital glaucoma: 2005 update. *J Pediatr Ophthalmol Strabismus.* 2005;42(6):333–341.

Childhood Cataracts and Other Pediatric Lens Disorders

Disorders of the pediatric lens include, in addition to cataract, abnormalities in lens shape, size, location, and development. Such abnormalities constitute a significant source of visual impairment in children. The incidence of lens abnormalities varies worldwide, ranging from 1:4000 to 1:10,000 per year. Pediatric lens abnormalities must be treated promptly if lifelong vision loss is to be avoided.

See BCSC Section 11, *Lens and Cataract,* for additional discussion.

Pediatric Cataracts

Cataracts are responsible for nearly 10% of all vision loss in children worldwide. Pediatric cataracts can be

- isolated or associated with a systemic condition
- congenital or acquired
- inherited or sporadic
- unilateral or bilateral
- partial or complete
- stable or progressive

General Features

Cataracts in children can be isolated, or they can be associated with a number of conditions, including chromosomal abnormalities, systemic syndromes and diseases, infection, trauma, and radiation exposure. In almost all cases of cataract associated with systemic disease, the cataracts are bilateral; not all bilateral cataracts, however, are associated with systemic disease (Table 23-1). Significant asymmetry can be present in bilateral cases.

Cataracts can also be associated with other ocular anomalies, including persistent fetal vasculature (discussed later), anterior segment dysgenesis, aniridia, retinal or optic nerve coloboma, and other retinal disorders.

Pediatric cataracts can be congenital or acquired. In general, the earlier the onset, the more amblyogenic the cataract will be. Lens opacities that are visually significant before 2–3 months of age are the most likely to be detrimental to vision.

Table 23-1 Etiology of Pediatric Cataracts

Bilateral cataracts
  Idiopathic
  Familial (hereditary), usually autosomal dominant; also X-linked; rarely autosomal recessive
  Chromosomal abnormality
    Trisomy 21 (Down), 13, 18
    Other translocations, deletions, and duplications
  Craniofacial syndromes
    Hallermann-Streiff, Rubinstein-Taybi, Smith-Lemli-Opitz, others
  Musculoskeletal disorders
    Conradi-Hünermann syndrome, Albright syndrome, myotonic dystrophy
  Renal syndromes
    Lowe syndrome, Alport syndrome
  Metabolic diseases
    Galactosemia, Fabry disease, Wilson disease, mannosidosis, diabetes mellitus
  After intrauterine infection
    Toxoplasmosis
    Rubella
    Cytomegalovirus
    Varicella
    Syphilis
  Ocular anomalies
    Aniridia
    Anterior segment dysgenesis syndrome
  Iatrogenic
    Corticosteroid use
    Radiation exposure (may also be unilateral)
Unilateral cataracts
  Idiopathic
  Ocular anomalies
    Persistent fetal vasculature (PFV)
    Retinal detachment (from any cause)
  Trauma (rule out child abuse)

Most hereditary cataracts are transmitted as an autosomal dominant trait, and they are almost always bilateral. X-linked and autosomal recessive inheritance may also occur. See the *Online Mendelian Inheritance in Man (OMIM)* website, which includes the most recent information on genetic disorders with significant involvement of the lens.

Morphology

Cataracts can involve the entire lens (total, or complete, cataract) or only part of the lens structure. The location in the lens and morphology of the cataract provide information about its etiology (Table 23-2), onset, and prognosis. The most common and important clinical morphologies of partial cataracts are discussed in the following subsections.

Anterior polar cataract

Anterior polar cataracts (APCs) are common and usually less than 3 mm in diameter, appearing as small white dots in the center of the anterior lens capsule (Fig 23-1). They are congenital, usually sporadic opacities. APCs can be unilateral or bilateral. They are usually nonprogressive and visually insignificant. However, unilateral APCs are associated with

Table 23-2 Morphology and Etiology of Select Pediatric Cataracts

Cataract Morphology	Etiology	Other Possible Findings
Spokelike	Fabry syndrome Mannosidosis	Corneal whorls Hepatosplenomegaly
Vacuolar	Diabetes mellitus	Increased blood glucose level
Multicolored flecks	Hypoparathyroidism Myotonic dystrophy	Low serum calcium level Characteristic facial features, tonic "grip"
Green "sunflower"	Wilson disease	Kayser-Fleischer corneal ring
Thin disciform	Lowe syndrome	Hypotonia, glaucoma

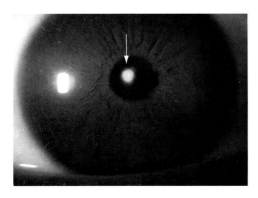

Figure 23-1 Anterior polar cataract *(arrow).* *(Courtesy of Gregg T. Lueder, MD.)*

anisometropia, which may cause amblyopia; thus, careful refraction and follow-up are indicated. *Anterior pyramidal cataracts,* as the name suggests, have a pyramidal shape and project into the anterior chamber. This cataract is a larger, more severe form of APC that can be progressive and amblyogenic, depending on its size.

Nuclear cataract

Nuclear cataracts are opacities that involve the center, or nucleus, of the lens. They are usually about 3 mm in diameter, but the irregularity of the lens fibers can extend more peripherally. Density and size, however, can vary. These opacities are usually stable, but they can progress. Nuclear cataracts can be unilateral but are more often bilateral. They can be inherited or sporadic. They are congenital but may not be significantly dense at birth (Fig 23-2). Eyes with nuclear cataracts may be smaller than normal and are at risk for developing glaucoma later in childhood.

Lamellar cataract

Identified by their discrete, round shape, lamellar *(zonular)* cataracts affect 1 or more of the layers of the developing lens cortex surrounding the nucleus. Larger in diameter than nuclear cataracts, these opacities are typically 5 mm or more in diameter (Fig 23-3). They can be unilateral but are more often bilateral. The size and corneal diameter of affected eyes are normal. Because onset is usually after the fixation reflex has been established, patients with lamellar cataracts have a better visual prognosis than patients with cataracts of earlier onset.

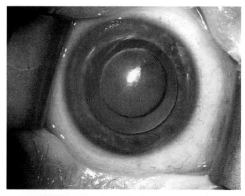

Figure 23-2 Nuclear cataract. *(Courtesy of Ken K. Nischal, MD.)*

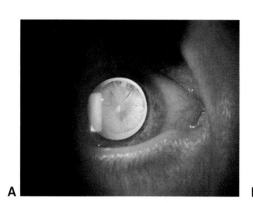

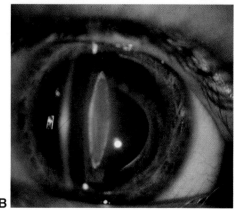

A

B

Figure 23-3 Lamellar cataract. **A,** Retroillumination shows size of the lamellar opacity. **B,** Slit-lamp view shows lamellar opacity surrounding clear nucleus. *(Courtesy of David A. Plager, MD.)*

Posterior lenticonus

Posterior lenticonus (lentiglobus) is caused by progressive thinning of the central posterior capsule (Fig 23-4A). This thinning initially causes the deformation to have an "oil droplet" appearance on red reflex examination. As the outpouching of the lens progresses, the cortical fibers gradually opacify in the area of the outpouching (Fig 23-4B). This process can take many years, but if the capsule develops a small tear, rapid, total opacification of the lens can occur (Fig 23-4C).

Posterior lenticonus opacities are almost always unilateral, and the affected eye is normal in size. Although the weakness in the posterior capsule may be congenital, the cataract does not usually form until later and therefore behaves like an acquired cataract. The visual prognosis after surgery is usually favorable.

Posterior subcapsular cataract

Posterior subcapsular cataracts (PSCs) are less common in children than in adults. They are usually acquired and bilateral, and they tend to be progressive. Causes of PSC include corticosteroid use, uveitis, retinal abnormalities, and radiation exposure. PSCs can be seen

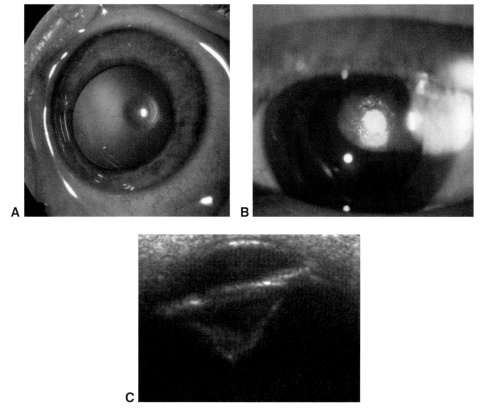

Figure 23-4 Posterior lenticonus/lentiglobus. **A,** Early clear defect in central posterior capsule and **(B)** early opacification of central defect. **C,** Ultrasound biomicroscopy of advanced posterior lenticonus. *(Part A courtesy of Edward L. Raab, MD; part B, David A. Plager, MD; part C, Ken K. Nischal, MD.)*

in association with neurofibromatosis 2 and may be the first observable manifestation of this disorder.

Sectoral cataract

Wedge-shaped cortical cataracts are occasionally seen in children. These opacities may be idiopathic, or they may be associated with occult posterior segment tumor, previous blunt trauma, or retinal coloboma with fibrous bands attached to the posterior lens capsule. Careful posterior segment examination is warranted to rule out these associated pathologies.

Peripheral vacuolar cataract

These asymptomatic peripheral lens vacuoles are sometimes seen in premature infants. The cataracts are most often encountered during examination for retinopathy of prematurity. They are rarely visually significant and usually resolve over time.

Persistent fetal vasculature

Persistent fetal vasculature (PFV; previously called *persistent hyperplastic primary vitreous*) is the most common cause of a unilateral cataract. It is typically an isolated, sporadic malformation of the eye, but bilateral cases may be associated with systemic or neurologic abnormalities. Usually, affected eyes are smaller than normal.

PFV has a spectrum of severity (Fig 23-5). Features of mild PFV are prominent hyaloid vessel remnants, a large Mittendorf dot, and a Bergmeister papilla. At the other end of the spectrum are microphthalmic eyes with dense retrolental plaques; a thick, fibrous persistent hyaloid artery; elongated ciliary processes (classic for PFV), which may be visible through the dilated pupil; and prominent radial iris vessels. Traction on the optic disc may cause distortion of the posterior retina. Varying degrees of lens opacification occur. The opacity usually consists of a retrolental plaque that is densest centrally and may contain cartilage and fibrovascular tissue.

The natural history of more severely affected eyes is usually one of progressive cataract formation and anterior chamber shallowing, causing secondary glaucoma. The glaucoma can occur acutely because of rapid, total lens opacification and swelling that develop over a few days, or it may develop gradually, over years. Congenital retinal nonattachment, ciliary body detachment, vitreous hemorrhage, and optic nerve dysmorphism are other features of severe PFV.

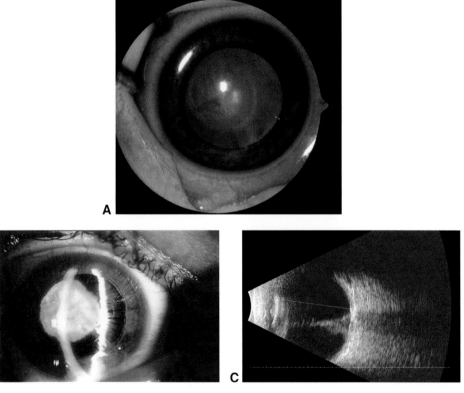

Figure 23-5   Persistent fetal vasculature (PFV). **A,** Mild variant with central retrolental membrane. **B,** Elongated ciliary processes are adherent to lens. Note the dense fibrous plaque on the posterior lens capsule. **C,** Ultrasonogram of eye with PFV. Note the dense stalk arising from the optic nerve and attaching to the posterior lens. *(Part A courtesy of David A. Plager, MD; part C courtesy of Edward L. Raab, MD.)*

Retinoblastoma may be part of the initial differential diagnosis of PFV. The presence of microphthalmos and cataract are important factors in the differentiation of these disorders, as retinoblastoma is rarely found in microphthalmic eyes, and cataracts are very unusual in retinoblastoma.

Evaluation

All newborns should have a screening eye examination, including an evaluation of the red reflex (see Chapter 1). Retinoscopy through an undilated pupil is helpful for assessing the potential visual significance of an axial lens opacity in a preverbal child. Any central opacity or surrounding cortical distortion measuring 3 mm or more in diameter is usually visually significant.

History

The clinician should obtain a detailed history of the child's growth, development, and systemic disorders, in addition to a family history. A slit-lamp examination of immediate family members can reveal previously undiagnosed lens opacities that are visually insignificant but that may indicate an inherited cause for the child's cataracts. Congenital posterior sutural cataracts, for example, develop in female carriers of X-linked Nance-Horan syndrome, and mild lenticular opacities develop in female carriers of Lowe syndrome by puberty.

Examination

Visual function

The mere presence of a cataract does not suggest that surgical removal is necessary. That determination requires assessment of the visual significance of the lens opacity.

In healthy infants aged 2 months or younger, the fixation reflex may not be fully developed; thus, its absence in this group of patients is not necessarily abnormal. In general, anterior capsule opacities are not visually significant unless they occlude the entire pupil. Central or posterior lens opacities of sufficient density that are greater than 3 mm in diameter are usually visually significant. Opacities that have a large area of surrounding normal red reflex or that have clear areas within them may allow for good visual development. Strabismus associated with a unilateral cataract and nystagmus associated with bilateral cataracts indicate that the opacities are visually significant. Although these signs may also indicate that the optimal time for treatment has passed, cataract surgery can still result in improvement of visual function.

In preverbal children older than 2 months, standard clinical assessment of fixation behavior, fixation preference, and objection to occlusion provide additional evidence of the visual significance of the cataract(s). For bilateral cataracts, assessment of the child's visual behavior and the family's observations of the child at home help determine the level of visual function. Preferential looking tests and visually evoked potentials can provide additional quantitative information (see Chapter 1). In older children, particularly those with lamellar or posterior subcapsular cataracts, glare testing may be useful for assessing decreased vision.

Ocular examination

Slit-lamp examination can help classify the morphology of the cataract and reveal associated abnormalities of the anterior segment. If the cataract allows some view of the posterior segment, careful examination of the optic nerve and fovea should be performed. If no such view is possible, B-scan ultrasonography is required in order to assess for gross anatomical abnormalities of the posterior segment. The presence of retinal or optic nerve abnormalities cannot be definitively ruled out, however, until the posterior pole can be visualized directly. See Table 23-3 for additional information.

Workup

Unilateral cataracts are not usually associated with occult systemic or metabolic disease; laboratory tests are therefore not warranted. In contrast, bilateral cataracts may be associated with many systemic and metabolic diseases. If the child has a positive family history of isolated congenital or childhood cataract or if examination of the parents shows lens opacities (and there are no associated systemic diseases to explain their cataracts), systemic evaluation and laboratory tests are not necessary. A basic laboratory evaluation for bilateral cataracts of unknown etiology in apparently healthy children is outlined in Table 23-3.

Further workup should be directed by the presence of other systemic abnormalities. Evaluation by a geneticist may be helpful for determining whether there are associated disorders and for counseling the patient's family regarding recurrence risks.

Table 23-3 Evaluation of Pediatric Cataracts

Family history (autosomal dominant, X-linked, autosomal recessive, reduced penetrance, variable
   expressivity; associated anomalies may be indicative of chromosomal translocation, balanced
   in the parent, unbalanced in the child)
Detailed history of the child's growth, development, and systemic disorders
Pediatric physical examination
Ocular examination, including
   Corneal diameter
   Iris configuration
   Anterior chamber depth
   Lens position
   Cataract morphology
   Posterior segment
      Rule out posterior mass.
      Rule out retinal detachment.
      Rule out optic nerve stalk to lens.
   Intraocular pressure
Laboratory studies for bilateral cataracts
   Disorders of galactose metabolism: urine for reducing substances; galactose-1-phosphate
      uridyltransferase; galactokinase
   Infectious diseases: TORCH and varicella titers, VDRL
   Metabolic diseases: urine amino acids test (Lowe syndrome); serum calcium (low in
      hypoparathyroidism), phosphorus (high in hypoparathyroidism), glucose (high in diabetes
      mellitus), and ferritin (high in hyperferritinemia)

Cataract Surgery in Pediatric Patients

Timing of the Procedure

Once a decision has been made to remove the cataract(s), the next issues to be resolved are (1) when to perform surgery and (2) whether to implant an intraocular lens (IOL). In general, the younger the child, the greater the urgency to remove the cataract, because of the risk of visual deprivation amblyopia. For optimal visual development in newborn and young infants, a visually significant unilateral cataract should be removed before age 6 weeks; visually significant bilateral cataracts, before age 10 weeks.

For older children with bilateral cataracts, surgery should be recommended when the level of visual function interferes with the child's visual needs. Although children with best-corrected visual acuity of roughly 20/70 may function relatively well in early grade school, their participation in important activities of daily living such as unrestricted driving will be restricted later in life in parts of the United States and elsewhere. Surgery should be considered when visual acuity decreases to 20/40 or worse. For teenaged patients, cataract surgery may be indicated when the visual requirements for obtaining a driver's license need to be met.

For older children with unilateral cataract, cataract surgery is suggested when optical treatment and amblyopia therapy cannot improve visual acuity beyond 20/40.

Intraocular Lens Use in Children

The choice of optical device for correction of aphakia depends primarily on the age of the patient and the laterality of the cataract. IOL implantation in children aged 1–2 years and older is widely accepted. The use of IOLs in younger infants, however, is controversial because of a higher rate of complications and the rapid shift in refractive error that occurs during the first 1–2 years of life. It has been shown that, compared with contact lens rehabilitation in aphakic patients, IOL implantation in infants aged 1–6 months is associated with a significantly higher rate of adverse events requiring further surgery, but it is not associated with a significant difference in grating visual acuity at age 1 year. In cases without significant posterior pole abnormalities, it is possible to obtain some degree of central vision and, occasionally, excellent vision if early surgical intervention is followed by consistent contact lens wear and patching of the uninvolved eye for treatment of amblyopia. In most infants who are left aphakic, secondary IOL implantation can be performed after 1–2 years of age.

The Infant Aphakia Treatment Study showed that aphakic infants with mild PFV treated with contact lenses had a higher incidence of adverse events after lensectomy compared with children with other forms of unilateral cataract. However, both groups had similar visual outcomes 1 year after surgery.

Lambert SR, Buckley EG, Drews-Botsch C, et al; Infant Aphakia Treatment Study Group. A randomized clinical trial comparing contact lens with intraocular lens correction of monocular aphakia during infancy: grating acuity and adverse events at age 1 year. *Arch Ophthalmol.* 2010;128(7):810–818.

Morrison DG, Wilson ME, Trivedi RH, Lambert SR, Lynn MJ; Infant Aphakia Treatment Study Group. Infant Aphakia Treatment Study: effects of persistent fetal vasculature on outcome at 1 year of age. *J AAPOS.* 2011;15(5):427–431.

Management of the Anterior Capsule

To allow access to the lens nucleus and cortex during cataract surgery, a *capsulorhexis* is performed. Because the tearing characteristics of the pediatric capsule are quite different from those of the adult capsule, lens removal techniques are modified for pediatric patients so that the risk of inadvertent extension of the tear is minimized. The elasticity of the capsule is greatest in younger patients, especially infants, making continuous curvilinear capsulorhexis more difficult in these patients. The pulling force should be directed nearly perpendicular to the direction of intended tear, and the capsule should be regrasped frequently to maintain optimal control over the direction of tear. The use of a 2-incision push-pull technique may be helpful (Fig 23-6). An alternative to capsulorhexis in infants is *vitrectorhexis,* the creation of an anterior capsule opening using a vitrectomy

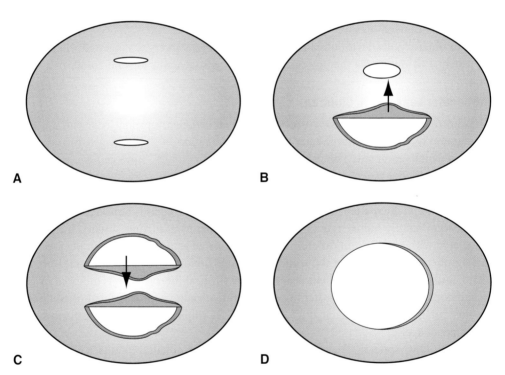

Figure 23-6 In the 2-incision push-pull rhexis technique, 2 small linear incisions are made in the superior and inferior lens capsule **(A),** and the center of the flap of the superior incision is grasped **(B);** pushing to the center of the pupil will result in a semicircular tear **(B).** The tear is extended to the center of the capsule, between the sites of the initial stab incisions **(B). C,** The flap of the inferior stab incision is then grasped and pulled to the center of the pupil, forming another semicircular tear. **D,** The semicircular tears are joined to form a complete, continuous curvilinear capsulorhexis. *(Redrawn with permission from Hamada S, Low S, Walters BC, Nischal KK. Five-year experience of the 2-incision push-pull technique for anterior and posterior capsulorrhexis in pediatric cataract surgery.* Ophthalmology. *2006;113(8):1309–1314.)*

instrument. In children with opaque capsules, visibility can be enhanced with application of trypan blue ophthalmic solution 0.06% to the capsule.

Lensectomy Without Intraocular Lens Implantation

In children who will be left aphakic, lensectomy is performed through a small limbal or pars plana incision with a vitreous-cutting instrument (vitrector). Irrigation can be provided by an integrated infusion sleeve or by a separate cannula. Ultrasonic phacoemulsification is not required, as the lens cortex and nucleus are generally soft in children of all ages. It is important to remove all cortical material because of the propensity for reproliferation of pediatric lens epithelial cells. Tough, fibrotic plaques such as those occasionally encountered in severe PFV may require manual excision with intraocular scissors and forceps.

Because posterior capsule opacification occurs rapidly in young children, a controlled posterior capsulectomy and anterior vitrectomy should be performed at the time of cataract surgery in children who are unlikely candidates for awake Nd:YAG capsulotomy, which would otherwise be necessary within 18 months of the primary surgery. This technique allows for rapid, permanent establishment of a clear visual axis for retinoscopy and prompt fitting and monitoring of the aphakic optical correction. If possible, sufficient peripheral lens capsule should be left to facilitate secondary posterior chamber IOL implantation at a later date.

Lensectomy With Intraocular Lens Implantation

Single-piece acrylic foldable IOLs, which can be placed through a 3-mm clear corneal or scleral tunnel incision, have become popular in pediatric cataract surgery, although larger single-piece polymethylmethacrylate (PMMA) lenses are also still used. Silicone lenses have not been well studied in children.

If an IOL is to be placed at the time of cataract extraction, 2 basic techniques can be used for the lensectomy, depending on whether the posterior capsule will be left intact. Many pediatric cataract surgeons leave the posterior capsule intact if the child is approaching the age when an awake Nd:YAG capsulotomy could be performed (usually 5 years of age). Primary capsulectomy is usually preferred for younger children. Studies have shown that in early childhood, the lens capsule opacifies, on average, within 18–24 months after surgery, but this can vary considerably.

Technique with posterior capsule intact

After the cortex is aspirated, the clear corneal or scleral tunnel incision is enlarged to allow placement of the IOL. Placement in the capsular bag is desirable, but ciliary sulcus fixation is an acceptable alternative. The surgeon should remove all viscoelastic material to prevent a postoperative spike in intraocular pressure (IOP). Closure of 3-mm clear corneal incisions with absorbable suture has been shown to be safe and does not induce astigmatism in children.

Techniques for primary posterior capsulectomy

Posterior capsulectomy/vitrectomy before IOL placement After lensectomy, the vitrector settings should be set to the low-suction, high-cutting rate appropriate for vitreous surgery. A posterior capsulectomy with anterior vitrectomy is then performed. The anterior capsule is enlarged, if necessary, to an appropriate size for the IOL, and the lens is implanted in the capsular bag, if possible, or in the ciliary sulcus as an alternative. The surgeon must take care to ensure that the capsulotomy does not extend, the IOL haptics do not go through the posterior opening, and vitreous does not become entangled with the IOL or enter the anterior chamber.

Posterior capsulectomy/vitrectomy after IOL placement Some pediatric cataract surgeons prefer to place the IOL in the capsular bag, close the anterior incision, and approach the posterior capsule through the pars plana. Irrigation can be maintained through the same anterior infusion cannula used during lensectomy. A small conjunctival opening is made over the pars plana, and a sclerotomy is made with a microvitreoretinal (MVR) blade 2.5–3.0 mm posterior to the limbus. This provides good access to the posterior capsule, and a wide anterior vitrectomy can be performed.

Intraocular lens implantation issues

Because the eye continues to elongate throughout the first decade of life and beyond, selecting an appropriate IOL power is complicated. Power calculations in infants and young children may be unpredictable for several reasons, including widely variable growth of the eye, difficulty obtaining accurate keratometry and axial length measurements, and use of power formulas that were developed for adults rather than children. Studies have shown that the refractive error of aphakic pediatric eyes undergoes a variable myopic shift of approximately 7.00–8.00 D from age 1 to age 10, with a wide standard deviation. This suggests that if a child is made emmetropic with an IOL at age 1 year, refraction at age 10 years would be up to –8.00 D or greater. Refractive change below age 1 year is even more unpredictable. This approach assumes that the presence of an IOL does not alter the normal growth curve of the aphakic eye, an assumption that may not be valid based on both animal and early human studies.

Lens implantation in children requires a compromise that accounts for the age of the child and the target refraction at the time of surgery. There are 2 approaches to this situation. Some surgeons implant IOLs with powers that are expected to be required in adulthood, allowing the child to grow into the selected lens power. Thus, the child is undercorrected and requires hyperopic spectacles or contact lenses of decreasing powers until the teenaged years. Other surgeons aim for emmetropia at the time of lens implantation, especially in unilateral cases, believing that this approach may reduce the risk of amblyopia and facilitate development of binocular function by decreasing anisometropia in the early childhood years. These children can be expected to become progressively more myopic with time, and they may eventually require a secondary procedure in order to eliminate the increasing anisometropia.

Postoperative Care

Medical therapy

If all cortical material is adequately removed, postoperative inflammation in children without a lens implant is usually mild. Postoperative topical antibiotics, corticosteroids, and cycloplegics are commonly applied for a few weeks. Topical steroids should be used more aggressively in children who have undergone IOL implantation. Some surgeons administer intracameral steroids postoperatively, and others use oral steroids, especially in very young children and children with heavily pigmented irides. Some surgeons administer intracameral antibiotics in addition to topical antibiotics.

Amblyopia management

Amblyopia therapy should begin as soon as possible after surgery. For aphakic patients, corrective lenses—in general, contact lenses for unilateral or bilateral aphakia, spectacles for bilateral aphakia—should be dispensed within 1 week of surgery.

For infants with bilateral aphakia, spectacles are the safest and simplest method of correction. They can be easily changed to accommodate the refractive shifts that occur with growth of the eye. Until the child can use a bifocal lens properly, the power selected should make the eye myopic, because most of an infant's visual activity occurs at near. Contact lenses may also be used in bilaterally aphakic patients, but they require more effort on the part of both the caregiver and the physician than do spectacles.

For infants with unilateral aphakia, contact lenses are the most popular method of correction. Advantages of contact lenses include relatively easy power changes and the potential for extended wear with certain lenses. Disadvantages include easy displacement by eye rubbing, the expense of replacement, and the risk of microbial keratitis. Aphakic spectacles are occasionally used in infants with unilateral aphakia who are unable to tolerate contact lenses, but these spectacles are suboptimal owing to the amblyogenic effect of aniseikonia and the difficulty of wearing glasses that are much heavier on one side.

After optical correction of aphakia, patching of the better eye is almost always necessary in patients with unilateral cataract and in some patients with bilateral cataracts if the visual acuity is asymmetric. The amount of patching is titrated based on the degree of amblyopia and the age of the child. Part-time occlusion in the neonatal period may allow stimulation of binocular vision and may help prevent associated strabismus.

Complications

The complications seen in children after lens extraction are different from those in adults. Retinal detachments, macular edema, and corneal abnormalities are rare in children. The incidence of postoperative infections and bleeding, however, is similar in children and adults. In children, strabismus is very commonly associated with cataracts. The risk of glaucoma is increased in children who have surgery in infancy, and glaucoma often develops many years after lens extraction (see Chapter 22).

Visual Outcome After Cataract Extraction

Visual outcome after cataract surgery depends on many factors, including age of onset and type of cataract, timing of surgery, choice of optical correction, and treatment of amblyopia. Early surgery by itself does not ensure a good outcome. Optimal vision requires careful, long-term postoperative management, particularly regarding amblyopia. But even when congenital cataracts are detected late (after age 4 months), cataract removal combined with a strong postoperative vision rehabilitation program can achieve good vision in some eyes.

Structural or Positional Lens Abnormalities

Congenital Aphakia

Congenital aphakia, the absence of the lens at birth, is rare. This condition is usually associated with a markedly abnormal eye.

Spherophakia

A lens that is spherical and smaller than normal is called *spherophakic*. This condition is usually bilateral. The lens may dislocate and prolapse into the anterior chamber (Fig 23-7), causing secondary glaucoma.

Coloboma

A lens coloboma (a misnomer) involves flattening or notching of the lens periphery. A lens coloboma can be associated with a coloboma of the iris, optic nerve, or retina, all of which are caused by abnormal closure of the embryonic fissure. Lens colobomas are usually located inferonasally. Zonular fibers are typically absent or stretched in the colobomatous area, resulting in a flattening of the lens in that location, without any dislocation. In more significant colobomatous defects, lens dislocations may occur superiorly and temporally (Fig 23-8). Most colobomatous lenses do not worsen progressively.

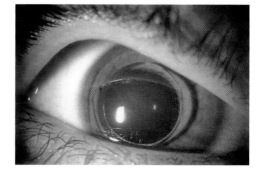

Figure 23-7 Spherophakia with lens dislocation into anterior chamber, left eye.

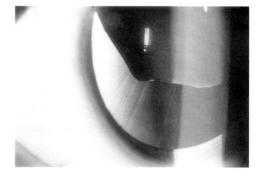

Figure 23-8 Flattening of the lens equator (with dislocation), which may be referred to as *lens coloboma*.

Dislocated Lenses in Children

When the lens is not in its normal anatomical position, it is said to be *dislocated, subluxed, subluxated, luxed, luxated,* or *ectopic.* Luxed or luxated lenses are completely detached from the ciliary body; they are free in the posterior chamber (Fig 23-9), or they have prolapsed into the anterior chamber. The amount of dislocation can vary from slight displacement with minimal *iridodonesis* (tremulousness of the iris) to severe displacement, with the lens periphery not visible through the pupillary opening. Lens dislocation can be familial or sporadic, or it can be associated with multisystem disease or an inborn error of metabolism (Table 23-4). Lens dislocation can occur with trauma, usually involving significant injury to the eye, but this is not common. Spontaneous lens dislocation has been reported rarely both in aniridia and in buphthalmos associated with congenital glaucoma.

Isolated Ectopia Lentis

In simple ectopia lentis, the lens is displaced superiorly and temporally. The condition is usually bilateral and symmetric. Most commonly, it is inherited as an autosomal dominant trait. Onset can be at birth or later in life. Glaucoma is common in the late-onset type.

Ectopia Lentis et Pupillae

Ectopia lentis et pupillae is a rare autosomal recessive condition in which there is bilateral displacement of the pupil, usually inferotemporally, and dislocation of the lens in the opposite direction (Fig 23-10A). Affected patients have small, round lenses (microspherophakia), miosis, and poor pupillary dilation with mydriatics. The condition may be the result of a membrane extending from a posterior origin to attach to the proximal pupil

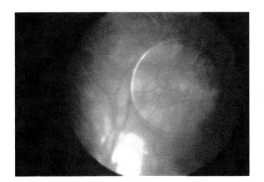

Figure 23-9 Lens dislocation into vitreous.

Table 23-4 Conditions Associated With Subluxated Lenses

Systemic conditions	Ocular conditions
Marfan syndrome	Aniridia
Homocystinuria	Iris coloboma
Weill-Marchesani syndrome	Trauma
Sulfite oxidase deficiency	Hereditary ectopia lentis

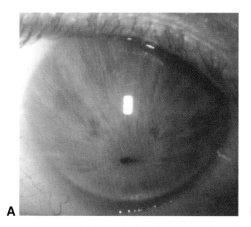
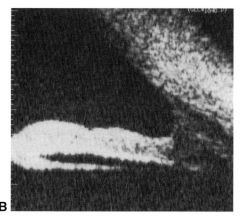

Figure 23-10 **A,** Ectopia lentis et pupillae. **B,** This 50-MHz ultrasonography scan shows a membrane posterior to the iris attaching at the pupil margin. *(Part A reproduced with permission from Byles DB, Nischal KK, Cheng H. Ectopia lentis et pupillae. A hypothesis revisited. Ophthalmology. 1998;105(7):1331–1336. Part B courtesy of Ken K. Nischal, MD.)*

margin (Fig 23-10B). Traction from the membrane may cause iris distortion and lens subluxation in the opposite direction due to disruption of zonules. Some family members may have subluxation only and no pupillary displacement. The condition is nonprogressive.

Marfan Syndrome

Marfan syndrome is the systemic disease most commonly associated with subluxated lenses. The syndrome consists of abnormalities of the cardiovascular, musculoskeletal, and ocular systems. It is inherited as an autosomal dominant trait, but family history is negative in 15% of cases. Marfan syndrome is caused by mutations in the fibrillin gene on chromosome 15, which is the major constituent of extracellular microfibrils. Affected patients are characteristically tall, with long limbs and fingers *(arachnodactyly)*; loose, flexible joints; scoliosis; and chest deformities. Cardiovascular abnormalities are a source of significant mortality and manifest as enlargement of the aortic root, dilation of the descending aorta, dissecting aneurysm, and floppy mitral valve. The life expectancy of patients with Marfan syndrome is about half that of the normal population.

Ocular abnormalities occur in more than 80% of affected patients, with lens dislocation being the most common. In approximately 75% of cases, the lens is subluxated superiorly. Typically, the zonules that are visible are intact and unbroken. Examination of the iris usually shows iridodonesis and may reveal transillumination defects that are more marked near the iris base. The pupil is small and dilates poorly. The corneal curvature is often decreased. The axial length is increased, and affected patients are frequently myopic. Retinal detachment can occur spontaneously, usually in the second and third decades of life.

Homocystinuria

Homocystinuria is a rare autosomal recessive condition that occurs in approximately 1 in 100,000 births. The classic form is caused by an abnormality in the enzyme cystathionine β-synthase, but it can be caused by other enzyme defects. This abnormality causes homocysteine to accumulate in the plasma and to be excreted in the urine.

The clinical manifestations of homocystinuria vary and can affect the eye, skeletal system, central nervous system, and vascular system. Most of the abnormalities develop after birth and become progressively worse with age. The skeletal features are similar to those of Marfan syndrome. Affected patients are usually tall, with osteoporosis, scoliosis, and chest deformities. Central nervous system abnormalities occur in approximately 50% of patients; intellectual disability and seizures are the most common.

Vascular complications are common and secondary to thrombotic disease, which affects large or medium-sized arteries and veins anywhere in the body. Partial or complete vascular obstruction is present in various organs. Hypertension and cardiomegaly are common. Anesthesia carries a higher risk for patients with homocystinuria because of thromboembolic phenomena; thus, this disorder should be identified before patients undergo general anesthesia.

The main ocular finding is lens subluxation, most frequently inferiorly, but the direction of subluxation can vary and is not diagnostic. Subluxation typically begins between the ages of 3 and 10 years. The lenses may dislocate into the anterior chamber, a finding suggestive of homocystinuria (Fig 23-11). The lens zonules are frequently broken, in contrast with those in Marfan syndrome.

Diagnosis is confirmed by the detection of disulfides, including homocystine, in the urine. The medical management of homocystinuria is directed toward normalizing the biochemical abnormality. Dietary management (low methionine and supplemental cysteine) has been attempted, and coenzyme supplements (pyridoxine) decrease systemic problems in approximately 50% of cases.

Weill-Marchesani Syndrome

Patients with Weill-Marchesani syndrome can be thought of as clinical opposites of patients with Marfan syndrome in that the former are characteristically short, with brachydactyly and short limbs. Inheritance can be autosomal dominant or recessive. The lenses are microspherophakic. With time, the lenses dislocate anteriorly into the anterior chamber, which may result in pupillary block glaucoma. For this reason, prophylactic laser peripheral iridectomy has been recommended; lensectomy may be required.

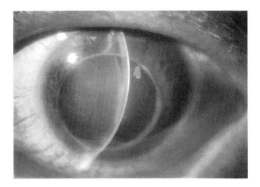

Figure 23-11 Homocystinuria. The lens may dislocate into the anterior chamber with acute pupillary block glaucoma.

Sulfite Oxidase Deficiency

Sulfite oxidase deficiency (molybdenum cofactor deficiency) is a very rare hereditary disorder of sulfur metabolism manifested by severe neurologic disorders and ectopia lentis. The enzyme deficiency interferes with conversion of sulfite to sulfate, resulting in increased excretion of sulfite in the urine. The diagnosis can be confirmed by the absence of sulfite oxidase activity in skin fibroblasts. Neurologic abnormalities include infantile hemiplegia, choreoathetosis, and seizures. Irreversible brain damage and death usually occur by age 5.

Treatment

Optical correction

Optical correction of the refractive error caused by lens dislocation is often difficult. With mild subluxation, the patient may be only myopic, and corrected visual function may be good. More severe dislocation causes optical distortion, because the patient is looking through the far periphery of the lens. Because the resultant myopic astigmatism is difficult to measure accurately by retinoscopy or automated refractometry, using an aphakic correction may provide the patient with superior vision. Predilation and postdilation refractions are often helpful for the ophthalmologist and patient in deciding on the best choice. If satisfactory visual function cannot be obtained with optical correction or if visual function worsens, lens removal should be considered.

Surgery

Subluxated lenses can be removed either from the anterior segment through a limbal incision or posteriorly through the pars plana. In most circumstances, complete lensectomy is indicated. Lens removal is easier when the lens is not severely subluxated.

In the United States, contact lenses or glasses are usually used for postoperative vision rehabilitation, with good visual results. Scleral-sutured IOLs should be used with caution because of the high rate of suture breakage. In the Netherlands, an iris-claw lens (Artisan, Ophtec BV, Groningen, the Netherlands) is widely used instead of scleral-sutured IOLs. This lens is currently available for compassionate use only in the United States.

Cleary C, Lanigan B, O'Keeffe M. Artisan iris-claw lenses for the correction of aphakia in children following lensectomy for ectopia lentis. *Br J Ophthalmol.* 2012;96(3):419–421.

CHAPTER 24

Uveitis in the Pediatric Age Group

This chapter discusses the features of uveitis occurring in children. See BCSC Section 9, *Intraocular Inflammation and Uveitis,* for a more detailed description of the clinical features and inflammatory mechanisms of the conditions discussed here.

Epidemiology and Genetics

The incidence of pediatric uveitis varies among studies, but pediatric cases account for 2%–14% of all uveitis cases. The distribution between the sexes is similar to that seen in adults, showing a slight female preponderance. The mean age of diagnosis is 8–9 years, and 75% of patients have bilateral disease. In the United States, approximately 62% of patients are Caucasian. The 2 major etiologies of uveitis in children are idiopathic (25%–54% of cases) and juvenile idiopathic arthritis (15%–47% of cases). Most types of uveitis are not inherited. Some are associated with various human leukocyte antigen (HLA) types; this chapter notes the HLA type in such cases.

Smith JA, Mackensen F, Sen HN, et al. Epidemiology and course of disease in childhood uveitis. *Ophthalmology.* 2009;116(8):1544–1551.

Classification

As in adults, uveitis in children can be classified according to several factors, including anatomical location (anterior, intermediate, posterior, or panuveitis), pathology (granulomatous or nongranulomatous), course (acute, chronic, or recurrent), or etiology (traumatic, immunologic, infectious [exogenous or endogenous], masquerade, or idiopathic). Anatomical location can be helpful in determining etiology (Table 24-1). Published studies of uveitis in children show that anterior uveitis accounts for 30%–50% of cases; intermediate uveitis, 12%–28%; posterior uveitis, 5%–30%; and panuveitis, 13%–21%.

Table 24-1 Differential Diagnosis of Uveitis in Children

Anterior uveitis
Juvenile idiopathic arthritis
Trauma
Sarcoidosis
Tuberculosis
Syphilis
Lyme disease
Herpes virus
Fuchs heterochromic iridocyclitis
Kawasaki disease
Tubulointerstitial nephritis and uveitis syndrome
Behçet disease
Inflammatory bowel disease
Granulomatosis with polyangiitis (Wegener granulomatosis)
Nonspecific orbital inflammation (orbital pseudotumor)
Idiopathic anterior uveitis

Intermediate uveitis
Sarcoidosis
Tuberculosis
Syphilis
Lyme disease
Multiple sclerosis
Idiopathic intermediate uveitis (pars planitis)

Posterior uveitis and panuveitis
Toxoplasmosis
Toxocariasis
Sarcoidosis
Tuberculosis
Syphilis
Lyme disease
Herpes virus
Rubella or measles
Sympathetic ophthalmia
Bartonella henselae infection (cat-scratch disease)
Candida albicans infection
Familial juvenile systemic granulomatosis (Blau syndrome)
Diffuse unilateral subacute neuroretinitis
Vogt-Koyanagi-Harada syndrome
Behçet disease
Idiopathic posterior uveitis or panuveitis

Anterior Uveitis

Juvenile Idiopathic Arthritis

Nomenclature

Juvenile idiopathic arthritis (JIA) (formerly *chronic arthritis* or *juvenile rheumatoid arthritis*) is defined as arthritis of at least 6 weeks' duration without any identifiable cause in children younger than 16 years. The subtypes of JIA are listed in Table 24-2.

Table 24-2 Subtypes of Juvenile Idiopathic Arthritis

Disease type
I. Systemic arthritis
II. Oligoarthritis
    A. Persistent
    B. Extended
III. Polyarthritis, RF-negative
IV. Polyarthritis, RF-positive
V. Psoriatic arthritis
VI. Enthesitis-related arthritis
VII. Undifferentiated arthritis

RF = rheumatoid factor.

Modified with permission from Kotaniemi K, Savolainen A, Karma A, Aho K. Recent advances in uveitis of juvenile idiopathic arthritis. *Surv Ophthalmol.* 2003;48(5):489–502.

Occurrence of uveitis in JIA

JIA is the most common identifiable etiology of childhood anterior uveitis. Overall, the prevalence of uveitis in JIA varies from 2% to 34%. The subtypes of JIA that are particularly associated with uveitis are oligoarthritis, rheumatoid factor (RF)–negative polyarthritis, psoriatic arthritis, and enthesitis-related arthritis. Uveitis almost never occurs in children with systemic arthritis and is very rare in those with RF-positive polyarthritis.

Oligoarthritis is the most frequent type of chronic arthritis in children in North America and Europe. Oligoarthritis occurs predominantly in young girls and affects 4 or fewer joints during the first 6 months of the disease. Anterior uveitis or iritis is most likely to occur with this type of arthritis. Uveitis has been reported in 10%–30% of children with oligoarthritis. Laboratory markers include a high prevalence of antinuclear antibodies (ANA). RF is almost always absent. HLA associations include HLA-A2, HLA-DR5, HLA-DR8, HLA-DR11, and HLA-DP2.1.

Children with *RF-negative polyarthritis* have more than 4 inflamed joints during the first 6 months of the disease. This disease is more common in girls, and its mean age of onset is later than in children with oligoarthritis. Uveitis occurs in about 10% of these children. ANA positivity may be present, but RF is absent. Strong HLA associations have not been consistently documented.

The pathogenesis of the anterior uveitis associated with JIA is unknown, but it is likely to have an immunologic basis. The risk for development of uveitis is highest during the first 4 years after diagnosis of JIA. Among patients with JIA in whom uveitis develops, 90% of uveitis cases develop within 7 years of the onset of arthritis. Occasionally, uveitis is diagnosed before or at the onset of joint symptoms. Unfortunately, these patients often have a poorer prognosis because the initially asymptomatic nature of their ocular inflammation often delays diagnosis. A shorter interval between the onsets of arthritis and uveitis is also associated with a more aggressive course.

JIA-associated uveitis is usually bilateral and nongranulomatous with fine to medium-sized keratic precipitates, but a minority of children, especially African Americans, may

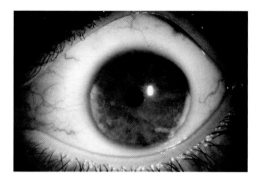

Figure 24-1 Slit-lamp photograph of a patient with uveitis associated with juvenile idiopathic arthritis. As is typical, the conjunctiva is "white." Band keratopathy is present. *(Courtesy of Amy Hutchinson, MD.)*

have granulomatous precipitates. Chronic inflammation may produce band keratopathy (Fig 24-1), posterior synechiae, ciliary membrane formation, hypotony, cataract, glaucoma, and phthisis. Vitritis and macular edema occur infrequently.

Recognition of the importance of screening for uveitis in children with JIA has resulted in an improved prognosis for this disorder. However, visual impairment has been reported in up to 40% of children with JIA-associated uveitis, and blindness may occur in as many as 10% of affected eyes. Screening guidelines continue to undergo revision but are based on 4 factors that are associated with an increased risk of uveitis:

1. category of arthritis
2. age at onset of arthritis
3. presence of ANA positivity
4. duration of the disease

Table 24-3 outlines the eye examination schedule for the first 4 years after diagnosis of JIA, as recommended by the American Academy of Pediatrics. After 4 years, the eye examinations become less frequent. Although female gender is associated with a higher incidence of uveitis, this factor is not incorporated into the guidelines. Initial ocular examination should occur within 6 weeks of diagnosis (see reference below).

Other arthritic diseases of childhood may also be associated with uveitis. *Psoriatic arthritis* is uncommon, but it may be underdiagnosed because the findings can resemble those of oligoarthritis and RF-negative polyarthritis. The diagnosis is suggested by the presence of arthritis and 2 of the following findings: nail changes (pitting or onycholysis), dactylitis, or a history of psoriasis in a first-degree relative. Insidious and chronic anterior uveitis, usually bilateral, is seen in 10% of affected children.

Enthesitis-related arthritis is a chronic arthritis that is associated with inflammation of entheses, which are the sites where the ligaments, tendons, fasciae, and capsules attach to the bone. This form of childhood arthritis, which has also been referred to as *juvenile ankylosing spondylitis,* usually has its onset at age 8–10 years and is more common in males. The uveitis is acute, symptomatic, and unilateral, but both eyes may be affected at different times. Most patients are HLA-B27–positive, and lumbosacral spine disease and sacroiliitis eventually develop in many.

Cassidy J, Kivlin J, Lindsley C, et al; Section on Rheumatology; Section on Ophthalmology. Ophthalmologic examinations in children with juvenile rheumatoid arthritis. *Pediatrics.* 2006;117(5):1843–1845.

Table 24-3 Frequency of Eye Examination in Patients With JIA

Age at Diagnosis	Frequency of Eye Examination, ANA-Positive Patient	Frequency of Eye Examination, ANA-Negative Patient
≤6 years of age	Every 3 months	Every 6 months
>6 years of age	Every 6 months	Every 12 months

ANA = antinuclear antibody; JIA = juvenile idiopathic arthritis; RF = rheumatoid factor.
Frequencies presented in this table are for eye examinations of patients with RF-negative oligoarthritis or polyarthritis within the first 4 years after diagnosis.

Tubulointerstitial Nephritis and Uveitis Syndrome

Tubulointerstitial nephritis and uveitis (TINU) syndrome is kidney disease associated with chronic or recurrent anterior uveitis in children. The etiology is unknown but may be associated with HLA-DRB1. The median age of onset is 15 years; early studies indicate that it is more common in females, while more recent studies indicate that it is more common in males. The renal disease is characterized by low-grade fever, fatigue, pallor, and weight loss. Elevated levels of β_2-microglobulin may be present in the urine. The uveitis is usually bilateral and may occur before, simultaneously with, or after the renal disease. Prognosis is generally good, although long-term follow-up is required because the inflammation may recur.

Mackensen F, Billing H. Tubulointerstitial nephritis and uveitis syndrome. *Curr Opin Ophthalmol.* 2009;20(6):525–531.

Kawasaki Disease

Kawasaki disease, also known as *mucocutaneous lymph node syndrome,* is a primary vasculitis mediated by immunoglobulin A (IgA) affecting children younger than 5 years. The cause is unknown, but recently, a locus at 19q13 was found to be associated with increased risk for the disease. Abnormalities include fever, conjunctival injection, mucous membrane changes, extremity changes involving the skin, rash, and cervical lymphadenopathy. The most significant complication of Kawasaki disease is coronary artery aneurysm, which occurs in 15%–25% of untreated children. Coronary artery evaluation by echocardiography is therefore indicated.

After conjunctivitis, anterior uveitis during the acute phase of the illness is the second most common ocular finding, occurring in approximately 10% of cases. This is generally self-limited. Rare ocular findings include keratitis, papilledema, optic neuritis, and conjunctival hemorrhage.

Treatment with aspirin and intravenous IgG reduces the incidence of coronary artery aneurysm formation.

Alves NR, Magalhães CM, Almeida R de F, Santos RC, Gandolfi L, Pratesi R. Prospective study of Kawasaki disease complications: review of 115 cases. *Rev Assoc Med Bras.* 2011;57(3):295–300.

Other Causes of Anterior Uveitis

Many cases of anterior uveitis are idiopathic or are caused by trauma. Other causes include a variety of infectious and noninfectious diseases (see Table 24-1).

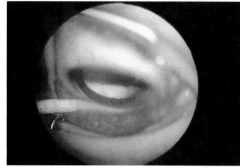

Figure 24-2 Intermediate uveitis with inferior snowbank formation, right eye.

Intermediate Uveitis

The term *intermediate uveitis* is an anatomically based description of the primary site of the ocular inflammation. The inflammation is localized to the vitreous base overlying the ciliary body, pars plana, and peripheral retina, as well as the anterior vitreous (Fig 24-2). Intermediate uveitis accounts for 5%–15% of all cases of uveitis and approximately 12%–28% of uveitis cases in the pediatric age group. In children, it may occur with a variety of conditions, including sarcoidosis, syphilis, Lyme disease, multiple sclerosis, and tuberculosis. Idiopathic disease, known as *pars planitis,* accounts for 85%–90% of cases. The distinction between pars planitis and intermediate uveitis is not always clear. The 2 terms are often used interchangeably.

Posterior Uveitis

Toxoplasmosis

Toxoplasmosis is the most common cause of posterior uveitis in children. It is discussed in Chapter 28.

Toxocariasis

Ocular toxocariasis is caused by the nematode larvae of a common intestinal parasite of dogs *(Toxocara canis)* or cats *(Toxocara cati).* This disease primarily affects children, as it is contracted through the ingestion of ascarid ova in soil contaminated by dog or cat feces. *Visceral larva migrans (VLM)* is an acute systemic infection produced by these organisms; it commonly occurs at approximately age 2 years. If symptomatic, it is associated with fever, cough, rashes, malaise, and anorexia. Laboratory testing reveals eosinophilia. VLM and ocular toxocariasis, for unknown reasons, seldom occur in the same patient.

Ocular toxocariasis is usually unilateral and is not associated with systemic illness or an elevated eosinophil count. The average age of onset is 11.5 years. The 3 major retinal forms of the disease include posterior pole granuloma, peripheral granuloma with

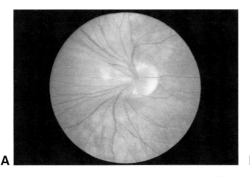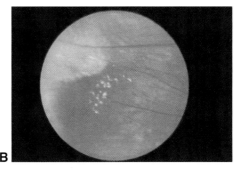

A B

Figure 24-3 Toxocariasis, right eye. **A,** Distortion of posterior pole vessels. **B,** Peripheral granuloma.

macular traction (Fig 24-3), and endophthalmitis. There is often little external evidence of inflammation. Patients may present with leukocoria, strabismus, or decreased vision. These are also common presenting symptoms of retinoblastoma, which must be differentiated from ocular toxocariasis. Although enzyme-linked immunosorbent assay (ELISA) titers for *Toxocara* species have a high sensitivity and specificity and are useful in diagnosing this disease, a positive laboratory finding does not eliminate the possibility of retinoblastoma, as elevated titers may be found in a significant percentage of the general pediatric population.

Treatment includes observation of peripheral lesions, periocular or systemic steroids for posterior lesions and endophthalmitis, or surgical intervention to address retinal traction, cataract, glaucoma, or cyclitic membranes. Systemic antihelmintics are not useful in treating ocular toxocariasis, as the organism producing the inflammation is already dead.

Woodhall D, Starr MC, Montgomery SP, et al. Ocular toxocariasis: epidemiologic, anatomic, and therapeutic variations based on a survey of ophthalmic subspecialists. *Ophthalmology.* 2012;119(6):1211–1217.

Panuveitis

Sarcoidosis

Sarcoidosis may present in 2 distinct forms in children. In young patients (<5 years), lung disease is rare and sarcoidosis is more often characterized by the triad of uveitis, arthritis, and rash. Early-onset sarcoidosis is considered a *pediatric granulomatous arthritis* and is phenotypically and genetically similar to Blau syndrome (see discussion in next section). Older children (8–15 years) have the pulmonary abnormalities and lymph node findings more commonly associated with the adult form of the disease and are at risk for uveitis. Although anterior uveitis (Fig 24-4) is the most common manifestation of ocular sarcoidosis in children, this disease can produce a panuveitis.

Diagnosis and treatment in children is similar to that in adults, but serum angiotensin-converting enzyme (ACE) levels in healthy children are higher than they are in adults and

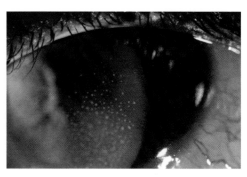

Figure 24-4 Keratic precipitates in sarcoid-osis. *(Courtesy of Ken K. Nischal, MD.)*

thus can be misleading when used to diagnose pediatric sarcoidosis. If this disorder is suspected, children should undergo careful evaluation for systemic disease.

> Shetty AK, Gedalia A. Childhood sarcoidosis: a rare but fascinating disorder. *Pediatr Rheumatol Online J.* 2008;6:16.

Familial Juvenile Systemic Granulomatosis

Familial juvenile systemic granulomatosis *(Blau syndrome)* is an autosomal dominant disease that may be identical to early-onset sarcoidosis; both are classified as *pediatric granulomatous arthritides.* Both diseases have mutations in the *NOD2* gene on chromosome 16, but in Blau syndrome other family members are affected. Both diseases present with granulomatous arthritis, uveitis, and rash during childhood. Pulmonary involvement and adenopathy are absent in Blau syndrome. Chronic panuveitis associated with multifocal choroiditis is the most common ocular presentation, but uveitis may be limited to the anterior segment in some cases, and the disease may be misdiagnosed as JIA. Ocular complications, including cataract, glaucoma, band keratopathy, and vision loss are common.

> Okafuji I, Nishikomori R, Kanazawa N, et al. Role of the *NOD2* genotype in the clinical phenotype of Blau syndrome and early-onset sarcoidosis. *Arthritis Rheum.* 2009;60(1):242–250.

Vogt-Koyanagi-Harada Syndrome

Vogt-Koyanagi-Harada syndrome is a chronic, progressive bilateral panuveitis that is associated with exudative retinal detachments and may be accompanied by meningeal irritation, auditory disturbances, and skin changes. It is rare in children, but those affected experience a higher frequency of ocular complications such as cataract and glaucoma and have a poorer visual prognosis than do adults.

> Martin TD, Rathinam SR, Cunningham ET Jr. Prevalence, clinical characteristics, and causes of vision loss in children with Vogt-Koyanagi-Harada disease in South India. *Retina.* 2010; 30(7):1113–1121.

Other Causes of Posterior Uveitis and Panuveitis

Other causes of posterior uveitis and panuveitis are listed in Table 24-1.

Table 24-4 Masquerade Syndromes

Disease	Age (Years)	Signs of Inflammation	Diagnostic Studies
Anterior segment			
Retinoblastoma	<15	Flare, cells, pseudohypopyon	Ultrasonography, MRI
Leukemia	<15	Flare, cells, hypopyon, heterochromia, hyphema	Bone marrow biopsy, peripheral blood smear
Intraocular foreign body	Any age	Flare, cells	X-ray, CT, ultrasonography
Malignant melanoma	Any age	Flare, cells	Fluorescein angiography, ultrasonography
Juvenile xanthogranuloma	<15	Flare, cells, hyphema	Examination of skin, iris biopsy
Peripheral retinal detachment	Any age	Flare, cells	Ophthalmoscopy
Posterior segment			
Retinitis pigmentosa	Any age	Cells in vitreous, waxy disc pallor, bone-spicule pigmentary changes in midperiphery	ERG, visual fields
Primary CNS lymphoma	≥15	Vitreous exudates, retinal hemorrhage or exudates, retinal pigment epithelium infiltrates	Cytology study of aqueous and vitreous, ultrasonography, MRI
Systemic lymphoma	≥15	Retinal hemorrhage or exudates, vitreous cells	Node biopsy, bone marrow biopsy, physical examination
Retinoblastoma	<15	Vitreous cells, retinal exudates	Ultrasonography, MRI
Malignant melanoma	≥15	Vitreous cells	Fluorescein angiography, ultrasonography
Multiple sclerosis	≥15	Periphlebitis, pars planitis	Neurologic examination

CNS = central nervous system; CT = computed tomography; ERG = electroretinogram; MRI = magnetic resonance imaging.

Masquerade Syndromes

Various conditions can simulate pediatric uveitis. Table 24-4 lists these masquerade syndromes and their diagnostic features.

Evaluation of Pediatric Uveitis

Establishing the correct diagnosis is important in managing a pediatric patient with uveitis, but some ophthalmologists defer the workup of isolated anterior uveitis unless it is recurrent or unresponsive to initial therapy. Accurate diagnosis requires a detailed history, thorough ophthalmic examination, and selected laboratory tests. An examination under anesthesia may be needed if the child is not cooperative enough for an office evaluation. Laboratory investigations are chosen based on the suspected diagnoses (Table 24-5; also see Table 24-4).

Table 24-5 Laboratory Tests for Various Types of Uveitis

Anterior uveitis
  Antinuclear antibody (JIA)
  ACE, serum lysozyme (sarcoidosis)
  Chest x-ray (sarcoidosis, tuberculosis)
  Tuberculin skin test, interferon-γ release assay (tuberculosis)
  FTA-ABS (syphilis)
  Lyme serology (Lyme disease)
  Complete blood count (leukemia)
  HLA-B27 and sacroiliac joint films (enthesitis-related arthritis, ankylosing spondylitis)
  Gastrointestinal series (if ulcerative colitis or regional enteritis [Crohn disease] is suspected)
  Urinalysis, blood urea nitrogen, serum creatinine, urine β_2-microglobulin (tubulointerstitial
    nephritis and uveitis syndrome)
  Antineutrophil cytoplasmic antibody (granulomatosis with polyangiitis)

Intermediate uveitis
  ACE, serum lysozyme (sarcoidosis)
  Chest x-ray (sarcoidosis, tuberculosis)
  Tuberculin skin test, interferon-γ release assay (tuberculosis)
  FTA-ABS (syphilis)
  Lyme serology (Lyme disease)

Posterior uveitis and panuveitis
  Toxoplasmosis PCR, ELISA
  Toxocariasis PCR, ELISA
  ACE, serum lysozyme (sarcoidosis)
  Chest x-ray (sarcoidosis, tuberculosis)
  Tuberculin skin test, interferon-γ release assay (tuberculosis)
  FTA-ABS (syphilis)
  Lyme serology (Lyme disease)
  PCR, blood cultures, viral cultures, or antibody levels if cytomegalovirus, herpes simplex, herpes
    zoster, rubella, measles, or *Bartonella henselae* infection is suspected

ACE = angiotensin-converting enzyme; ELISA = enzyme-linked immunosorbent assay; FTA-ABS = fluorescent treponemal antibody absorption test; HLA = human leukocyte antigen; JIA = juvenile idiopathic arthritis; PCR = polymerase chain reaction.

Treatment of Pediatric Uveitis

The goals of uveitis treatment in children are to eliminate the inflammation of the eye before ocular complications occur and to monitor for ocular and systemic adverse effects of the treatment. It is important to note that although the presence of cells in the anterior chamber indicates active inflammation, flare (protein) may chronically persist even after the inflammation has been successfully treated.

Infectious diseases and malignancies producing uveitis should be identified and treated appropriately. Treatment of noninfectious uveitis is discussed in the following sections.

Management of Inflammation

Anterior segment inflammation is initially treated with topical corticosteroid and mydriatic/cycloplegic agents. Because topical corticosteroids do not penetrate well into the vitreous or posterior segment, sub-Tenon injections of a corticosteroid may be useful in the treatment of intermediate or posterior uveitis. Short courses of oral corticosteroids may be used, but long-term use is usually avoided because of the potential for significant ocular and systemic adverse effects. Recently, steroid intravitreal implants containing either fluocinolone acetonide or dexamethasone have been used successfully to treat posterior uveitis in children.

Glaucoma and cataract formation are the most serious ocular complications of any corticosteroid therapy. In general, more-potent topical corticosteroids are more likely to increase intraocular pressure. Periocular injections of corticosteroids can elevate intraocular pressure for weeks to months after injection. Cataracts and glaucoma are reported adverse effects of intravitreal steroid implants. Risks of long-term systemic corticosteroid use in children include growth retardation, osteoporosis and bone fractures, cushingoid appearance, diabetes mellitus, peptic ulcers, myopathy, hypertension, altered mental status, idiopathic intracranial hypertension, and increased risk of infection. Patients may also require increased doses of corticosteroids during times of stress to avoid an addisonian crisis.

Naproxen and tolmetin are nonsteroidal anti-inflammatory drugs (NSAIDs) that are commonly used to treat arthritis in children and may have some efficacy in treating uveitis. Potential adverse effects of NSAIDs include gastrointestinal irritation, renal toxicity, rashes, and central nervous system reactions.

Systemic immunosuppressive therapy may be beneficial in treating both uveitis and arthritis. It can sometimes reduce or eliminate the need for steroids. The therapy should be undertaken in cooperation with a pediatric specialist familiar with the use of immunosuppressive and immunomodulatory medications and their adverse effects. In patients with JIA, use of immunosuppressive drugs is associated with a reduced risk of vision loss from uveitis.

Methotrexate is the most common antimetabolite used to treat arthritis and uveitis in children. Less commonly used antimetabolites include azathioprine and mycophenolate mofetil. These agents inhibit nucleic acid synthesis by a variety of mechanisms. Gastrointestinal disturbance is the most common adverse effect of methotrexate; it can be alleviated by switching from oral methotrexate to subcutaneous injections. Oral folic acid supplementation is often recommended for patients using methotrexate. Hepatic toxicity, interstitial pneumonitis, and cytopenia are rare but serious adverse effects of methotrexate use.

Biologic drugs for the treatment of refractive uveitis have been used with increasing frequency to suppress the immune system in children. The 2 classes of biologic medications are tumor necrosis factor α (TNF-α) inhibitors and cell-specific antibodies. The TNF-α inhibitors most commonly used to treat uveitis are infliximab and adalimumab, which are monoclonal IgG antibodies against TNF-α. Commonly used cell-specific antibodies include abatacept (antibody to CD80 and CD86) and rituximab (antibody to interleukin-2), with abatacept being the preferred drug. In general, TNF-α inhibitors are used before cell-specific antibodies. All these biologic drugs used to treat uveitis require intravenous infusion, except for adalimumab, which can be given subcutaneously. There is concern that children and adolescents treated with TNF-α blockers may be at increased risk for malignancies; however, a recent study showed that children with JIA are at increased risk for malignancies unrelated to the use of biologic drugs.

Beukelman T, Haynes K, Curtis JR, et al. Rates of malignancy associated with juvenile idiopathic arthritis and its treatment. *Arthritis Rheum.* 2012;64(4):1263–1271. Epub 2012 Feb 10.

Biester S, Deuter C, Michels H, et al. Adalimumab in the therapy of uveitis in childhood. *Br J Ophthalmol.* 2007;91(3):319–324.

Gregory AC II, Kempen JH, Daniel E, et al. Risk factors for loss of visual acuity among patients with uveitis associated with juvenile idiopathic arthritis: the Systemic Immunosuppressive Therapy for Eye Diseases Study. *Ophthalmology.* 2013;120(1):186–192.

Tugal-Tutkun I, Ayranci O, Kasapcopur O, Kir N. Retrospective analysis of children with uveitis treated with infliximab. *J AAPOS.* 2008;12(6):611–613.

Surgical Treatment of Uveitis Complications

Band keratopathy can be treated by removal of corneal epithelium followed by calcium chelation with ethylenediaminetetraacetic acid (EDTA). Treatment may have to be repeated. Phototherapeutic keratectomy has also been used to treat band keratopathy.

Cataract surgery for patients with uveitis can be complicated by hypotony, glaucoma, synechiae formation, cystoid macular edema, and retinal detachment. In patients with JIA, combined lensectomy and vitrectomy appears to produce better results than cataract extraction alone. Uveitis must be aggressively treated so that it is under control both before and after surgery. Intraocular lens implantation is usually not considered in children with uveitis until after a prolonged period of quiescence.

Glaucoma surgery may become necessary in children with uveitis. Many techniques have been used, and long-term success rates vary. Standard trabeculectomy is associated with a high rate of failure due to scarring. Goniotomy or trabeculotomy is effective in many children and can be the initial surgery if the angle is visible. Glaucoma drainage devices can be used when goniotomy fails or if the angle is closed.

Bohnsack BL, Freedman SF. Surgical outcomes in childhood uveitic glaucoma. *Am J Ophthalmol.* 2013;155(1):134–142.

CHAPTER 25

Disorders of the Retina and Vitreous

This chapter focuses on retinal diseases that are most often diagnosed in the first 2 decades of life. These include retinopathy of prematurity, Leber congenital amaurosis, and retinoblastoma, as well as systemic diseases with retinal manifestations (eg, diabetes mellitus). Many of the topics covered in this chapter are also discussed in BCSC Section 12, *Retina and Vitreous*. See BCSC Section 4, *Ophthalmic Pathology and Intraocular Tumors*, for detailed discussion of tumors.

Congenital and Developmental Abnormalities

Persistent Fetal Vasculature

Persistent fetal vasculature (PFV) is covered in Chapter 23.

Retinopathy of Prematurity

Retinopathy of prematurity (ROP) is a vasoproliferative retinal disorder unique to premature infants. It was first described in the 1950s in association with attempts to save premature infants with high doses of supplemental oxygen. Retinal vascular development begins during week 16 of gestation. Mesenchymal tissue (the source of retinal vessels) grows centrifugally from the optic disc, reaching the nasal ora serrata by 36 weeks' gestation and the temporal ora serrata by 40 weeks' gestation. ROP results from abnormal growth of these retinal blood vessels in a premature infant due to a complex interaction between vascular endothelial growth factor (VEGF) and insulin-like growth factor I (IGF-I) (Table 25-1).

Classification

The International Classification of Retinopathy of Prematurity (ICROP) describes the disease by stage, zone, and extent (Table 25-2; Figs 25-1 through 25-5). The higher the stage or the lower the zone, the worse the ROP.

Plus disease is diagnosed by comparison with a standard photograph and refers to marked arteriolar tortuosity and venous engorgement of the posterior pole vasculature. It implies vascular shunting through the new vessels and signifies severe disease (Fig 25-6).

Table 25-1 Interaction Between VEGF and IGF-I in Development of ROP

Phase I
   Occurs at 22–30 weeks' gestational age
   Retina is hyperoxic (relative to intrauterine oxygen levels)
   VEGF levels are low
   Retinal blood vessels stop growing; this arrested growth is
   • worsened by high oxygen levels
   • worsened by low levels of IGF-I
   • correlated with poor weight gain

Phase II
   Occurs at 31–44 weeks' gestational age
   Avascular retina is hypoxic
   VEGF levels rise (due to the hypoxic avascular retina)
   Neovascularization occurs

Treatment of ROP
   Laser therapy destroys hypoxic avascular retina, so VEGF levels fall
   Bevacizumab inhibits VEGF

IGF-I = insulin-like growth factor I; ROP = retinopathy of prematurity; VEGF = vascular endothelial growth factor.

Table 25-2 International Classification of Acute Stages of Retinopathy of Prematurity

Location—Zones II and III are based on convention rather than strict anatomy (see Fig 25-1)
   Zone I (posterior pole)—Circle with radius of 30°, twice the disc–macula distance
   Zone II—From edge of zone I to point tangential to nasal ora serrata and around to area near the temporal equator
   Zone III—Residual crescent anterior to zone II

Extent—Specified as hours of the clock as observer looks at each eye

Staging the disease
   Stage 0—Immature vascularization, no ROP
   Stage 1—Demarcation line (see Fig 25-2)
   Stage 2—Ridge, with or without small tufts of fibrovascular proliferation ("popcorn") (see Fig 25-3)
   Stage 3—Ridge with extraretinal fibrovascular proliferation (see Fig 25-4)
   • Mild fibrovascular proliferation
   • Moderate fibrovascular proliferation
   • Severe fibrovascular proliferation
   Stage 4—Subtotal retinal detachment (see Fig 25-5)
   A. Extrafoveal retinal detachment
   B. Retinal detachment including fovea
   Stage 5—Total retinal detachment
   Funnel: Anterior   Posterior
                 Open   Open
                 Narrow   Narrow

Plus disease—Plus (+) is added when vascular shunting is so marked that the posterior pole veins are enlarged and the arteries are tortuous (see Fig 25-6).

Data from the Committee for Classification of Retinopathy of Prematurity: an international classification of retinopathy of prematurity. *Arch Ophthalmol.* 1984;102(8):1130–1134.

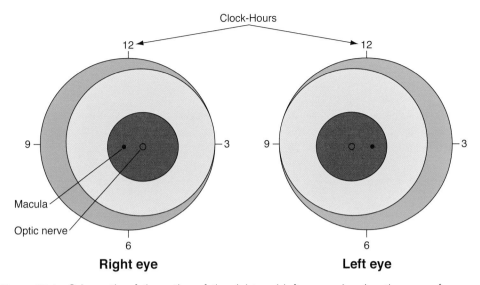

Figure 25-1 Schematic of the retina of the right and left eyes, showing the area of zones I *(red)*, II *(yellow)*, and III *(green)*, as well as clock-hours, which are used to describe the location of retinopathy of prematurity (ROP).

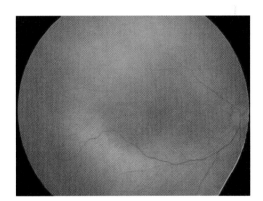

Figure 25-2 Stage 1 ROP. The demarcation line has no height. *(Courtesy of Daniel Weaver, MD.)*

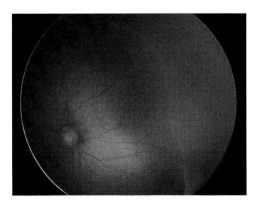

Figure 25-3 Stage 2 ROP. The demarcation line has height and width, creating a ridge. *(Courtesy of Andrea Molinari, MD.)*

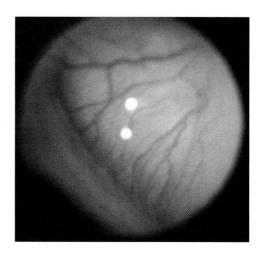

Figure 25-4 Stage 3 ROP. Ridge with extra-retinal fibrovascular proliferation. *(Reproduced with permission from Lueder GT. Pediatric Practice Oph-thalmology. New York: McGraw-Hill; 2011:232.)*

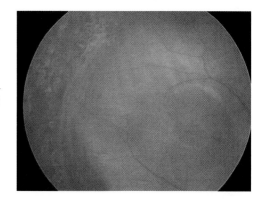

Figure 25-5 Subtotal extrafoveal retinal de-tachment in a patient with stage 4A ROP. *(Courtesy of Philip J. Ferrone, MD.)*

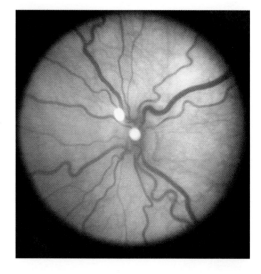

Figure 25-6 Plus disease. *(Reproduced with per-mission from Lueder GT. Pediatric Practice Ophthalmology. New York: McGraw-Hill; 2011:231.)*

Pre–plus disease refers to dilation and tortuosity that is abnormal but less than that seen in the standard photograph (Fig 25-7). *Aggressive posterior ROP* is a severe form of ROP found in some babies with zone I disease (Fig 25-8). The Cryotherapy for Retinopathy of Prematurity (CRYO-ROP) trial defined *threshold* disease as 5 contiguous or 8 total clock-hours of stage 3 in zone I or II with plus disease. The Early Treatment for Retinopathy of Prematurity (ETROP) trial further classified ROP into *type 1* and *type 2* disease to delineate which babies would benefit from treatment before the development of threshold disease (Table 25-3).

> Committee for Classification of Retinopathy of Prematurity. An international classification of retinopathy of prematurity. *Arch Ophthalmol.* 1984;102(8):1130–1134.

Risk factors for development of ROP

Gestational age and weight at birth, 2 of the strongest risk factors for ROP, are inversely correlated with the development of ROP: smaller babies and those born at an earlier gestational age are at higher risk. The incidence of ROP requiring treatment is lower among African American than non–African American babies.

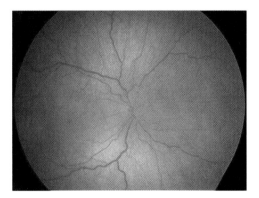

Figure 25-7   Pre–plus disease. *(Courtesy of Daniel Weaver, MD.)*

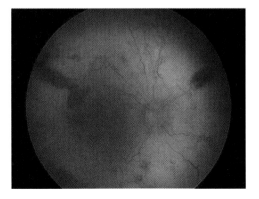

Figure 25-8   Aggressive posterior ROP in an infant born at 31 weeks' gestation and weighing 1375 g. *(Courtesy of Gregg T. Lueder, MD.)*

Table 25-3 ETROP Classification of ROP

Type 1 ROP
Zone I, any stage with plus disease
Zone I, stage 3 without plus disease
Zone II, stage 2 or 3 with plus disease

Type 2 ROP
Zone I, stage 1 or 2 without plus disease
Zone II, stage 3 without plus disease

ETROP = Early Treatment for Retinopathy of Prematurity.

Modified from Wallace DK. Retinopathy of prematurity. *Focal Points: Clinical Modules for Ophthalmologists.* San Francisco: American Academy of Ophthalmology; 2008, module 12:p 4.

Use of supplemental oxygen is a risk factor, as shown in the 1960s when ROP markedly decreased (and death and cerebral palsy markedly increased) with the severe limitation of oxygen for premature infants. However, the exact role that oxygen plays is still not well understood. Despite many studies, the optimal amount of supplemental oxygen to give to premature infants to promote normal development and limit ROP remains elusive. Even though some studies have shown that maintaining oxygen saturation levels at a lower level than was customary prior to 34 weeks' corrected age can lower the incidence of ROP, it is unclear whether the benefit is significant enough to warrant the systemic risks to the infant. Low early levels of IGF-I are associated with slower-than-expected weight gain and more severe ROP. The *w*eight, *I*GF-I, *n*eonatal *ROP* (WINROP) algorithm (Premacure AB, Uppsala, Sweden) is a surveillance system that identifies babies at high risk for development of type 1 ROP. This algorithm—which uses the gestational age, serum IGF-I levels, and tracking of the infant's weight gain—may allow for targeted, cost-effective screening of infants at high risk for severe ROP.

International Committee for the Classification of Retinopathy of Prematurity. The International Classification of Retinopathy of Prematurity revisited. *Arch Ophthalmol.* 2005;123(7):991–999.

Löfqvist C, Hansen-Pupp I, Andersson E, et al. Validation of a new retinopathy of prematurity screening method monitoring longitudinal postnatal weight and insulinlike growth factor I. *Arch Ophthalmol.* 2009;127(5):622–627.

Diagnosis

Dilated fundus examinations should be performed to screen for ROP in infants who were born at a gestational age of 30 weeks or earlier or had a birth weight of less than 1500 g. They should also be performed in premature infants with an unstable course if the pediatrician believes that the child is at high risk for ROP. The first examination should be done at 4 weeks' chronologic (postnatal) age or at a corrected gestational age of 30–31 weeks, whichever is later (but not later than 6 weeks' chronologic age). Current recommendations can be found on the website of the American Academy of Pediatrics (http://pediatrics.aappublications.org/content/131/1/189.full.pdf+html?sid=1db1246f -7f4d-48d9-8692-17301d5808d8).

Cyclomydril (0.2% cyclopentolate and 1.0% phenylephrine) is recommended for the examination of premature infants. Alternatively, tropicamide 0.5% or 1.0% and phenylephrine 2.5% can be used. Sterile instruments should be used to examine the infant.

A nurse should be present for examinations in the neonatal intensive care unit because the infant may experience apnea and bradycardia during examination. If an examination must be postponed, the postponement and medical reason should be documented in the patient's medical record. Follow-up examinations should be performed according to Table 25-4.

Currently, the incidence of ROP is rising in developing countries, echoing the epidemic that occurred in the United States and the United Kingdom in the 1940s and early 1950s. Affected infants in developing countries are larger and of older gestational age than infants in the United States in whom ROP develops, suggesting that screening criteria for ROP should be modified in developing countries.

Digital retinal photography is highly accurate for detecting clinically significant ROP. Therefore, telemedicine involving retinal image–based screening has been used in underserved areas to identify infants at high risk of requiring treatment.

Chiang MF, Melia M, Buffenn AN, et al. Detection of clinically significant retinopathy of prematurity using wide-angle digital retinal photography: a report by the American Academy of Ophthalmology. *Ophthalmology*. 2012;119(6):1272–1280. Epub 2012 Apr 27.

Fierson WM; American Academy of Pediatrics Section on Ophthalmology; American Academy of Ophthalmology; American Association for Pediatric Ophthalmology and Strabismus; American Association of Certified Orthoptists. Screening examination of premature infants for retinopathy of prematurity. *Pediatrics*. 2013;131(1):189–195.

Treatment

Treatment guidelines have been created based on the results of several multicenter ROP trials. These guidelines indicate which level of disease requires treatment to decrease the risk of adverse visual sequelae. In the CRYO-ROP trial, cryotherapy applied to the

---

Table 25-4 Recommended Intervals of Follow-Up Eye Examinations for ROP Without Plus Disease

1 Week or Less
Immature vascularization: zone 1 or posterior zone II
Stage 1 or 2 ROP: zone I
Stage 3 ROP: zone II
Presence or suspected presence of aggressive posterior ROP

1 to 2 Weeks
Immature vascularization: posterior zone II
Stage 2 ROP: zone II
Unequivocally regressing ROP: zone I

2 Weeks
Stage 1 ROP: zone II
Immature vascularization: zone II
Unequivocally regressing ROP: zone II

2 to 3 Weeks
Stage 1 or 2 ROP: zone III
Regressing ROP: zone III

Modified from Fierson WM; American Academy of Pediatrics Section on Ophthalmology; American Academy of Ophthalmology; American Association for Pediatric Ophthalmology and Strabismus; American Association of Certified Orthoptists. Screening examination of premature infants for retinopathy of prematurity. *Pediatrics*. 2013;131(1):189–195.

avascular peripheral retina at threshold resulted in a 50% lower rate of retinal detachment compared with observation. In later studies, laser therapy was used following the same guidelines as those in the CRYO-ROP trial; it was shown to be equally effective in inducing regression of the new vessels and more effective in preventing adverse visual sequelae (Fig 25-9). More recently, the ETROP trial found that earlier treatment in high-risk eyes classified as type 1 resulted in better structural and visual outcomes than conventional treatment at threshold. Laser treatment is strongly recommended for any eye with type 1 ROP. Eyes with type 2 ROP should be closely observed for progression to type 1 disease.

Aggressive posterior ROP is often difficult to treat and has a poor prognosis (see Fig 25-8). The stages of ROP do not progress in the typical fashion, and stage 3 can often appear as flat neovascularization.

The study Bevacizumab Eliminates the Angiogenic Threat of Retinopathy of Prematurity (BEAT-ROP) evaluated the use of antiangiogenic (anti-VEGF) medications in the treatment of ROP. This study showed a significant structural outcome benefit for zone I eyes compared with laser treatment. However, recurrence of ROP requiring retreatment occurred a mean of 16 weeks after initial treatment with bevacizumab, which was significantly later than recurrence of ROP in laser-treated eyes (mean of 6 weeks), and late-onset retinal detachments have been reported. There is also concern about the effects of antiangiogenic drugs on the developing vasculature in other areas of the body. A reduction in serum VEGF has been demonstrated in infants after intravitreal injections.

Early Treatment for Retinopathy of Prematurity Cooperative Group. Revised indications for the treatment of retinopathy of prematurity: results of the Early Treatment for Retinopathy of Prematurity randomized trial. *Arch Ophthalmol.* 2003;121(12):1684–1694.

Early Treatment for Retinopathy of Prematurity Cooperative Group; Good WV, Hardy RJ, Dobson V, et al. Final visual acuity results in the Early Treatment for Retinopathy of Prematurity study. *Arch Ophthalmol.* 2010;128(6):663–671.

Mintz-Hittner HA, Kennedy KA, Chuang AZ; BEAT-ROP Cooperative Group. Efficacy of intravitreal bevacizumab for stage 3+ retinopathy of prematurity. *N Engl J Med.* 2011;364(7): 603–615.

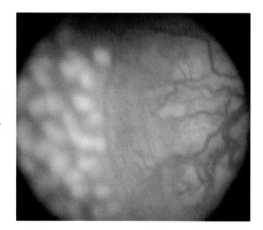

Figure 25-9 Laser photocoagulation applied to avascular retina. Note the thick band of neovascularization and plus disease. *(Courtesy of Philip J. Ferrone, MD.)*

Patel RD, Blair MP, Shapiro MJ, Lichtenstein SJ. Significant treatment failure with intravitreous bevacizumab for retinopathy of prematurity. *Arch Ophthalmol.* 2012;130(6):801–802.

Sato T, Wada K, Arahori H, et al. Serum concentrations of bevacizumab (Avastin) and vascular endothelial growth factor in infants with retinopathy of prematurity. *Am J Ophthalmol.* 2012;153(2):327–333.

Sequelae and complications

One of the most common sequelae of significant ROP, whether treated or spontaneously resolved, is myopia, which may be severe. Amblyopia may result from high myopia, especially if asymmetric, or strabismus. Dragging of the macula can occur, giving rise to pseudostrabismus and the appearance of an exotropia as a result of a large positive angle kappa (Figs 25-10, 25-11). Eyes that have undergone treatment may also experience late retinal detachments at the border of the treated and untreated retina. Therefore, a child who has had ROP requires periodic ophthalmic examinations beyond the newborn period. Late changes associated with stage 5 ROP include cataract, glaucoma, and phthisis bulbi.

When laser treatment, cryotherapy, or bevacizumab has not prevented the progression of ROP to stage 4 or 5 (retinal detachment), scleral buckling and vitrectomy may be indicated if there is reasonable hope of successful reattachment. Anatomical success varies depending on many factors, but visual acuity results have been disappointing, particularly with stage 5 eyes.

Unfortunately, even with the current screening guidelines and recommended treatment of ROP, many babies are blinded by this disease each year.

Repka MX, Tung B, Good WV, Capone A Jr, Shapiro MJ. Outcome of eyes developing retinal detachment during the Early Treatment for Retinopathy of Prematurity study. *Arch Ophthalmol.* 2011;129(9):1175–1179.

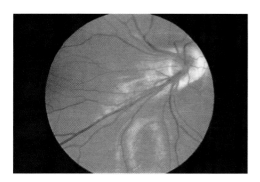

Figure 25-10 Posterior pole traction and dragging of the macula, a sequela of ROP, right eye.

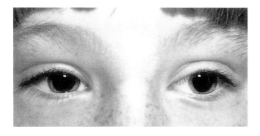

Figure 25-11 Pseudoexotropia in a fixating left eye in ROP. The patient has a positive angle kappa as a result of macular dragging.

Hereditary Retinal Disease

Nystagmus is the most common presenting sign of hereditary retinal disorders. The onset of nystagmus typically occurs between 8 and 12 weeks of age and indicates limited visual potential (see Chapter 13). Although most diseases that present with nystagmus in infancy have visible structural abnormalities of the eyes, 3 of the diseases discussed here (Leber congenital amaurosis, achromatopsia, and X-linked congenital stationary night blindness) can present with a normal retinal appearance. Nystagmus does not develop in all patients with hereditary retinal disease; for example, it might not develop in those with less severe retinal damage. Poor visual function or failed vision screening may be the presenting abnormality in older children with retinal disease. Paradoxical pupils (pupils that initially constrict in the dark) are common in hereditary retinal dystrophies (Table 25-5).

Many important tests necessary for diagnosis of hereditary retinal disorders (eg, electroretinogram [ERG], electro-oculogram [EOG], color vision testing, visual field testing, dark adaptation tests) are difficult to perform in young children. Sedation or general anesthesia may be required for an ERG. The ERG response matures in the first year of life. Thus, an ERG can appear highly abnormal in an infant who will later develop a normal response. It is often advisable to either delay the ERG until age 6 months or repeat the ERG after 6 months of age.

Hereditary retinal diseases with onset late in childhood are much like adult hereditary retinal diseases and are not covered here.

Leber congenital amaurosis

Leber congenital amaurosis (LCA) is a group of hereditary (usually autosomal recessive) retinal diseases that affect both rod and cone photoreceptors. LCA is characterized by severe vision loss in infancy, nystagmus, poorly reactive pupils, and an extinguished ERG. Visual acuity ranges from 20/200 to bare light perception in most patients. Funduscopic appearance varies highly, depending on the genotype. It ranges from a normal appearance, particularly in infancy; to pigment clumping in the retinal pigment epithelium (RPE); to resemblance of classic retinitis pigmentosa, with bone spicules, attenuation of arterioles, and disc pallor. Other reported but less common fundus findings include extensive chorioretinal atrophy, macular coloboma, white dots (similar to those seen in retinitis punctata albescens), and marbleized retinal appearance (Fig 25-12). Histologic examination shows diffuse absence of photoreceptors.

Table 25-5 Differential Diagnosis of Paradoxical Pupils

Congenital stationary night blindness
Achromatopsia (complete, incomplete, or blue-cone monochromatism)
Leber congenital amaurosis
Retinitis pigmentosa
Best disease
Albinism
Optic nerve hypoplasia

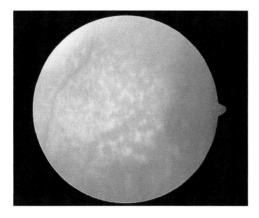

Figure 25-12 Leber congenital amaurosis with marbleized fundus.

Additional ocular manifestations include the oculodigital reflex (eye poking), photoaversion, cataracts, keratoconus, and keratoglobus. High refractive errors, usually high hyperopia, are common.

LCA-like phenotypes can also be found in a number of systemic diseases, including peroxisomal diseases (Zellweger syndrome, neonatal adrenoleukodystrophy, and infantile Refsum disease) and the ciliopathies (Alström syndrome, Joubert syndrome, Senior-Loken syndrome, and Bardet-Biedl syndrome). The ciliopathies are a group of disorders that affect the function and/or structure of the cilia, manifesting in brain, renal, and eye disease.

Diagnosis An ERG is usually required to diagnose LCA. Genetic testing is important and can be used to counsel the patient's family, confirm the diagnosis, distinguish LCA from other retinal diseases, and predict prognosis. Molecular diagnosis of LCA is hindered by the fact that the disease is heterogeneous. Currently, there are 15 genetic mutations known to cause LCA; the most frequent involve *CEP290* (15%), *GUCY2D* (12%), and *CRB1* (10%). Mutations cannot be identified in approximately 30% of cases.

Treatment Currently, gene therapy is available in human clinical trials only for the *RPE65* gene. These studies have demonstrated improvement in subjective and objective vision after subretinal injections of the gene promoter attached to an adeno-associated viral particle.

Jacobson SG, Cideciyan AV, Ratnakaram R, et al. Gene therapy for Leber congenital amaurosis caused by *RPE65* mutations: safety and efficacy in 15 children and adults followed up to 3 years. *Arch Ophthalmol.* 2012;130(1):9–24.

Achromatopsia

Complete achromatopsia, also known as *rod monochromatism,* is an autosomal recessive congenital disorder of the cone photoreceptors in which patients have no color vision, poor central vision, nystagmus, and photophobia. These patients see the world in shades of gray. The photophobia actually represents a desire to avoid bright light rather than true pain or discomfort; it may be manifested by squinting or fluttering of the eyelids in normal indoor illumination. Hemeralopia, the inability to see clearly in bright light, occurs in these patients.

Findings on retinal examination are usually normal, with the possible exception of a poor or absent foveal reflex. Although achromatopsia was initially thought to be a stationary disorder, recent studies have shown deterioration of visual acuity, macular appearance, and cone function on ERG.

Diagnosis Results of color vision testing are markedly abnormal, as is the ERG, which shows extinguished cone or photopic responses but normal rod responses. To date, 3 autosomal recessive genes have been linked to achromatopsia: *CNGA3*, *CNGB3*, and *GNAT2*; the *CNGB3* mutation is the most common.

Other cone dystrophies causing early-onset visual impairment and nystagmus include *incomplete achromatopsia* and *blue-cone monochromatism*. In both disorders, patients usually have better vision than do those with complete achromatopsia. Incomplete achromatopsia is an autosomal recessive disorder that shows some residual cone function on ERG testing. Blue-cone monochromatism is an X-linked disorder; on ERG testing, the blue (short-wavelength) cones show normal function but the photopic response is usually extinguished.

Treatment Dark glasses or red glasses that exclude short wavelengths may help. Gene therapy has been used in animal models.

Thiadens AA, Slingerland NW, Roosing S, et al. Genetic etiology and clinical consequences of complete and incomplete achromatopsia. *Ophthalmology.* 2009;116(10):1984–1989.

Congenital stationary night blindness

Congenital stationary night blindness (CSNB) refers to a group of nonprogressive retinal disorders characterized predominantly by abnormal function of the rod system. The condition may be X-linked (the most common form), autosomal recessive, or autosomal dominant. The X-linked form has been mapped to the locus Xp11.

CSNB, especially the autosomal recessive and X-linked forms, usually presents in early infancy with nystagmus and normal fundi. These forms are often also associated with myopia and decreased visual acuity of roughly 20/200. However, the range of vision in these patients is wide, and occasionally, patients have normal vision. The retina usually appears normal, but the optic nerve may show myopic tilt and temporal pallor.

Diagnosis An ERG is necessary for diagnosis. The most common ERG pattern seen in CSNB is the "negative" dark-adapted ERG: a large a-wave and a reduced-amplitude (negative) b-wave. Dark adaptation is abnormal in all patients with CSNB. Infants with CSNB may have a flat ERG until approximately 6 months of age, when it converts to the classic negative configuration.

Treatment Bright illumination should be used for visual tasks and refractive errors corrected.

Foveal hypoplasia

Foveal hypoplasia, or incomplete development of the fovea, is another cause of nystagmus in early infancy. Although this condition is most often associated with albinism or aniridia, it may also be isolated or familial and may be related to a defect in the *PAX6* gene. On ophthalmoscopic examination, the foveal reflex is poor or absent and the macula exhibits hypoplasia to varying degrees, which can also be seen in patients with complete achromatopsia.

Diagnosis Fundus examination showing foveal hypoplasia is diagnostic. Optical coherence tomography may be useful.

Treatment No treatment is currently available.

> Al-Saleh AA, Hellani A, Abu-Amero KK. Isolated foveal hypoplasia: report of a new case and detailed genetic investigation. *Int Ophthalmol.* 2011;31(2):117–120.

Aicardi syndrome

Aicardi syndrome is an X-linked autosomal dominant disorder characterized by the clinical triad of widespread round or oval depigmented chorioretinal lacunae, infantile spasms, and agenesis of the corpus callosum (Fig 25-13). Chorioretinal lacunae occur in 88% of patients, and optic nerve abnormalities occur in 81%. Colobomas, persistent pupillary membranes, and microphthalmos may also occur. Aicardi syndrome is typically lethal in males.

Diagnosis The clinical picture provides the foundation for diagnosis.

Treatment No treatment is currently available.

> Fruhman G, Eble TN, Gambhir N, Sutton VR, Van den Veyver IB, Lewis RA. Ophthalmologic findings in Aicardi syndrome. *J AAPOS.* 2012;16(3):238–241.

Hereditary Macular Dystrophies

Macular abnormalities are seen in a number of hereditary disorders. The abnormality can be associated with a hereditary systemic disease (eg, the cherry-red spot seen in generalized gangliosidosis) or can reflect a primary retinal disorder, such as Stargardt disease or Best disease. Only primary retinal disorders are discussed here.

Stargardt disease

Stargardt disease (juvenile macular degeneration) is the most common hereditary macular dystrophy. Inheritance is usually autosomal recessive; in rare cases, it is autosomal dominant. Most cases are caused by mutations in the retina-specific adenosine

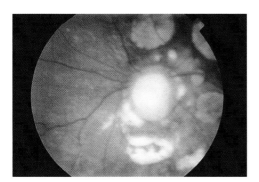

Figure 25-13 Aicardi syndrome. Fundus photograph showing optic disc coloboma and chorioretinal lacunae.

triphosphate–binding transporter gene *(ABCA4)*. It usually presents between ages 8 and 15 years with a decrease in vision. It is a bilateral, symmetric, progressive condition; visual acuity levels off at approximately 20/50–20/200.

Diagnosis The disease often progresses through stages. Initially, the fundus appears normal even when vision is decreased, and the patient may be misdiagnosed as having functional vision loss. The first ophthalmoscopic changes observed are loss of foveal reflex, followed by development of a characteristic macular bull's-eye atrophy with surrounding round or pisciform yellow flecks, which develop in the posterior pole at the level of the RPE. If the flecks are scattered throughout the fundus, the condition may be referred to as *fundus flavimaculatus*. Before the flecks develop, the macula often appears atrophic due to diseased RPE, inducing a peculiar light-reflecting quality that resembles that of beaten bronze (Fig 25-14).

The "dark choroid" sign on fluorescein angiography is distinctive and helps confirm the diagnosis of Stargardt disease. This phenomenon is due to the accumulation of lipofuscin-like pigment throughout the RPE, which blocks the choroidal fluorescence on fluorescein angiography; it is present in 80% of patients with Stargardt disease.

ERGs are often normal in the early stages of Stargardt disease. Stargardt disease can be associated with a progressive cone–rod dystrophy that has a much worse visual prognosis and an extinguished ERG.

Genetic testing for *ABCA4* mutations may be diagnostic.

Treatment Gene therapy for Stargardt disease has been used in animal models and is being studied in phase 1 clinical trials in humans.

Han Z, Conley SM, Makkia RS, Cooper MJ, Naash MI. DNA nanoparticle-mediated *ABCA4* delivery rescues Stargardt dystrophy in mice. *J Clin Invest.* 2012;122(9):3221–3226.

Best disease

Best disease, or *juvenile-onset vitelliform macular dystrophy (VMD)*, is an autosomal dominant retinal disorder with variable penetrance and expressivity. The condition is caused by mutations in the *BEST1* gene on chromosome 11, which encodes for the protein bestrophin. Patients usually present asymptomatically in childhood with the classic retinal appearance or later in life with decrease in vision.

Diagnosis The retina may appear normal at first, but between 4 and 10 years of age, the "egg yolk," or vitelliform, stage begins. A yellow-orange cystlike structure is seen, usually in the

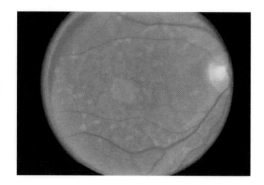

Figure 25-14 Stargardt disease. The macula has an atrophic, beaten-metal appearance.

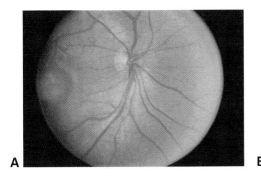 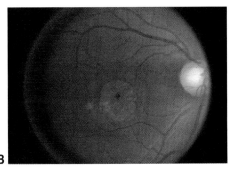

A   B

Figure 25-15 Best disease. **A,** Early disease, or "yolk" stage. **B,** Advanced disease, or "scrambled egg" stage. *(Part B courtesy of Richard A. Lewis, MD.)*

macula; however, the lesion may occur elsewhere, and occasionally there are multiple lesions (Fig 25-15A). The lesions are usually 1.5–5.0 disc diameters in size. The egg yolk–like appearance is associated with good central vision. With time, the cystic material may become granular, giving rise to the "scrambled egg" stage (Fig 25-15B). At this stage, central vision usually remains good, with visual acuity often being roughly 20/30. The cyst may rupture and become partially resorbed; a pseudohypopyon may form from cystic contents. Subretinal neovascularization and serous detachment of the RPE develop in 20% of patients. Subretinal hemorrhage may occur, and visual acuity may deteriorate to 20/100 or worse.

The EOG is usually abnormal in affected patients and carriers. This disorder is one of the few in which the EOG is abnormal and the ERG is normal. *BEST1* gene mutations are found in 60%–83% of affected patients. Carriers can be identified by the presence of an abnormal EOG with a normal retina or a *BEST1* gene mutation.

Treatment No treatment is indicated unless subretinal neovascularization occurs.

> Meunier I, Sénéchal A, Dhaenens CM, et al. Systematic screening for *BEST1* and *PRPH2* in juvenile and adult vitelliform macular dystrophies: a rationale for molecular analysis. *Ophthalmology.* 2011;118(6):1130–1136.

Hereditary Vitreoretinopathies

Hereditary vitreoretinopathies include a broad range of disease entities. The ones discussed here characteristically present in childhood.

Juvenile retinoschisis

Juvenile retinoschisis (splitting of the retina) is an X-linked disease caused by mutations in the *RS1* gene, which encodes for the retinal protein retinoschisin, an adhesion protein that is believed to be essential to the health of Müller cells. Males usually present in early childhood with decreased vision. Visual acuity varies but usually deteriorates to roughly 20/200.

Diagnosis Foveal retinoschisis is present in almost all cases. Approximately 50% of patients also have peripheral retinoschisis (Fig 25-16). The retinoschisis occurs in the nerve fiber layer. The fovea has a star-shaped or spokelike configuration that may resemble cystoid macular edema; it becomes less distinct over time. Vitreous veils or strands are

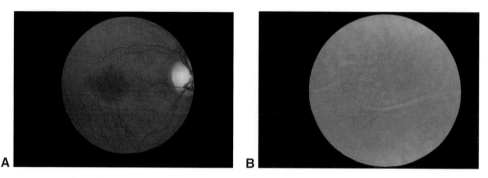

Figure 25-16 Juvenile retinoschisis. Central (macular) schisis **(A)** and peripheral schisis **(B)** may be present. *(Part A courtesy of Richard A. Lewis, MD.)*

common, and vitreal syneresis, or liquefaction, is prominent. Complications include vitreous hemorrhage and retinal detachment. The ERG shows a reduction of the scotopic b-wave with preservation of the a-wave. Optical coherence tomography scans show schisis spaces in the middle layers of the macula.

Treatment Contact sports should be avoided since the retina is more susceptible to trauma. Gene replacement has had some success in mouse models.

> Molday RS, Kellner U, Weber BH. X-linked juvenile retinoschisis: clinical diagnosis, genetic analysis, and molecular mechanisms. *Prog Retin Eye Res.* 2012;31(3):195–212.

Stickler syndrome

Stickler syndrome is the most common of the hereditary hyaloideoretinopathies. A hallmark of all such conditions is vitreous liquefaction that results in an optically empty vitreous cavity, except for vitreous veils that may be attached to the retina. There are many types of Stickler syndrome, which may present with ocular findings only, systemic findings only, or both ocular and systemic findings. The most common type of Stickler syndrome is autosomal dominant, has ocular and systemic findings, and is caused by a mutation in *COL2A1,* the gene that encodes for type II procollagen.

Diagnosis The diagnosis is made based on the clinical features as well as the results of genetic testing. In addition to the optically empty vitreous, common ocular abnormalities include high myopia, a high incidence of retinal detachment secondary to retinal breaks, lattice degeneration, and proliferative vitreoretinopathy. Anterior chamber angle anomalies, ectopia lentis, cataracts, ptosis, and strabismus are less common.

The systemic abnormalities are characterized by a flat midface, progressive hearing loss, cleft palate, Pierre Robin sequence, mitral valve prolapse, and progressive arthropathy with spondyloepiphyseal dysplasia. Although the arthropathy may not be symptomatic initially, children with Stickler syndrome often show radiographic abnormalities of long bones and joints.

Treatment The retinal detachments are often difficult to repair because the patient may have large retinal breaks posteriorly and the incidence of proliferative vitreoretinopathy is high. The incidence of vitreous loss during cataract surgery is high, as is the rate of subsequent retinal detachment. Retinal folds and breaks should be treated before cataract extraction. Prophylactic retinopexy may be appropriate in certain patients.

Snead MP, McNinch AM, Poulson AV, et al. Stickler syndrome, ocular-only variants and a key diagnostic role for the ophthalmologist. *Eye (Lond).* 2011;25(11):1389–1400.

Norrie disease

Norrie disease is an X-linked recessive disorder of retinal dysplasia caused by a mutation in the *NDP* gene, which encodes for the protein norrin.

Diagnosis Affected boys are typically born blind and have varying degrees of hearing impairment and intellectual disability. The condition is characterized by a distinctive retinal appearance: a globular, severely dystrophic retina with pigmentary changes in the avascular periphery. During the first few days or weeks of life, a bilateral, yellowish retinal detachment appears, followed by a whiter mass behind the clear lens. Over time, the lenses, and later the cornea, opacify; phthisis bulbi may ensue by age 10 years or earlier. Female carriers show peripheral retinal abnormalities.

Treatment No treatment exists.

Familial exudative vitreoretinopathy

Familial exudative vitreoretinopathy (FEVR) is a disease of abnormal retinal vascularization similar to that seen in ROP (discussed earlier in the chapter). Type 1 FEVR is autosomal dominant and is caused by a mutation on chromosome 11. Type 2 FEVR is an X-linked recessive disorder caused by a mutation in the *NDP* gene, the same gene involved in Norrie disease

Diagnosis Posterior pole findings in FEVR include retinal traction, folds, breaks, and detachment secondary to vitreous traction; posterior vitreous detachment; avascular peripheral retina; and thick peripheral intraretinal and subretinal exudates. The disease is bilateral and can mimic ROP but affects infants born at full term. Fluorescein angiography shows areas of retinal nonperfusion. Examination of family members is important in the diagnosis of FEVR. Affected family members can show marked variation in severity, from minimal straightening of retinal vessels and peripheral nonperfusion to total retinal detachment.

Treatment Cryopexy, photocoagulation, retinal detachment surgery, vitrectomy, and cataract surgery have all been used to manage this disorder.

Infections

Herpes Simplex Virus and Cytomegalovirus

Herpes simplex virus and cytomegalovirus are discussed in Chapter 28.

Human Immunodeficiency Virus

The ocular complications of HIV infection have been observed only rarely since the advent of highly active antiretroviral therapy (HAART). Such complications typically occur only in children with advanced HIV infection who are severely immunocompromised. For more information, see BCSC Section 9, *Intraocular Inflammation and Uveitis,* and Section 12, *Retina and Vitreous.*

Tumors

Choroidal and Retinal Pigment Epithelial Lesions

A pigmented fundus lesion in a child is usually benign. Flat choroidal nevi are common and are not a cause for concern. Malignant melanoma of the choroid is extremely rare in children. Choroidal osteoma is a benign bony tumor of the uveal tract that may occur in childhood, usually presenting with decreased vision. Diffuse hemangioma of the choroid associated with Sturge-Weber syndrome is discussed in Chapter 28. Patients with neurofibromatosis 1 often have flat, tan-colored spots in the choroid (see Chapter 28).

Congenital hypertrophy of the retinal pigment epithelium (CHRPE) is a sharply demarcated, flat, hyperpigmented lesion that may be isolated or multifocal (Fig 25-17). Such lesions are sometimes grouped, in which case they are also known as *bear tracks.*

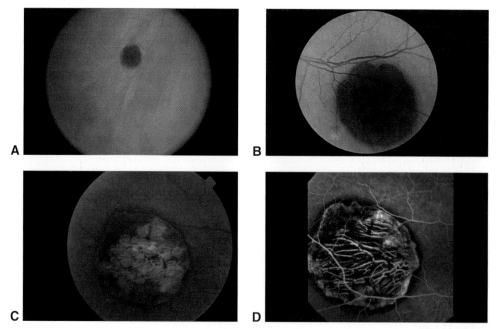

Figure 25-17 Congenital hypertrophy of the retinal pigment epithelium (CHRPE). Examples of varying clinical appearances. **A,** Small CHRPE. **B,** Medium-sized CHRPE; note the homogeneous black color and well-defined margins of this nummular lesion. **C,** Color fundus photograph. **D,** Corresponding fluorescein angiogram of a large CHRPE. Note the loss of retinal pigment epithelium architecture and highlighted choroidal vasculature. *(Parts A, C, and D courtesy of Timothy G. Murray, MD.)*

Pigmented lesions similar to CHRPE have been associated with Gardner syndrome. Gardner syndrome is autosomal dominant and is caused by a mutation in the *APC* gene located on 5q21. Patients with Gardner syndrome have many polyps of the colon and are at very high risk for adenocarcinoma of the colon in early adulthood. They may also have skeletal hamartomas and various other soft-tissue tumors. The pigmented retinal lesions associated with Gardner syndrome are different from CHRPE in that they have a surrounding halo and tail of depigmentation that is oriented radially and directed toward the optic nerve. The presence of 4 or more pigmented retinal lesions not restricted to 1 sector of the fundus or bilateral involvement should raise suspicion of Gardner syndrome.

Combined hamartoma of the retina and retinal pigment epithelium is an ill-defined, elevated, variably pigmented tumor that may be juxtapapillary or located in the retinal periphery. The tumor is often minimally elevated and has retinal traction and tortuous retinal vessels. In peripheral tumors, dragging of the retinal vessels is a prominent feature. The tumors have a variable composition of glial tissue and RPE. This condition can be associated with neurofibromatosis types 1 and 2, incontinentia pigmenti, X-linked retinoschisis, and facial hemangiomas.

Retinoblastoma

Retinoblastoma is the most common malignant intraocular tumor of childhood and one of the most common pediatric solid tumors, with an incidence of 1:14,000–1:20,000 live births. It is equally common in both sexes and has no racial predilection. Retinoblastoma is a neuroblastic tumor and is therefore biologically similar to neuroblastoma and medulloblastoma. The tumor can be unilateral or bilateral; 30%–40% of cases are bilateral. Retinoblastoma is typically diagnosed during the first year of life in familial and bilateral cases and between ages 1 and 3 years in sporadic unilateral cases. Approximately 90% of cases are diagnosed before 3 years of age; onset later than age 5 is rare but can occur. The most common initial sign is leukocoria (white pupil), which is usually first noticed by the family and described as a glow, glint, or cat's-eye appearance (Fig 25-18). The differential diagnosis of leukocoria is shown in Table 25-6. Approximately 25% of cases present with strabismus (esotropia or exotropia). Less common presentations include vitreous hemorrhage, hyphema, ocular or periocular inflammation, glaucoma, proptosis, and pseudohypopyon.

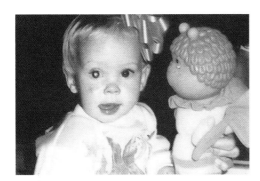

Figure 25-18 Leukocoria of the right eye, which is visible in this family photograph of a 1-year-old girl with retinoblastoma. *(Courtesy of A. Linn Murphree, MD.)*

Table 25-6 Differential Diagnosis of Leukocoria

Retinoblastoma
Persistent fetal vasculature
Retinopathy of prematurity
Cataract
Coloboma of choroid or optic disc
Uveitis
Toxocariasis
Congenital retinal fold
Coats disease
Organizing vitreous hemorrhage
Retinal dysplasia
Corneal opacity
Familial exudative vitreoretinopathy (FEVR)
High myopia or anisometropia
Myelinated nerve fibers
Norrie disease
Retinal detachment
Photographic artifact

Diagnosis

Diagnosis of retinoblastoma is usually based on its ophthalmoscopic appearance. Intraocular retinoblastoma can exhibit a variety of growth patterns. With endophytic growth, it appears as a white to cream-colored mass that breaks through the internal limiting membrane (Fig 25-19). Endophytic retinoblastoma is sometimes associated with vitreous seeding, in which individual cells or fragments of tumor tissue become separated from the main mass, as shown in Figure 25-20. Vitreous seeds may be few and localized or so extensive that the clinical picture resembles endophthalmitis. Occasionally, malignant cells enter the anterior chamber and form a pseudohypopyon.

Exophytic tumors are usually yellow-white and occur in the subretinal space; the overlying retinal vessels are commonly larger in caliber and more tortuous (Fig 25-21). Exophytic retinoblastoma growth is often associated with subretinal fluid accumulation, which can obscure the tumor and closely mimic the appearance of an exudative retinal detachment suggestive of advanced Coats disease. Retinoblastoma cells have the potential to implant on previously uninvolved retinal tissue and grow, thereby creating an impression of multicentricity in an eye with only a single primary tumor.

Large tumors often show signs of both endophytic and exophytic growth. Small retinoblastoma lesions appear as a grayish mass and are frequently confined between the internal and external limiting membranes. A third pattern, diffuse infiltrative retinoblastoma, is usually unilateral and nonhereditary. It is found in children older than 5 years. The tumor presents with conjunctival injection, anterior chamber seeds, pseudohypopyon, large clumps of vitreous cells, and retinal infiltration of tumor. Because no distinct tumor mass is present, diagnostic confusion with inflammatory conditions is common.

Spontaneous regression of retinoblastoma is possible. It can be asymptomatic, resulting in the development of a benign retinocytoma, or it can be associated with inflammation

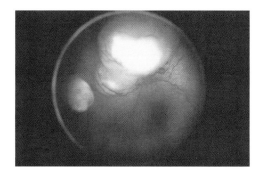

Figure 25-19 Wide-angle fundus photograph showing multiple endophytic retinoblastoma lesions, left eye. *(Courtesy of A. Linn Murphree, MD.)*

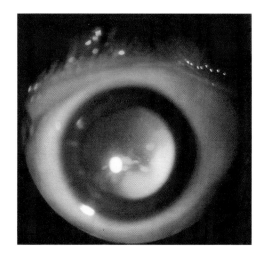

Figure 25-20 Endophytic retinoblastoma with vitreous seeding.

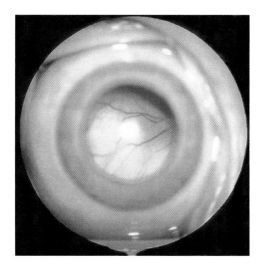

Figure 25-21 Exophytic retinoblastoma with overlying detached retina.

and, ultimately, phthisis bulbi. In either case, the genetic implications are the same as for an individual with an active retinoblastoma.

The most common retinal lesion simulating retinoblastoma is seen in Coats disease. The presence of crystalline material, extensive subretinal fluid, and peripheral vascular abnormalities—combined with the absence of calcium—suggests Coats disease. *Astrocytic hamartomas* and *hemangioblastomas* are benign retinal tumors that may simulate the appearance of small retinoblastomas. Both are usually associated with neurocutaneous syndromes (see Chapter 28).

Evaluation of a patient with presumed retinoblastoma requires imaging of the head and orbits, which can confirm the diagnosis and evaluate for extraocular extension and intracranial disease. In the past, computed tomography (CT) was used to facilitate the diagnosis by demonstrating intraocular calcification. However, CT is no longer recommended by the European Retinoblastoma Imaging Collaboration because of the increased risk of secondary tumors in many patients being evaluated for retinoblastoma. Magnetic resonance imaging and ultrasonography, which avoid the use of radiation, are recommended. Other, more invasive tests are reserved for atypical cases. Aspiration of ocular fluids for diagnostic testing should be performed only under the most unusual circumstances because such procedures can disseminate malignant cells.

The characteristic histologic features of retinoblastoma include Flexner-Wintersteiner rosettes, which are usually present, and fleurettes, which are less common. Both represent limited degrees of retinal cellular differentiation. Homer Wright rosettes are also frequently present but are less specific for retinoblastoma because they are common in other neuroblastic tumors. Calcification of varying extent is usually present.

Genetics The retinoblastoma gene *(RB1)* maps to a locus within the q14 band of chromosome 13 and codes for a protein, pRB, that suppresses tumor formation. For retinoblastoma to occur, both *RB1* genes must have a mutation. Approximately 60% of retinoblastoma cases arise from somatic nonhereditary mutations of both alleles of *RB1* in a retinal cell. These mutations generally result in unifocal and unilateral tumors. In the other 40% of patients, a germline mutation in 1 of the 2 alleles of *RB1* either is inherited from an affected parent (10% of all retinoblastoma cases) or occurs spontaneously in one of the gametes. A second somatic mutation in a retinal cell is all that is necessary for retinoblastoma to develop; such cases are often multicentric and bilateral.

Genetic counseling for families of retinoblastoma patients is complex (Table 25-7). Both parents and all siblings should be examined. In approximately 1% of cases, a parent may be found to have an unsuspected fundus lesion that represents a spontaneously regressed retinoblastoma (retinocytoma).

Genetic testing for retinoblastoma is important to aid in determining the risk of subsequent cancers (both retinoblastoma and other primary neoplasms) in the affected child and the risk of retinoblastoma in other family members. The probability of detection of the *RB1* gene depends on many factors, including the capabilities of the molecular diagnostic laboratory, the presence of tumor tissue, and the ability to test other affected family members.

Table 25-7 Genetic Counseling for Retinoblastoma

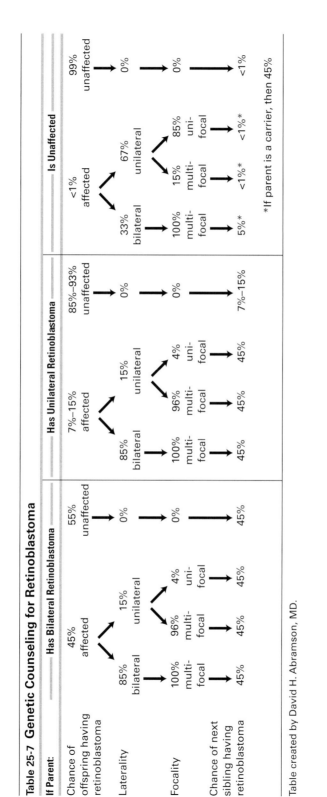

If Parent:	Has Bilateral Retinoblastoma		Has Unilateral Retinoblastoma		Is Unaffected	
Chance of offspring having retinoblastoma	45% affected	55% unaffected	7%–15% affected	85%–93% unaffected	<1% affected	99% unaffected
Laterality	85% bilateral → ; 15% unilateral →	0%	85% bilateral → ; 15% unilateral →	0%	33% bilateral → ; 67% unilateral →	0%
Focality	100% multifocal; 96% multifocal; 4% unifocal	0%	100% multifocal; 96% multifocal; 4% unifocal	0%	100% multifocal; 15% multifocal; 85% unifocal	0%
Chance of next sibling having retinoblastoma	45%; 45%; 45%	45%	45%; 45%; 45%	7%–15%	5%*; <1%*; <1%*	<1%

*If parent is a carrier, then 45%

Table created by David H. Abramson, MD.

Preimplantation genetic testing can be performed, and in vitro fertilization techniques have been successfully used to select embryos that are free from the germinal *RB1* mutation.

de Graaf P, Göricke S, Rodjan F, et al; European Retinoblastoma Imaging Collaboration. Guidelines for imaging retinoblastoma: imaging principles and MRI standardization. *Pediatr Radiol.* 2012;42(1):2–14.

Dhar SU, Chintagumpala M, Noll C, Chévez-Barrios P, Paysse EA, Plon SE. Outcomes of integrating genetics in management of patients with retinoblastoma. *Arch Ophthalmol.* 2011;129(11): 1428–1434.

Classification of retinoblastoma The Reese-Ellsworth classification (Table 25-8) was originally developed to predict globe salvage after external-beam radiation. Although it is still useful for comparing contemporary treatment modalities with older ones, the International Classification of Retinoblastoma (Table 25-9) is more useful for predicting the response to chemotherapy. The American Joint Committee on Cancer (AJCC) also has a staging system for retinoblastoma that addresses both intraocular and extraocular disease (see BCSC Section 4, *Ophthalmic Pathology and Intraocular Tumors*).

Shields CL, Mashayekhi A, Au AK, et al. The International Classification of Retinoblastoma predicts chemoreduction success. *Ophthalmology.* 2006;113(12):2276–2280.

Treatment

The management of retinoblastoma has changed dramatically over the past decade and continues to evolve. Many specialists may be involved, including ocular oncologists, pediatric ophthalmologists, geneticists, genetic counselors, pediatric oncologists, and radiation oncologists. External-beam radiation is seldom used to treat intraocular retinoblastoma because of its high association with development of craniofacial deformity and secondary tumors in the field of radiation. When the likelihood of salvaging vision is low, primary enucleation of eyes with advanced unilateral retinoblastoma is recommended to avoid the adverse effects of systemic chemotherapy. To prevent extraocular spread of the

---

Table 25-8 **Reese-Ellsworth Classification of Retinoblastoma**

Group I
    a. Solitary tumor, <4 disc diameters in size, at or behind the equator
    b. Multiple tumors, none >4 disc diameters in size, all at or behind the equator
Group II
    a. Solitary tumor, 4–10 disc diameters in size, at or behind the equator
    b. Multiple tumors, 4–10 disc diameters in size, behind the equator
Group III
    a. Any lesion anterior to the equator
    b. Solitary tumors >10 disc diameters behind the equator
Group IV
    a. Multiple tumors, some >10 disc diameters
    b. Any lesion extending anterior to the ora serrata
Group V
    a. Massive seeding involving more than half the retina
    b. Vitreous seeding

Table 25-9 International Classification of Retinoblastoma

Group A	Small tumors (≤3 mm) confined to the retina; >3 mm from the fovea; >1.5 mm from the optic disc
Group B	Tumors (>3 mm) confined to the retina in any location, with clear subretinal fluid ≤6 mm from the tumor margin
Group C	Localized vitreous and/or subretinal seeding (<6 mm total from tumor margin) If there is more than 1 site of subretinal or vitreous seeding, the total of these sites is <6 mm
Group D	Diffuse vitreous and/or subretinal seeding (≥6 mm total from tumor margin) If there is more than 1 site of subretinal or vitreous seeding, the total of these sites is ≥6 mm Subretinal fluid >6 mm from tumor margin
Group E	No visual potential or Presence of any of the following: • tumor in the anterior segment • tumor in or on the ciliary body • neovascular glaucoma • vitreous hemorrhage obscuring the tumor or significant hyphema • phthisical or prephthisical eye • orbital cellulitis-like presentation

Modified from Shields CL, Mashayekhi A, Au AK, et al. The International Classification of Retinoblastoma predicts chemoreduction success. *Ophthalmology.* 2006;113(12):2276–2280.

tumor, the surgeon should minimize manipulation of the globe and obtain a long segment of optic nerve. Small retinoblastoma tumors can often be treated with either laser photocoagulation or cryotherapy.

Primary systemic chemotherapy (chemoreduction) followed by local therapy (consolidation) has been used to spare vision for larger tumors (Fig 25-22) and is often used in cases of bilateral retinoblastoma. Most studies of chemoreduction for retinoblastoma have employed vincristine, carboplatin, and an epipodophyllotoxin. Others have added cyclosporine. Chemotherapy is rarely successful when used alone and often requires local therapy (cryotherapy, laser photocoagulation, thermotherapy, or plaque radiotherapy) as well. Adverse effects of chemoreduction treatment include low blood count, hair loss, hearing loss, renal toxicity, neurologic and cardiac disturbances, and possible increased risk for acute myelogenous leukemia.

Intra-arterial chemotherapy has recently been reported as an alternative to systemic chemoreduction for unilateral retinoblastoma in group B, C, D, or E eyes. Chemotherapy is delivered via cannulation of the ophthalmic artery in single or multiple sessions. Many chemotherapy agents have been used; melphalan is the most common. Overall, the results show higher rates of globe salvage in eyes treated initially and in those that did not respond to prior treatments. Systemic complications include neutropenia and metastasis. Ocular complications include vascular occlusion, blepharoptosis, cilia loss, temporary dysmotility, and periocular edema in the distribution of the supratrochlear artery. There is concern about the radiation that is delivered during the procedure, especially for patients with germline *RB1* gene mutations, who are at higher risk for malignant tumors.

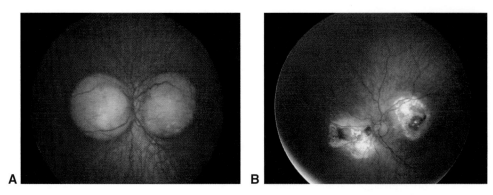

Figure 25-22 **A,** Left eye of infant with bilateral retinoblastoma; 2 tumors straddle the optic nerve. **B,** After chemoreduction and laser consolidation, the tumors are nonviable. The child's visual acuity was 20/25 at age 5 years.

Intravitreal chemotherapy has been used for refractory and recurrent vitreous seeding from retinoblastoma. Periocular injections of chemotherapy have been used as an adjuvant to other treatments.

Treated retinoblastoma sometimes disappears altogether, but more often it persists as a calcified mass (type 1, or "cottage cheese," pattern) or a noncalcified, translucent grayish lesion (type 2, or "fish flesh," pattern), which may be difficult to distinguish from untreated tumor. Type 3 regression has elements of both types 1 and 2, and type 4 regression is a flat, atrophic scar. A child with treated retinoblastoma must be observed closely for new or recurrent tumor formation, with frequent examinations under anesthesia if necessary.

Extraocular retinoblastoma, though uncommon in the United States, is still problematic in developing countries, primarily because of delay in diagnosis. The 4 major types are optic nerve involvement, orbital invasion, central nervous system involvement, and distant metastasis. Treatment of extraocular retinoblastoma includes intensive multimodality chemotherapy, autologous hematopoietic stem cell rescue, and external-beam radiation. Long-term disease-free survival is possible if the central nervous system is not involved; otherwise, the prognosis is usually poor.

Patients with trilateral retinoblastoma have a primitive neuroectodermal tumor of the pineal gland or parasellar region, in addition to retinoblastoma. The risk of trilateral retinoblastoma has been less than 0.5% and 5%–15% in patients with unilateral and bilateral retinoblastoma, respectively. However, the rate of trilateral retinoblastoma appears to be lower in patients treated with chemoreduction. Treatment usually involves a multimodal approach, and the prognosis is poor.

Abramson DH, Dunkel IJ, Brodie SE, Marr B, Gobin YP. Superselective ophthalmic artery chemotherapy as primary treatment for retinoblastoma (chemosurgery). *Ophthalmology.* 2010;117(8):1623–1629.

Shields CL, Bianciotto CG, Jabbour P, et al. Intra-arterial chemotherapy for retinoblastoma: report no. 2, treatment complications. *Arch Ophthalmol.* 2011;129(11):1407–1415.

Monitoring Identification of *RB1* mutations is very useful in determining how frequently to monitor patients. Patients with unilateral tumors who have somatic mutations are not at risk for development of additional tumors (ocular or systemic). Patients with bilateral tumors and patients with unilateral tumors who carry germline *RB1* mutations are at high risk, and frequent monitoring is crucial. The risk of additional eye tumors decreases with age and is low after age 24 months. Genetic testing can also help determine the need to monitor siblings. If genetic testing is not available, siblings should be monitored routinely during the first 2 years of life.

Nonocular tumors are common in patients with germinal mutations; the estimated incidence rate is 1% per year of life (eg, 10% prevalence by age 10, 30% by age 30). The incidence is higher among patients treated with external-beam radiation before 1 year of age. The most common secondary tumors (and the mean age at diagnosis) are pinealoma (2.7 years), sarcoma (13 years), melanoma (27 years), and carcinomas (29 years). Patients in whom second, nonocular tumors develop are at even greater risk for additional malignant tumors.

Woo KI, Harbour JW. Review of 676 second primary tumors in patients with retinoblastoma: association between age at onset and tumor type. *Arch Ophthalmol.* 2010;128(7):865–870.

Acquired Disorders

Coats Disease

The classic findings in Coats disease are yellow subretinal and intraretinal lipid exudates associated with retinal vascular abnormalities—most often telangiectasia, tortuosity, aneurysmal dilatations, and retinal capillary nonperfusion. The clinical presentation varies, ranging from mild changes to total retinal detachment (Fig 25-23).

Males are affected more frequently than females, and the condition is usually, but not always, unilateral. The average age at diagnosis is 6–8 years, but the disease has also been observed in infants. The etiology of Coats disease is unknown. Associations with various gene deletions have been reported, but the disease is isolated in most cases.

Diagnosis

The diagnosis of Coats disease requires the presence of abnormal retinal vessels, which occasionally are small and difficult to find. The subretinal exudate is thought to come from the leaking anomalous vessels. Fluorescein angiography may be helpful in identifying leakage from the telangiectatic vessels and in assessing the effectiveness of therapy.

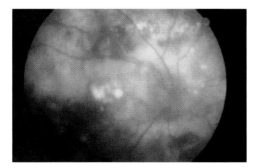

Figure 25-23 Coats disease. Affected right eye. Note extensive subretinal exudate and exudative retinal detachment.

The differential diagnosis includes PFV, ROP, toxocariasis, familial exudative vitreoretinopathy, Norrie disease, retinal dysplasia, endophthalmitis, leukemia, and retinoblastoma. Calcium is frequently detected by ultrasonography in retinoblastoma but is distinctly rare in Coats disease. Coats disease often presents with xanthocoria (yellow pupil reflex), whereas retinoblastoma presents with leukocoria (white pupil reflex).

Treatment

Treatment is directed at obliterating the abnormal leaking vessels and includes cryotherapy or laser photocoagulation. Exudative retinal detachments and subretinal fibrosis develop in eyes with progressive disease. Once the fovea is detached and the subretinal exudate becomes organized, the prognosis for restoration of central vision is poor. Use of intravitreal bevacizumab in addition to laser treatment has been reported, but one study found that this approach was associated with a higher incidence of vitreoretinal fibrosis and tractional retinal detachment.

Mulvihill A, Morris B. A population-based study of Coats disease in the United Kingdom II: investigation, treatment, and outcomes. *Eye (Lond).* 2010;24(12):1802–1807.

Ramasubramanian A, Shields CL. Bevacizumab for Coats disease with exudative retinal detachment and risk of vitreoretinal traction. *Br J Ophthalmol.* 2012;96(3):356–359.

Systemic Diseases and Disorders With Retinal Manifestations

Diabetes Mellitus

Type 1, or insulin-dependent, diabetes mellitus was formerly called *juvenile-onset diabetes mellitus.* The prevalence of retinopathy in this condition is directly proportional to the duration of diabetes after puberty. Retinopathy rarely occurs less than 5 years after the onset of diabetes mellitus. Proliferative diabetic retinopathy is rare in pediatric cases.

A variety of nonproliferative changes may occur in the pediatric age group. Microaneurysms are the first ophthalmoscopic sign; they may be followed by retinal hemorrhages, areas of retinal nonperfusion, cotton-wool spots, hard exudates, intraretinal microvascular abnormalities, and venous dilation.

A rapid rise of blood glucose may produce myopia, and sudden reduction of blood glucose can induce hyperopia, because of osmotic changes in the lens and alteration of its refractive status. Several weeks may be required before acuity returns to normal. True diabetic cataracts are uncommon, occurring most often in patients with poorly controlled disease. Such cataracts resemble a snowstorm that affects the anterior and posterior cortices of young patients.

Diabetes mellitus, especially in young children, may be part of *DIDMOAD syndrome* (*d*iabetes *i*nsipidus, *d*iabetes *m*ellitus, *o*ptic *a*trophy, and *d*eafness). This condition, which is also known as *Wolfram syndrome,* is associated with congenital cataracts as well.

Diagnosis

To screen for diabetic retinopathy, the American Academy of Ophthalmology recommends annual ophthalmic examinations beginning 5 years after the onset of diabetes mellitus (www.aao.org/ppp). The American Academy of Pediatrics (AAP) recommends an initial ophthalmic examination 3–5 years after diagnosis if the patient is older than 9 years, with annual follow-up examinations thereafter (www.aap.org). Specifically, the AAP states that children younger than 9 years do not require screening examinations, because the incidence of diabetic retinopathy is negligible in this age group.

Lueder GT, Silverstein J; American Academy of Pediatrics Section on Ophthalmology and Section on Endocrinology. Screening for retinopathy in the pediatric patient with type 1 diabetes mellitus. *Pediatrics.* 2005;116(1):270–273.

Treatment
Treatment is discussed in BCSC Section 12, *Retina and Vitreous.*

Albinism

Albinism is a group of conditions that involve the synthesis of melanin in the skin and eye *(oculocutaneous albinism [OCA])* or the eye alone *(ocular albinism [OA]).*

Diagnosis
The major ophthalmic findings in all types of OCA and OA are iris transillumination from decreased pigmentation, foveal aplasia or hypoplasia, and a characteristic deficit of pigment in the retina, especially peripheral to the posterior pole (Fig 25-24A, B). Nystagmus,

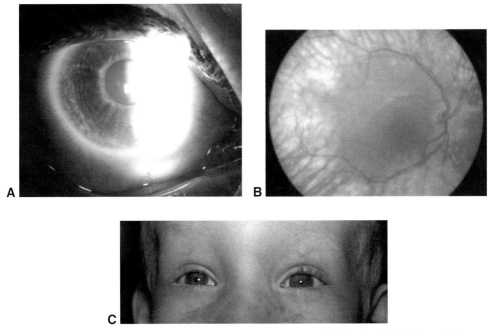

Figure 25-24 **A,** Transillumination of iris in albinism, right eye. **B,** Fundus in albinism, right eye, demonstrating complete lack of pigment and macular hypoplasia. **C,** Child with oculocutaneous albinism type 2 (OCA2). Note white hair, eyebrows, and lashes and light-colored irides and freckles. *(Parts A and C courtesy of Edward L. Raab, MD.)*

light sensitivity, high refractive errors, and reduced central visual acuity are often present, and visual acuity ranges from 20/25 to 20/200. If a child has significant foveal hypoplasia, nystagmus will begin at 2–3 months of age. The severity of the visual impairment tends to be proportional to the degree of nystagmus and foveal hypoplasia. Optical coherence tomography has demonstrated that the size of the photoreceptor outer segment is the strongest predictor of visual acuity. An abnormally large number of crossed fibers appear in the optic chiasm of patients and animals with albinism, precluding stereopsis and often inducing strabismus. Asymmetric visually evoked potentials are often seen in affected patients and may be helpful in diagnosis.

There are 4 major types of OCA, all of which exhibit various degrees of skin and hair pigmentation (Fig 25-24C). They are autosomal recessive and are caused by different genes (Table 25-10).

Ocular albinism (OA1), also called *Nettleship-Falls albinism,* is usually caused by a mutation in the *GPR143* gene on the X chromosome. This gene controls melanosome number and size; the mutation results in macromelanosomes, which may be revealed by skin biopsy. An autosomal recessive form of OA has also been reported. Affected individuals appear to have decreased pigment in the eyes but not the skin. Patches of decreased pigment in the fundus and iris transillumination are apparent in many female carriers.

Albinism can be part of a broader syndrome, such as Hermansky-Pudlak syndrome or Chédiak-Higashi syndrome, both of which are autosomal recessive. *Hermansky-Pudlak syndrome* occurs with higher frequency in Puerto Rico and is characterized by pulmonary interstitial fibrosis and bleeding abnormalities. *Chédiak-Higashi syndrome* is a rare

Table 25-10 Classification of Oculocutaneous Albinism (OCA)

Type of OCA	Defective Gene	Chromosome	Associated Findings
OCA1A	Tyrosinase gene *(TYR)*	11q14–q21	White skin and hair; no tyrosinase; poorest vision
OCA1B	Tyrosinase gene *(TYR)*	11q14–q21	"Yellow variant"; some tyrosinase activity
OCA minimal pigment (MP)	Tyrosinase gene *(TYR)*	11q14–q21	Some tyrosinase activity
OCA temperature-sensitive	Tyrosinase gene *(TYR)*	11q14–q21	Tyrosine function in cooler areas of body only
OCA2	*OCA2* gene	15q11.2–q12	Most prevalent worldwide; seen frequently in African Americans
OCA3	Tyrosinase-related protein 1 gene *(TYRP1)*	9p23	"Red rufous" type; reddish hair; seen in persons of African descent; mild visual abnormalities
OCA4	Membrane-associated transporter protein gene *(MATP)*	5p13.3	Common in Japanese population

condition characterized by increased susceptibility to bacterial infections. Whenever a patient is diagnosed with albinism, the clinician should inquire about bleeding or bruising tendencies and frequent infections.

Treatment

Tinted glasses may be used for patients with photophobia. Patients with OCA are at risk for skin cancer and should be counseled.

Levin AV, Stroh E. Albinism for the busy clinician. *J AAPOS.* 2011;15(1):59–66.

Mohammad S, Gottlob I, Kumar A, et al. The functional significance of foveal abnormalities in albinism measured using spectral-domain optical coherence tomography. *Ophthalmology.* 2011;118(8):1645–1652.

CHAPTER 26

Optic Disc Abnormalities

Developmental Anomalies

Optic Nerve Hypoplasia

Optic nerve hypoplasia (ONH) is the most common optic disc anomaly encountered by ophthalmologists. Histologically, optic nerve hypoplasia is characterized by a decreased number of optic nerve axons. Clinically, the disc is pale or gray and smaller than normal. This condition can be unilateral or bilateral and is often asymmetric (Fig 26-1). It may be associated with a yellow to white ring around the disc (double-ring sign). The edge of the outer ring corresponds with the normal junction between the sclera and the lamina cribrosa; the outer ring itself corresponds with the abnormal extension of the retina and pigment epithelium over the outer portion of the lamina cribrosa; and the inner ring corresponds to the hypoplastic optic nerve. Because the size of the outer ring often corresponds to the normal disc diameter, careful observation is necessary to avoid interpreting the hypoplastic disc/ring complex as a normal-sized optic nerve with normal cup–disc ratio. The vascular pattern is also abnormal and can be associated with too few or too many disc vessels. Retinal vascular tortuosity is common.

Visual acuity ranges from normal to no light perception and is related to the integrity of the macular fibers; it often does not correlate with the overall size of the disc. Localized visual field defects and visual field constriction are common. Children with bilateral ONH often present with congenital sensory nystagmus, and those affected unilaterally often present with sensory strabismus. Because patients with ONH can have strabismus,

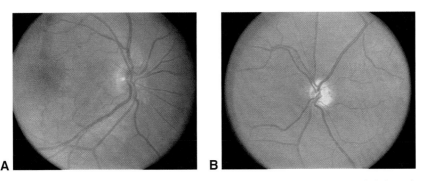

A   **B**

Figure 26-1   Optic nerve hypoplasia. **A,** Normal right optic nerve. **B,** Hypoplastic left optic nerve.

unilateral vision loss may partially result from superimposed amblyopia and may improve with patching therapy.

Midline central nervous system (CNS) anomalies are associated with unilateral and bilateral ONH; thus, magnetic resonance imaging (MRI) is indicated. *Septo-optic dysplasia (de Morsier syndrome)* denotes the association of ONH with absence of the septum pellucidum and agenesis of the corpus callosum (Figs 26-2, 26-3). These abnormalities are not associated with neurodevelopmental defects or endocrinologic dysfunction.

Patients with ONH may also have cerebral hemisphere or pituitary gland abnormalities. Cerebral hemisphere abnormalities include schizencephaly, periventricular leukomalacia, and encephalomalacia. They occur in approximately 45% of patients with ONH and are associated with neurodevelopmental defects.

Approximately 15% of patients with ONH have pituitary gland abnormalities. MRI in these patients reveals an ectopic posterior pituitary bright spot at the upper infundibulum.

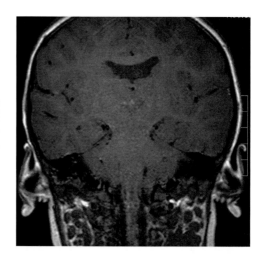

Figure 26-2 Coronal T1-weighted magnetic resonance (MR) image through the lateral ventricles: the septum pellucidum (interventricular septum) is absent. *(Courtesy of Jane L. Weissman, MD.)*

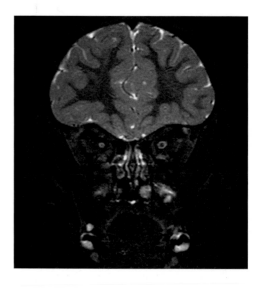

Figure 26-3 Coronal T2-weighted MR image through the orbits: the right optic nerve is smaller and more T2 hyperintense than the left optic nerve. *(Courtesy of Jane L. Weissman, MD.)*

This finding is associated with pituitary hormone abnormalities, including growth hormone deficiency, hypothyroidism, hyperprolactinemia, panhypopituitarism, and diabetes insipidus. A history of neonatal jaundice suggests hypothyroidism; neonatal hypoglycemia or seizures indicate possible panhypopituitarism. Patients with ONH and diabetes insipidus can have problems with thermal regulation and must be monitored carefully during febrile illnesses. Referral to a pediatric endocrinologist is indicated for patients with either clinical signs of endocrinologic dysfunction or pituitary abnormalities on MRI.

ONH denotes injury to the optic nerve prior to complete development and can occur from any prenatal or perinatal injury. Frequently, the etiology is unknown. ONH has been associated with maternal ingestion of phenytoin, quinine, and LSD, as well as with fetal alcohol syndrome. Segmental hypoplasia may occur in children whose mothers have type 1 diabetes mellitus.

Children with periventricular leukomalacia (PVL) display an unusual form of ONH. The optic nerves demonstrate a large cup within a normal-sized optic disc. This form of ONH occurs secondary to transsynaptic degeneration of optic axons, which is caused by bilateral lesions in the optic radiations.

Brodsky MC, Glasier CM. Optic nerve hypoplasia. Clinical significance of associated central nervous system abnormalities on magnetic resonance imaging. *Arch Ophthalmol.* 1993; 111(1):66–74.

Garcia-Filion P, Borchert M. Optic nerve hypoplasia syndrome: a review of the epidemiology and clinical associations. *Curr Treat Options Neurol.* 2013;15(1):78–89.

Morning Glory Disc Anomaly

Morning glory disc anomaly is caused by either an abnormal closure of the embryonic fissure or abnormal development of the distal optic stalk at its junction with the primitive optic vesicle. The anomaly is a funnel-shaped excavation of the posterior fundus that incorporates the optic disc. The surrounding retinal pigment epithelium is elevated, with an increased number of blood vessels looping at the edges of the disc (Fig 26-4). A central core of white glial tissue occupies the normal position of the cup. This tissue may have contractile elements, and the optic cup can sometimes be seen to open and close with some periodicity. Morning glory disc anomaly occurs more frequently in females and is typically unilateral. Visual acuity ranges from 20/20 to no light perception, but it is usually 20/100–20/200. Serous retinal detachments occur in approximately one-third of affected

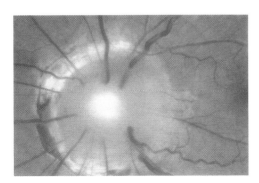

Figure 26-4 Morning glory disc anomaly, left eye.

patients. Morning glory disc anomaly has been associated with basal encephalocele in patients with midfacial anomalies, PHACE syndrome (*posterior fossa malformations, hemangiomas, arterial lesions, cardiac and eye anomalies*), and abnormalities of the carotid circulation (moyamoya disease). Therefore, MRI and MR angiography of the brain should be obtained in patients with morning glory disc anomaly.

Coloboma of the Optic Nerve

Coloboma of the optic nerve may be part of a chorioretinal coloboma that involves the entire embryonic fissure, or the coloboma may involve only the optic disc. Mild optic disc colobomas resemble deep physiologic cupping and may be confused with glaucomatous damage. More-extensive defects appear as an enlargement of the peripapillary area with a deep central excavation lined by a glistening white tissue; blood vessels overlie this deep cavity (Fig 26-5). The defects usually extend inferonasally and are often associated with retinal coloboma in the periphery. Nonrhegmatogenous or rhegmatogenous retinal detachments may occur. Optic nerve coloboma can be unilateral or bilateral; if bilateral, it can be very asymmetric. Visual acuity is difficult to predict from the optic disc appearance; it is related to involvement of the papillomacular/foveal region. Ocular colobomas may be associated with multiple systemic abnormalities, such as the CHARGE syndrome (*c*oloboma, *h*eart defects, choanal *a*tresia, mental *r*etardation, *g*enitourinary abnormalities, and *e*ar abnormalities) and the papillorenal syndrome (renal anomalies and optic nerve defects).

Optic nerve pits or holes

Considered by many authors to be a variant of optic nerve coloboma, optic nerve pits (Fig 26-6) are usually unilateral and typically appear in the inferotemporal quadrant or central portion of the disc. A pit may be shallow or very deep. It is often covered with a gray veil of tissue. Cilioretinal arteries often emerge from pits. Optic nerve pits are associated with serous retinal detachments occurring mainly during the second and third decades of life.

Myelinated Retinal Nerve Fibers

Normal myelination (medullation) starts at the lateral geniculate ganglion and stops at the lamina cribrosa. Occasionally, some of the fibers in the retina acquire a myelin sheath. Clinically, this appears as a white superficial retinal area whose frayed and feathered edges tend to follow the same orientation as that of the normal retinal nerve fibers (Fig 26-7).

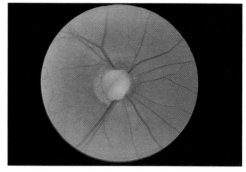

Figure 26-5 Optic nerve coloboma, right eye.

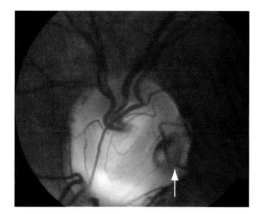

Figure 26-6 Left optic nerve with temporal optic nerve pit *(arrow)* and mild inferonasal disc coloboma. Cilioretinal vessels emanate from the optic nerve pit. *(Courtesy of Paul Phillips, MD.)*

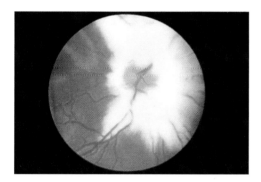

Figure 26-7 Myelinated nerve fibers of optic nerve and retina, right eye.

Retinal vessels that pass within the superficial layer of the nerve fibers are obscured. The myelinated fibers may occur as a single spot or as several noncontiguous patches. The most common location is along the disc margin. Vision loss can occur from macular involvement or from anisometropic amblyopia. In these cases, the macula can also be hypoplastic. Treatment of amblyopia should be attempted but may be unsuccessful. Scotomata may correspond to the area of the myelination.

Tilted Disc Syndrome

Tilted disc syndrome is a nonhereditary, typically bilateral condition in which the superior pole of the optic disc appears elevated, with posterior displacement of the inferior nasal disc; or the disc is horizontally tilted, resulting in an oval-appearing optic disc with an obliquely oriented long axis (Fig 26-8). This condition is often accompanied by a scleral crescent located inferiorly or inferonasally, situs inversus, and by posterior ectasia of the inferior nasal fundus. Many affected eyes are myopic and astigmatic.

Patients may demonstrate a bitemporal hemianopia, which is typically incomplete and preferentially involves the superior quadrants. The hemianopia can usually be distinguished from a chiasmal lesion because it does not respect the vertical midline. Refractive correction often results in elimination of the visual field defect. Tilted discs, myopic astigmatism, bilateral decreased vision, and visual difficulty at night suggest the possibility of X-linked congenital stationary night blindness (see Chapter 25). Acquired tilted

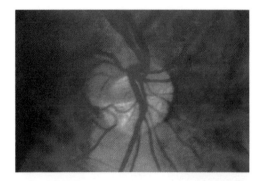

Figure 26-8 Tilted disc syndrome, right eye.

disc and peripapillary crescent formation have been documented in children with myopic progression.

Kim TW, Kim M, Weinreb RN, et al. Optic disc changes with incipient myopia of childhood. *Ophthalmology.* 2012;119(1):21–26.

Bergmeister Papilla

To varying extents, the hyaloid artery may not be resorbed before birth. The entire artery may remain as a fine thread or cord extending from the optic disc to the lens and can be associated with persistent fetal vasculature. The hyaloid artery may be patent and contain blood where it attaches to the posterior lens capsule. In mild cases, the attachment to the posterior lens capsule is located inferonasally (Mittendorf dot) and is usually visually insignificant. Bergmeister papilla is a benign prepapillary glial remnant of the hyaloid artery.

Megalopapilla

Megalopapilla features an abnormally large optic disc diameter and is often associated with an increased cup–disc ratio that can be confused with normal-tension glaucoma. Visual acuity is usually normal or slightly decreased, and visual fields may demonstrate a slightly enlarged blind spot. Megalopapilla can be unilateral or bilateral. The cause is unknown. In rare cases, megalopapilla has been associated with optic nerve glioma.

Peripapillary Staphyloma

Peripapillary staphyloma is a posterior bulging of the sclera in which the optic disc occupies the "bottom of the bowl." It is nonhereditary and usually unilateral, with rare bilateral cases. The disc may be normal, but it is surrounded by stretched choroid, thereby exposing the white sclera encircling the disc. Visual acuity is usually poor.

Optic Nerve Aplasia

Optic nerve aplasia is rare. The affected eye lacks optic nerve axons and retinal blood vessels, making the choroidal pattern clearly visible. Unilateral optic nerve aplasia may occur

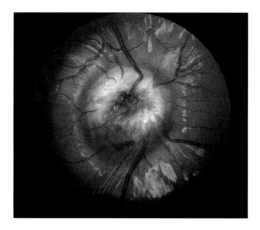

Figure 26-9 Melanocytoma of the optic disc and adjacent retina. *(Courtesy of Scott Lambert, MD.)*

with normal brain development. Bilateral optic nerve aplasia is usually associated with other CNS abnormalities.

Melanocytoma

Melanocytoma is a darkly pigmented tumor with little or no growth potential that usually involves the optic disc and adjacent retina (Fig 26-9). Malignant melanoma of the choroid is extremely rare in children.

Optic Atrophy

Optic atrophy in children usually results from anterior visual pathway disease such as inflammation (optic neuritis), hereditary optic atrophy (autosomal dominant, autosomal recessive, X-linked, and mitochondrial), perinatal asphyxia, hydrocephalus, or optic nerve tumors. Table 26-1 lists causes of acquired optic atrophy. Neuroimaging should be considered for all patients with optic atrophy of undetermined etiology, because tumor or hydrocephalus is present in over 40% of these cases. Specific underlying gene defects may be inferred from coexisting systemic features.

Dominant Optic Atrophy, Kjer Type

Bilateral slow loss of central vision in childhood may be due to dominant optic atrophy. This condition usually begins before the age of 10 years, with visual acuity ranging from 20/40 to 20/100. Visual fields show central or cecocentral scotomata with normal peripheral isopters. Color vision testing may be diagnostic, revealing a blue dyschromatopsia. Clinically, the optic disc shows temporal pallor with an area of triangular excavation (Fig 26-10). Inheritance is autosomal dominant, although family pedigrees may be hard to elicit. The long-term visual prognosis is fair, with visual function rarely reduced to the 20/200 level.

Table 26-1 Causes of Acquired Optic Atrophy in Childhood

Craniopharyngioma
Hereditary optic atrophy
Hydrocephalus
Optic nerve/chiasmal glioma
Optic neuritis
Postpapilledema
Retinal degenerative disease

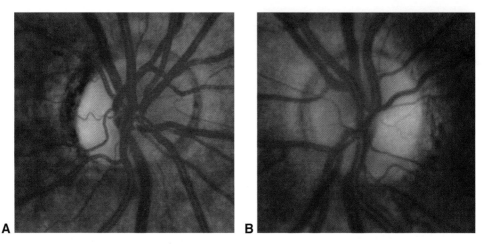

A   B

Figure 26-10 Dominant optic atrophy. Bilateral temporal pallor with excavated appearance. Right eye **(A)** and left eye **(B)**. *(Reproduced with permission from Lueder GT. Pediatric Practice Ophthalmology. New York: McGraw-Hill Professional; 2011:263.)*

Recessive Optic Atrophy

Recessive optic atrophy is a rare condition characterized by severe bilateral vision loss before age 5 years. Nystagmus is present in approximately 50% of these patients. Fundus examination reveals a pale optic disc with vascular attenuation of the type characteristically seen in retinal degeneration. Electroretinogram results are normal, however.

Behr Optic Atrophy

A hereditary disorder, Behr optic atrophy occurs mainly in males, with onset in childhood. This condition is associated with increased deep tendon reflexes, cerebellar ataxia, bladder dysfunction, intellectual disability, hypotonia of the extremities, and external ophthalmoplegia.

Leber Hereditary Optic Neuropathy

A maternally inherited (mitochondrial) disease, Leber hereditary optic neuropathy (LHON) is characterized by acute or subacute bilateral loss of central vision, acquired

red-green dyschromatopsia, and central or cecocentral scotomata in otherwise healthy patients (usually males) in their second to fourth decade of life. See BCSC Section 5, *Neuro-Ophthalmology,* for further discussion.

Optic Neuritis

Optic neuritis in childhood frequently presents after systemic infections such as viral illnesses. It can also be associated with immunizations and bee stings. The cause of the postinfectious form of viral optic neuritis is unknown. It has been speculated that an autoimmune process, triggered by a previous viral infection, results in a demyelinative injury.

Optic neuritis in children, in contrast with that in adults, is more frequently bilateral and associated with disc edema. Vision loss can be severe. Over half of affected children have systemic symptoms, including headache, nausea, vomiting, lethargy, or malaise.

Optic neuritis in children can occur as an isolated neurologic deficit or as a component of more generalized neurologic disease, such as acute disseminated encephalomyelitis, neuromyelitis optica, or multiple sclerosis. The relationship between optic neuritis and the development of multiple sclerosis, which is common in adults, is less clear in children. A small subset of children with optic neuritis develop signs and symptoms consistent with multiple sclerosis. Older age and MRI findings extrinsic to the visual system are associated with increased risk for MS. Most of the neurologic deficits are minor, but disability can be severe.

Treatment of optic neuritis in children is controversial. As vision loss is often bilateral, treatment with intravenous steroids should be considered in order to hasten visual recovery. The Optic Neuritis Treatment Trial did not specifically address the issue of treatment in children, so it is difficult to apply the results of this study to children. See also BCSC Section 5, *Neuro-Ophthalmology.*

Neuroretinitis denotes inflammatory disc edema associated with a stellate pattern of exudates in the macula (macular star; Fig 26-11). The etiology is most commonly *Bartonella henselae* infection (cat-scratch disease). Other infectious etiologies include mumps,

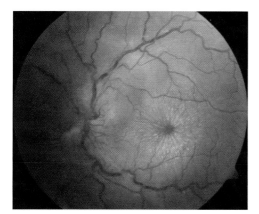

Figure 26-11 Neuroretinitis. Inflammatory optic disc edema with a macular star. *(Courtesy of Paul Phillips, MD.)*

Toxocara, tuberculosis, and syphilis. Patients with neuroretinitis are not at risk for developing multiple sclerosis.

Waldman AT, Stull LB, Galetta SL, Balcer LJ, Liu GT. Pediatric optic neuritis and risk of multiple sclerosis: meta-analysis of observational studies. *J AAPOS.* 2011;15(5):441–446.

Papilledema

Papilledema refers to optic disc edema secondary to elevated intracranial pressure (ICP). It is frequently bilateral. Typically, visual acuity, color vision, and pupillary reactions are initially normal. However, visual dysfunction may occur from severe or chronic papilledema.

Increased ICP in children can be caused by a number of conditions (eg, hydrocephalus, mass lesions, meningitis, idiopathic intracranial hypertension; Table 26-2). A full evaluation, including neuroimaging followed by lumbar puncture, is indicated. In infants, increased ICP results in firmness and distension of the open fontanelles. Significantly elevated pressure is usually accompanied by nausea, vomiting, and headaches. Older children may describe transient visual obscurations. Esotropia and diplopia may result from sixth nerve palsy. The esotropia usually resolves once ICP is reduced.

Table 26-2 Conditions Associated With Pediatric Optic Disc Swelling

Papillitis
Optic neuritis (postinfectious)
Toxoplasmosis
Lyme disease
Bartonella infection
Neuroretinitis
Toxocara infection of disc
Leber hereditary optic neuropathy
Papilledema
  Intracranial mass
  Meningitis
  Idiopathic intracranial hypertension
  Dural sinus thrombosis
  Cranial synostosis
  Hydrocephalus
    Chiari malformation
    Aqueductal stenosis
    Dandy-Walker syndrome
    Infection
Hypertension
Optic nerve glioma
Leukemic infiltrate
Pseudopapilledema
  Astrocytoma of optic disc (tuberous sclerosis)
  Optic disc drusen
  Hyperopia
  Prominent glial tissue

Idiopathic Intracranial Hypertension

Idiopathic intracranial hypertension (IIH), or *pseudotumor cerebri,* is characterized by increased ICP with normal-sized or small ventricles on neuroimaging, and normal cerebrospinal fluid. IIH is uncommon in childhood but can occur at any age. It may be associated with viral infections, drug use (tetracycline, corticosteroids, vitamin A, nalidixic acid, thyroid medications, and growth hormone), and cerebral venous sinus thrombosis. *Prepubescent* children with IIH have a lower incidence of obesity compared with adult IIH patients, and the male to female ratio is approximately equal. *Postpubescent* children with IIH have a clinical profile similar to that of adults, with a higher incidence of obesity and female sex preponderance. Down syndrome is also associated with IIH.

Common presenting symptoms are headache, vision loss, transient visual obscurations, and diplopia. Papilledema may be noted on routine examination of an asymptomatic child. Ocular examination frequently reveals excellent visual acuity with bilateral papilledema. Unilateral or bilateral sixth nerve palsy may be present. The patient should be monitored closely for decreased visual acuity, visual field loss, and worsening headaches. Visual field tests can be difficult to interpret in children but should be obtained if possible.

Treatment of IIH begins with discontinuation of any causative medications. Medical treatment includes acetazolamide and topiramate. Surgical treatment options include optic nerve sheath fenestration or shunting procedures (lumbar or ventriculoperitoneal), both of which can reduce the incidence of vision loss. Shunting procedures are preferred for patients with good visual function and severe headaches unresponsive to medical management. With treatment the visual prognosis is excellent for most patients, although vision loss can occur secondary to chronic papilledema. In most cases, spontaneous resolution occurs within 12–18 months after initial treatment.

Pseudopapilledema

Pseudopapilledema refers to any elevated anomaly of the optic disc that resembles papilledema (see Table 26-2). Disc anomalies that are frequently confused with papilledema in children include drusen, hyperopia, and prominent glial tissue. Pseudopapilledema can be differentiated from true papilledema by the absence of disc hyperemia and retinal hemorrhages and exudates and by the lack of systemic findings associated with increased ICP (Fig 26-12A). Pseudopapilledema is associated with anomalous branching of the large retinal vessels.

Most children with pseudopapilledema do not have other related ophthalmic or systemic abnormalities. However, pseudopapilledema is associated with Down syndrome, Alagille syndrome, and retinitis pigmentosa. Down syndrome is associated with IIH as well; thus, an elevated optic disc in a child with Down syndrome should not be assumed to be benign. If there are clinical symptoms and signs of elevated ICP (headaches, sixth nerve palsy, true papilledema), neuroimaging followed by lumbar puncture should be obtained.

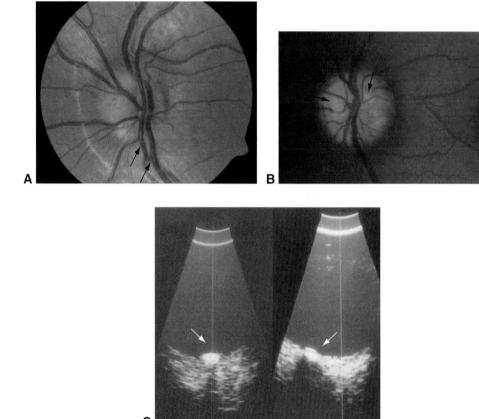

Figure 26-12 A, Pseudopapilledema. There is anomalous branching *(arrows)* of the large retinal vessels without disc hyperemia, retinal hemorrhages, or exudates. **B,** Optic nerve head drusen seen as refractile opacities on disc surface *(arrows)*. **C,** Ultrasonographic image of bright spot in nerve *(arrows)* consistent with drusen. *(Parts A and B courtesy of Paul Phillips, MD; part C courtesy of Edward G. Buckley, MD.)*

Drusen

Intrapapillary drusen, the most common cause of pseudopapilledema in children, can appear within the first or second decade of life (Fig 26-12B). Drusen are frequently inherited (autosomal dominant); thus, examination of the parents is helpful when drusen are suspected in children.

Clinically, the elevated disc does not obscure the retinal arterioles lying anteriorly and often has an irregular border suggesting the presence of drusen beneath the surface. There is no dilation of the papillary network, and superficial retinal hemorrhages and exudates are absent. Peripapillary subretinal hemorrhages and subretinal neovascular membranes rarely occur. When drusen are not buried, they appear as shiny refractile bodies visible on the disc surface, with a gray-yellow translucent appearance. Visual field defects are frequently associated; inferior nasal field defects are common. Concentric narrowing, an arcuate scotoma, and central defects can also occur. These defects can be slowly progressive. Central visual acuity is rarely affected.

In some patients, fundus evaluation can identify drusen as the cause of the swollen disc appearance. Occasionally, however, such identification cannot be made with certainty, and B-scan ultrasonography can be helpful in detecting bright calcific reflections at the optic nerve head (Fig 26-12C). Computed tomography can also detect these drusen.

Most children with optic disc drusen do not have other related ophthalmic or systemic abnormalities. However, children with pseudoxanthoma elasticum or retinitis pigmentosa have a higher incidence of optic disc drusen compared with the general population.

CHAPTER 27

Ocular Trauma in Childhood

Trauma is one of the most important causes of ocular morbidity in childhood. Only amblyopia is responsible for more early monocular vision loss. Management of eye trauma in very young patients requires several special considerations in response to issues specific to this patient group. One issue is the often-difficult nature of evaluation and treatment of accidental and nonaccidental trauma because of inadequate patient cooperation or unreliable history. If the physician uses force to examine the child's eye, there is a risk of exacerbating the damage caused by penetrating wounds or blunt impact. When preliminary assessment indicates that prompt surgical treatment may be necessary, it is appropriate to defer detailed physical examination of the eye until the patient is in the operating room and under general anesthesia.

Another issue in the care of children with eye trauma is the potential for the injury to lead to vision loss from amblyopia. In children younger than 5–7 years, deprivation amblyopia associated with traumatic cataract or other media opacity may cause severe, long-term reduction of visual acuity that is worse than the original physical damage. Minimizing the interval between the injury and the restoration of optimal media clarity and optics, including adequate aphakic refractive correction, must be a high priority. Monocular occlusion following injury should be kept to a minimum; the expected benefit from an occlusive dressing must be weighed against the risk of disturbing binocular function or inducing amblyopia in a very young child.

Accidental Trauma

In younger children, most accidental ocular trauma occurs during casual play with other children. Older children and adolescents are most likely to be injured while participating in sports. A majority of serious childhood eye injuries could therefore, in principle, be prevented by appropriate adult supervision and by regular use of protective eyewear during sports activities. Fireworks and BB guns are less frequent causes of pediatric ocular trauma, but they are likely to cause severe injuries.

Children aged 11–15 years have a particularly high incidence of severe eye injury compared with other age groups. Injured boys outnumber girls by a factor of 3 or 4 to 1.

American Academy of Pediatrics, Committee on Sports Medicine and Fitness; American Academy of Ophthalmology, Eye Health and Public Information Task Force. Protective eyewear for young athletes. *Ophthalmology.* 2004;111(3):600–603.

Superficial Injury

Corneal abrasion is one of the most common ocular injuries in children and adults. Topical cycloplegic drops and antibiotic ointment may help reduce discomfort and risk of infection, respectively. Traumatic corneal epithelial defects usually heal within 1–2 days. Use of a pressure patch to keep the eyelids closed is not necessary for most abrasions, since many children find this uncomfortable and patching does not decrease the time required for the abrasion to heal.

Cigarette burns of the cornea are the most common thermal injuries to the ocular surface in childhood. Usually, these occur in toddlers and are accidental, not manifestations of abuse. These burns result from the child running into a cigarette held at eye level by an adult. Despite the alarming initial white appearance of coagulated corneal epithelium, cigarette burns typically heal in a few days and without scarring. Treatment is the same as for mechanical abrasions.

Chemical burns in childhood are generally caused by organic solvents or soaps in household cleaning agents. Even burns involving almost total loss of corneal epithelium are likely to heal in a week or less with or without patching. Acid and alkali burns in children, as in adults, can be much more serious. The initial and most important step in management of all chemical injuries is immediate copious irrigation and meticulous removal of any particulate matter from the conjunctival fornices. See also BCSC Section 8, *External Disease and Cornea.*

Corneal foreign bodies in children can sometimes be dislodged with a forceful stream of irrigating solution. After topical anesthetic is placed, a cotton swab or blunt spatula can often be used to remove the corneal foreign body, with or without a slit lamp; sharp instruments should be avoided. If these methods are unsuccessful, the child may require sedation in order to facilitate removal of the foreign body.

Penetrating Injury

Unless an adult has witnessed the traumatic incident, the history cannot be relied on to exclude the possibility of penetrating injury to the globe. The anterior segment and fundus must be thoroughly inspected and general anesthesia used, if necessary, when a penetrating injury is suspected. An area of subconjunctival hemorrhage or chemosis or a small break in the skin of the eyelid may be the only surface manifestation of scleral perforation by a sharp-pointed object, such as a pencil or scissors blade (Fig 27-1). Distortion of the pupil may be the most evident sign of a small corneal or limbal perforation. Imaging should be considered if there is any reason to suspect an intraocular or orbital foreign body.

Corneoscleral lacerations in children are repaired according to the same principles as for adults (see BCSC Section 8, *External Disease and Cornea*). Corneal wounds heal relatively rapidly in very young patients; thus, sutures should be removed correspondingly earlier. Small conjunctival lacerations are often self-sealing.

Fibrin clots may form quickly in the anterior chamber of a child's eye after a penetrating injury to the cornea, and these can simulate the appearance of fluffy cataractous lens cortex to a remarkable degree. To avoid unnecessarily rendering the eye aphakic (and thereby compromising vision rehabilitation), the clinician should not perform lens removal in the course of primary wound repair unless absolutely certain that the anterior

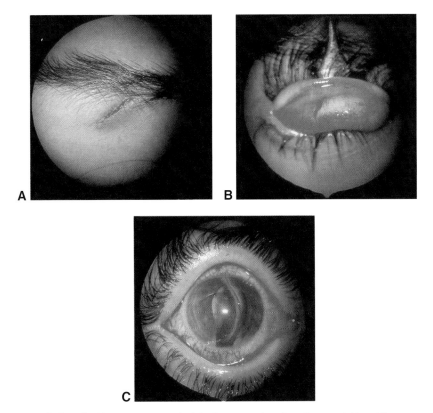

Figure 27-1 **A,** Small skin entry wound, right brow region, in a 7-year-old boy. The wound was created by a thrown dart. **B,** Conjunctival exit wound indicates complete perforation of the eyelid. **C,** Extensive injury to the anterior segment of the same eye.

capsule has been ruptured. Even if lens cortex is exposed, postponing cataract surgery for 1–2 weeks, until severe posttraumatic inflammation has quieted down, may result in a smoother postoperative recovery and reduced risk of complications without significantly worsening the visual prognosis. See also BCSC Section 11, *Lens and Cataract.*

Full-thickness eyelid lacerations should be repaired meticulously, especially those involving a canaliculus, and sedation or general anesthesia may be required, even in older children. Working near the eyes with sharp instruments and draping the face to create a sterile field are likely to frighten an awake child and add to the difficulty of the repair. Clearly superficial wounds can be repaired in the emergency department. Use of an absorbable suture is acceptable if the physician wishes to avoid the need for removal of nonabsorbable sutures.

Blunt Injury

Hyphema

As with all forms of pediatric trauma, the precise occurrence that led to the hyphema may be difficult to determine. The possibility of abuse must be considered, as must the possibility of a nontraumatic etiology: retinoblastoma, juvenile xanthogranuloma of the iris, and bleeding diathesis resulting from leukemia or other blood dyscrasia are relatively rare but important causes of spontaneous hyphema during the early years of life. Ultrasonography or magnetic resonance imaging should be performed to rule out intraocular tumor when the findings are suspicious and the iris and fundus cannot be adequately seen. A complete blood count should be performed with coagulation studies if a bleeding disorder is suspected.

Intraocular pressure (IOP), an important parameter for therapeutic decision making with traumatic hyphema, is often difficult to monitor in the pediatric patient. The risks of inaccurate measurements and of further traumatizing the injured eye may outweigh the potential value of obtaining measurements in uncooperative children. With small hyphemas (Fig 27-2), concern about pressure is greatest in patients with sickle cell trait or disease. Sickling may develop in the anterior chamber, elevating IOP and retarding resorption of blood, or in the retinal circulation, causing vascular occlusion. All African American children with traumatic hyphema require sickle cell screening to evaluate for these conditions.

It was once common practice to admit all patients with hyphema to the hospital and place them on bed rest with bilateral patching of the eyes. These restrictions have never been shown to improve prognosis and are likely to be unproductive in children. However, some decrease in normal childhood activity is reasonable, as is placing a protective metal shield over the affected eye. If parental cooperation is questionable or if the patient has sickle trait, hospitalization for several days after injury, when risk of rebleeding is greatest, remains justifiable. Outpatient management with close follow-up is acceptable.

Medical management of hyphema remains as controversial in children as it is in adults. Many ophthalmologists routinely use cycloplegic and corticosteroid drops to facilitate fundus examination, improve comfort, and reduce the risk of inflammatory complications and possibly of rebleeding as well. The value of these topical agents is unproven, however, and some clinicians prefer to use them selectively for control of pain or obvious inflammation, or to avoid them altogether to minimize manipulation of the eye. Pressure-lowering medication is appropriate for eyes known or strongly suspected to have increased IOP. Aspirin-containing compounds should be avoided because of their

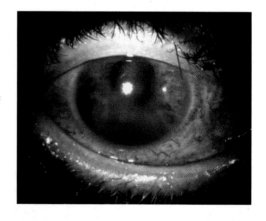

Figure 27-2 Small hyphema. Note layering of blood inferiorly. *(Courtesy of Edward L. Raab, MD.)*

antiplatelet action. Nonsteroidal anti-inflammatory drugs can also increase the risk of rebleeding and should be avoided.

Many treatments have been proposed to prevent rebleeding in traumatic hyphema, although none is universally accepted. They include an antifibrinolytic agent (aminocaproic acid or tranexamic acid) administered orally, topical aminocaproic acid, and oral prednisolone.

Surgical evacuation of hyphema is usually performed in adults when early corneal blood staining is detected or when significant IOP elevation has persisted for 5–7 days. The difficulty of detecting early blood staining in a child and the risk that corneal staining may cause severe deprivation amblyopia, coupled with the problems of accurately measuring IOP, justify earlier surgical intervention whenever a total hyphema persists for 4–5 days. Even earlier surgery may be necessary if elevated pressures occur in a patient with sickle cell trait or disease. Various operative techniques have been employed; none has been shown to offer particular advantages in children.

Late glaucoma is a potential complication of traumatic hyphema in children, as in adults, and may present with no symptoms. Gonioscopy can be performed after the eye has healed and the child can cooperate. Annual follow-up should be continued in children who are found to have angle recession.

Orbital Fractures

Orbital floor fractures

Blunt facial trauma is the usual cause of orbital floor fractures. When the rim remains intact, this is termed *blowout fracture.* Orbital floor fracture is thought to be caused by an acute increase in intraorbital pressure from direct impact that closes the orbital entrance, or by compression of the rim, which results in buckling of the floor. Orbital floor fracture can be part of more extensive fractures of the orbit and midface. In some cases, the mechanism causing floor fractures extends to include the medial wall as well.

Injury to the inferior rectus muscle or to its nerve, with resulting weakness, may be caused by hemorrhage or ischemia, in addition to restriction. It can occur either at the time of injury or during repair of the fracture.

Clinical features Injury to the inferior rectus muscle can present as either limited elevation or depression. Hypoesthesia in the cutaneous distribution of the infraorbital nerve can also occur.

In a patient with limited elevation, a positive forced-duction test indicates the presence of restriction. Bradycardia, heart block, nausea, or syncope can occur as a vagal response to entrapment. When the entrapment involves the more anterior portion of the orbital floor or when there is associated injury to the inferior rectus muscle or its nerve, there can also be limited depression. Reduced saccadic velocity and force generation on attempted downgaze suggest weak muscle action. Orbital computed tomography and high-resolution, multipositional magnetic resonance imaging are useful for revealing the presence and extent of the injury.

A special presentation, the *white-eyed blowout fracture,* is characterized by marked restriction (in both directions) of vertical ocular motility despite minimal signs of soft-tissue injury. This restriction is due to entrapment of the inferior rectus muscle either beneath a trapdoor fracture or, in the case of children, in a linear opening caused by flexion deformity of the floor. Early surgery, rather than observation, is required in order to minimize permanent muscle and nerve damage.

Criden MR, Ellis FJ. Linear nondisplaced orbital fractures with muscle entrapment. *J AAPOS.* 2007;11(2):142–147

Management There are several approaches to the management of orbital floor fractures. Some clinicians advocate surgical exploration in all cases, irrespective of the results of forced-duction testing. The justification for this approach is that, especially with large bony defects, progressive herniation of orbital contents into the adjacent maxillary sinus can occur, resulting in disfiguring enophthalmos. Others recommend waiting for a few days to 2 weeks to allow orbital ecchymosis to subside. For these surgeons, the main indication to operate is evidence of restriction with nonresolving diplopia in primary position. Diplopia immediately after the injury is common and is not necessarily an indication for urgent intervention. Management of persistent diplopia is covered in Chapter 11.

Orbital roof fractures

Though rare in older patients, orbital roof fractures are common in early childhood (<10 years of age). Isolated roof fractures typically result from impact to the brow region in a fall, often from a height of only a few feet. The principal external manifestation is hematoma in the upper eyelid (Fig 27-3). These fractures often heal without treatment.

For further discussion of diagnosis and management of orbital trauma, see BCSC Section 7, *Orbit, Eyelids, and Lacrimal System.*

Traumatic Optic Neuropathy

The optic nerve may be damaged by trauma to the head, orbit, or globe. Vision loss is usually immediate and severe with an afferent pupillary defect present. Initially, the optic nerve appears normal, but it becomes atrophic within 1–2 months of injury. Management is controversial and includes high-dose intravenous steroids and optic canal decompression.

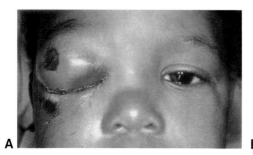
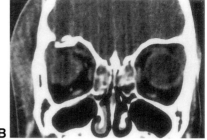

Figure 27-3 Orbital roof fracture in a child from direct impact from a fall. **A,** Marked right upper eyelid swelling from hematoma originating in the superior orbit, adjacent to a linear fracture. **B,** Coronal computed tomography shows a bone fragment displaced into the right orbit.

For further discussion of diagnosis and management of traumatic optic neuropathy, see BCSC Section 5, *Neuro-Ophthalmology*.

Nonaccidental Trauma

Although most eye injuries in childhood are accidental or innocently caused by other children, a significant portion of them result from physical abuse by adults. The terms used for intentional physical abuse of a child include *nonaccidental trauma* and *child abuse*. Child abuse includes emotional abuse, sexual abuse, and neglect as well as physical abuse. It is a pervasive problem, with an estimated 750,000 victims per year in the United States.

A reliable history is often difficult to obtain when nonaccidental trauma has occurred. Suspicion of nonaccidental trauma should be aroused when repeated accounts of the circumstances of injury or histories obtained from different individuals are inconsistent or when the events described do not correlate with the injuries (eg, bruises on multiple aspects of the head after a fall) or with the child's developmental level (eg, a 1-month-old rolling off a bed or a 4-month-old climbing out of a high chair).

Any physician who suspects child abuse is required by law in every US state and Canadian province to report the incident to a designated governmental agency. Once this obligation has been discharged, full investigation of the situation by appropriate specialists and authorities is usually performed. Physicians should be familiar with the regulations in their own country. If possible, ocular abnormalities should be documented photographically or with a detailed drawing to use as evidence in court.

Abusive Head Trauma

A unique complex of ocular, intracranial, and sometimes other injuries occurs in infants who have been abused by violent shaking. This is recognized as one of the most important manifestations of child abuse. Although the term *shaken baby syndrome* is still occasionally used, it has largely been replaced with the terms *abusive head trauma (AHT)* and *inflicted childhood neurotrauma* because these infants may sustain impact injury as well as shaking injury involving the head.

Patients with AHT are usually younger than 5 years and most often younger than 12 months. When a reliable history is available, it typically involves a parent or other caregiver who shook an inconsolably crying baby in anger or frustration. Often, however, the only information provided is that the child's mental status deteriorated or that a seizure or respiratory difficulty developed. The involved caregiver may relate that an episode of relatively minor trauma occurred, such as a fall from a bed. Even without a supporting history, the diagnosis of AHT can still be made with confidence on the basis of characteristic clinical findings. It must be kept in mind, however, that answers to important questions concerning the timing and circumstances of injury and the identity of the perpetrator frequently cannot be inferred from medical evidence alone.

Intracranial injury in AHT frequently includes subdural hematoma (typically bilateral over the cerebral convexities or in the interhemispheric fissure) and subarachnoid hemorrhage. Displacement of the brain in relation to the skull and dura mater ruptures bridging vessels, and compression against the cranial bones produces further damage. Neuroimaging may also acutely show intracranial edema, ischemia, or contusion and in later stages atrophy. These findings are thought to result from repetitive abrupt deceleration of the child's head as it whiplashes back and forth during the shaking episode. The infant's head is particularly vulnerable to the effects of repeated acceleration-deceleration because of its relatively large mass in relation to the body and poor stabilization by neck muscles. Some authorities, citing the frequency with which patients with AHT also show evidence of having received blows to the head, think that impact is an essential component, although in many cases no sign of impact is found.

Ocular involvement

The most common ocular manifestation of AHT, present in approximately 85% of cases, is retinal hemorrhage. Preretinal, nerve-fiber-layer, deep-retinal, or subretinal localization may be seen. The hemorrhages may be unilateral or bilateral. They tend to be concentrated in or near the macular region, but sometimes they are so extensive that they occupy nearly the entire fundus (Fig 27-4). Vitreous hemorrhage may also develop, usually as a secondary phenomenon resulting from migration of blood that was initially preretinal. Occasionally, the vitreous becomes almost completely opacified by dispersed hemorrhage within a few days of injury. Retinal hemorrhages in shaken infants cannot be dated with precision and usually resolve over a period of weeks to months. Vitrectomy should be considered if there is a risk of amblyopia due to persistent vitreous hemorrhage.

Some eyes show evidence of retinal tissue disruption in addition to hemorrhage. Full-thickness perimacular folds in the neurosensory retina, typically with circumferential orientation around the macula that creates a craterlike appearance, are highly characteristic. Splitting of the retina (traumatic retinoschisis), either deep to the nerve fiber layer or superficial (involving only the internal limiting membrane), may create cavities of considerable extent that are partially filled with blood, also usually in the macular region (Fig 27-5). Full-thickness retinal breaks and detachment are rare. Retinal folds usually flatten out within a few weeks of injury, but schisis cavities can persist indefinitely.

A striking feature of AHT is the typical lack of external evidence of trauma. The ocular adnexa and anterior segment may appear entirely normal. Occasionally, the trunk or

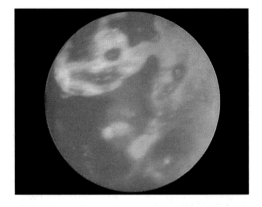

Figure 27-4 Extensive retinal hemorrhages in a 2-month-old infant suspected to have been violently shaken.

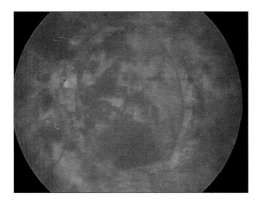

Figure 27-5 Traumatic retinoschisis. *(Courtesy of Ken K. Nischal, MD.)*

extremities show bruises representing the imprint of the perpetrator's hands. In a minority of cases, broken ribs or characteristic metaphyseal fractures of the long bones result from forces generated during shaking. It must be kept in mind, however, that these patients may have been subjected to other forms of abuse.

When extensive retinal hemorrhage accompanied by perimacular folds and schisis cavities is found in association with intracranial hemorrhage or other evidence of trauma to the brain in an infant, AHT can usually be diagnosed with confidence regardless of other circumstances. Severe accidental head trauma (eg, sustained in a fall from a second-story level or in a motor vehicle collision) is not frequently accompanied by retinal hemorrhage, which is not extensive when present. Retinal hemorrhage is rare and has never been documented to be extensive following cardiopulmonary resuscitation by trained personnel. Severe, fatal, acute head-crush injury rarely causes hemorrhagic retinopathy with perimacular folds, which can be differentiated from AHT by the associated injuries.

Extensive retinal hemorrhage without other ocular findings strongly suggests that intracranial injury has been caused by AHT, but alternative possibilities such as a co-agulation disorder must be considered as well. Retinal hemorrhages resulting from birth trauma are common in newborns, but they seldom persist beyond the age of 1 month. Other possible causes of retinal hemorrhage in children include anemia, hypertension, increased intracranial pressure, leukemia, meningitis, glutaric aciduria, and retinopathy of prematurity.

American Academy of Ophthalmology. Information Statement. *Abusive Head Trauma/ Shaken Baby Syndrome.* San Francisco: American Academy of Ophthalmology; 2010. Available at http://one.aao.org/guidelines-browse?filter=clinicalstatement. Accessed February 19, 2014.

Christian CW, Block R; Committee on Child Abuse and Neglect; American Academy of Pediatrics. Abusive head trauma in infants and children. *Pediatrics.* 2009;123(5):1409–1411.

Prognosis

In one large study, 29% of children with AHT died of their injuries. Poor visual and pupillary responses were correlated with a higher risk of mortality. Survivors often had permanent impairment ranging from mild learning disability and motor disturbances to severe cognitive impairment and quadriparesis. The most common cause of vision loss is from cortical injury followed by optic atrophy. Dense vitreous hemorrhage, usually associated with deep traumatic retinoschisis, carries a poor prognosis for both vision and life.

Ocular Injury Secondary to Nonaccidental Trauma

The presenting sign of child abuse involves the eye in approximately 5% of cases. Blunt trauma inflicted with fingers, fists, or implements such as belts or straps is the usual mechanism of nonaccidental injury to the ocular adnexa or anterior segment. Periorbital ecchymosis, subconjunctival hemorrhage, and hyphema should raise suspicion of recent abuse if the explanation provided is implausible (see the section "Hyphema" earlier in this chapter). Cataract and lens dislocation may be a sign of repeated injury or trauma inflicted earlier. Child abuse should also be suspected with rhegmatogenous retinal detachment in a child without a history of injury or an apparent predisposing factor, such as high myopia.

CHAPTER 28

Ocular Manifestations of Systemic Disease

This chapter focuses on systemic disorders with multiple types of ocular involvement. Systemic disorders associated with one primary ocular abnormality are discussed in other chapters in this volume (eg, Marfan syndrome is covered in Chapter 23, Childhood Cataracts and Other Pediatric Lens Disorders).

Diseases due to Chromosomal Abnormalities

Chromosomal disorders are classified as abnormalities in number (aneuploidy: trisomy or monosomy), structure (duplications, deletions, translocations, inversions, or rings), or type (autosomal or sex chromosome). Their incidence is approximately 1 in 150 live births.

Common trisomy syndromes are 13, 18, and 21. Turner syndrome is monosomy X. The most common deletions are 4p, 5p, 18p, and 18q. Table 28-1 describes the ocular findings associated with these disorders.

Inborn Errors of Metabolism

Nearly 500 genes that contribute to inherited eye diseases have been identified. The overall incidence of inborn errors of metabolism is estimated to be 1 in 1400 births.

Inborn errors of metabolism are characterized by the genetic absence, either physical or functional, of 1 or more enzymes. Such errors may cause eye abnormalities in 1 of several ways: direct toxicity of abnormal metabolic products, accumulation of abnormal (or normal) metabolites, errors of synthetic pathways, or deficient production of energy. Inborn errors of metabolism are usually inherited as recessive disorders, either autosomal or X-linked. Germline mutations may also occur. Carriers of inborn errors of metabolism possess half the normal quantity of an enzyme, as would be expected in persons with 1 normal gene and 1 defective gene. This deficiency usually results in adequate metabolic function but subnormal serum levels. Measurements of enzyme levels in fetal cells obtained through amniocentesis may enable prenatal detection of many of these conditions.

Table 28-1 Chromosomal Anomalies With Ocular Associations

Chromosomal Abnormality	Associated Ocular Findings
Trisomy 13, Patau syndrome	*More common:* microphthalmia, coloboma, retinal dysplasia with frequent islands of intraocular cartilage *Less common:* cataract, corneal opacification, cyclopia, persistent fetal vasculature, shallow supraorbital ridges, upward-slanting palpebral fissures, absent eyebrows, hypotelorism, hypertelorism, anophthalmia, glaucoma
Trisomy 18, Edwards syndrome	*More common:* short palpebral fissures, hypertelorism, epicanthus, hypoplastic supraorbital ridge *Less common:* cataract, microcornea, corneal opacification, congenital glaucoma, retinal depigmentation, colobomatous microphthalmia, cyclopia
Trisomy 21, Down syndrome (most common trisomy)	*More common:* epicanthus with upward-slanting palpebral fissures, blepharitis, Brushfield spots, congenital or acquired cataract, myopia, congenital nasolacrimal duct obstruction and difficulty with probings, ectropion, strabismus, hypoaccommodation, nystagmus, increased number of vessels at optic disc margin *Less common:* infantile glaucoma, keratoconus
Deletion 4p, Wolf-Hirschhorn syndrome	*More common:* colobomatous microphthalmia, epicanthus, downward-slanting palpebral fissures, hypertelorism, strabismus, ptosis, corneal opacification (Peters anomaly) *Less common:* anterior segment anomalies, cataract
Deletion 5p, cri-du-chat syndrome	*More common:* upward- or downward-slanting palpebral fissures, hypotelorism or hypertelorism, epicanthus, strabismus *Less common:* ptosis, decreased tear production, myopia, cataract, glaucoma, tortuous retinal vessels, foveal hypoplasia, optic atrophy, colobomatous microphthalmia
Deletion 18p	*More common:* hypertelorism, ptosis, epicanthus, and strabismus *Less common:* cataracts, retinal dysplasia, colobomatous microphthalmia, synophthalmia/cyclopia
Deletion 18q	*More common:* epicanthus, hypertelorism, downward-slanting palpebral fissures, strabismus, dysplastic or atrophic optic nerve, nystagmus *Less common:* corneal abnormalities, cataracts, blue sclera, myopia, colobomatous microphthalmia
Monosomy X, Turner syndrome	*More common:* strabismus, ptosis *Less common:* cataracts, refractive errors, corneal scars, blue sclera Incidence of color blindness similar to that of unaffected males

The age of onset of eye problems in inborn errors of metabolism is variable; some are present at birth and others emerge in early childhood. Consultation with a geneticist is warranted for any patient with ocular findings that suggest an inborn error of metabolism. Table 28-2 summarizes the common ophthalmic manifestations of the major inborn errors of metabolism.

Inborn errors of metabolism can be categorized according to the processes and biochemical pathways affected by enzyme deficiencies (examples of specific disorders are in parentheses):

- carbohydrate synthesis (galactosemia)
- amino acid metabolism (homocystinuria)
- organic acid metabolism (methylmalonic aciduria)
- mitochondrial metabolism (Kearns-Sayre syndrome)
- urea cycle (ornithine transcarbamylase deficiency)
- peroxisome function (adrenoleukodystrophy, Zellweger disease)
- steroid pathway (Smith-Lemli-Opitz syndrome)
- lipid storage (Tay-Sachs disease, Gaucher disease)
- transport (cystinosis)
- lysosomal storage (mucopolysaccharidoses, cystinosis, neuronal ceroid lipofuscinosis, galactosialidosis)
- metal metabolism (Wilson disease)

These disorders can also be categorized according to the affected ocular structure.

Poll-The BT, Maillette de Buy Wenniger-Prick CL. The eye in metabolic diseases: clues to diagnosis. *Eur J Paediatr Neurol.* 2011;15(3):197–204.

Cornea

Metabolic diseases cloud the cornea via accumulation of a pathway product. If the product is produced in the cornea, the clouding may be found throughout the cornea. If the level of the product is elevated in the blood, the peripheral cornea alone may be involved. Diseases that affect the cornea include the mucopolysaccharidoses (MPS; types I H, I S, I H/S, II, IV, VI, and VII) (Fig 28-1), cystinosis, and Wilson disease. Cystinosis causes crystal-like deposits throughout the cornea and symptoms of photophobia. Wilson disease may present with a peripheral brown Kayser-Fleischer ring. See also Chapter 20.

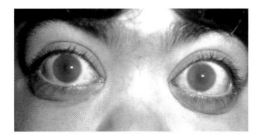

Figure 28-1 Mucopolysaccharidosis VI. *(Courtesy of Edward L. Raab, MD.)*

Table 28-2 Ocular Findings in Mucopolysaccharidoses, Mucolipidoses, Lipidoses, Gangliosidoses, and Miscellaneous Disorders

Disease (code)*	Enzyme Deficiency	Corneal Clouding	Motility Disorders	Cherry-Red Spot	RPE Degeneration	Optic Atrophy	Other	Inheritance
Mucopolysaccharidoses (MPS)								
MPS I H, I S Hurler (607014) Scheie (607016)	α-L-Iduronidase	+++	–	–	+++	+	Glaucoma; plus papilledema (I H only)	AR
MPS II Hunter (309900)	Iduronate 2-sulfatase	–	–	–	++	+	–	XR

MPS III
Sanfilippo syndrome
  A (252900)
  B (252920)
  C (252930)
  D (252940)
	A: Heparan N-sulfatase
	B: α-N-Acetyl-glucosaminidase
	C: Acetyl-CoA:α-glucosaminide N-acetyltransferase
	D: N-Acetylglucosamine-6-sulfatase
		–	–	–	++	Rare	Late blindness	AR

MPS IV Morquio A (253200) Morquio B (253010)	A: N-Acetyl-galactosamine-6-sulfatase B: β-Galactosidase	++	–	–	Rare	Rare	–	AR AR AR
MPS VI Maroteaux-Lamy (253200)	Arylsulfatase B	++	–	–	–	+	Papilledema, glaucoma	AR
MPS VII Sly (253220)	β-Glucuronidase	+	–	–	–	–	–	AR
Mucolipidoses								
Type I (256550) Sialidosis (glycoproteinosis) "Cherry-red spot myoclonus syndrome"	Neuraminidase	–	+	+	+	–	Hearing loss	AR
Type II (252500) I-Cell disease	Multiple lysosomal enzymes	++	–	–	–	–	Hurler-like	AR
Type III (252600) Pseudo-Hurler polydystrophy	Multiple lysosomal enzymes	+++	–	–	–	–	Hurler-like puffy eyelids	AR
Type IV (252650) Gangliosidosis	Mucolipin-1 defect	+++	–	–	++	+	Photophobia	AR
Lipidoses								
Niemann-Pick disease (257220)	Sphingomyelinase	+	Nystagmus	+	–	+	Eventual vision loss	AR
Fabry disease (301500)	α-Galactosidase A	Whorl-like	–	–	–	–	Angiokeratoma, spokelike cataract, aneurysmal conjunctival vessels	XR
Gaucher disease Type I (230800) Type II (230900) Type III (231005)	Acid β-glucosidase	–	Paralytic strabismus, looped saccades	–	+	–	Pinguecula, conjunctival pigmentation	AR
Metachromatic leukodystrophy (250100)	Arylsulfatase A	–	Nystagmus	+	–	+	Blindness, decreased pupil reaction	AR
Krabbe disease (245200)	Galactosylceramidase	–	Nystagmus	Rare	–	+	Cortical blindness	AR
Fucosidosis (230000)	α-L-Fucosidase	–	–	–	+	–	Hurler-like features, angiokeratoma, tortuous conjunctival vessels	AR

Disease (code)*	Enzyme Deficiency	Conjunctival Tortuosity	Corneal Clouding	Motility Disorders	Cherry-Red Spot	RPE Degeneration	Optic Atrophy	High Myopia	Blindness	Inheritance
Gangliosidoses										
Generalized (GM$_1$) gangliosidoses										
Type I (230500)	β-Galactosidase-1	+	±	ET, nystagmus	50% of patients	–	+	+	+	AR
Type II (230600)	β-Galactosidase-1	–	–	ET, nystagmus	–	+	±	+	Late	AR
Derry disease Juvenile GM$_1$										
Type III (230650)	β-Galactosidase-1	±	Rare	–	–	–	–	–	–	AR
Adult GM$_1$										
GM$_2$ gangliosidoses										
Tay-Sachs disease (272800)										
Type I, Classic infantile	Hexosaminidase A	–	–	Nystagmus, ophthalmoplegia	+	–	+		+	AR
B1 variant, Late infantile	HEXA defect									AR
Type III, Juvenile subacute	Hexosaminidase A or B		+	Strabismus	+	+	+	+	+	AR
Chronic adult	HEXA defect			Ocular motor defects						AR
Type II (268800)	Hexosaminidase A and B	–	Rare	ET	+	–	±	–	+	AR
Sandhoff disease										
Type AB, Hexosaminidase activator deficiency	HEXA or HEXB mutation			Strabismus	+	+	+		Late	AR

Disease (code)*	Enzyme Deficiency	Corneal Clouding	Motility Disorders	Cherry-Red Spot	RPE Degeneration	Optic Atrophy	Other	Inheritance
Miscellaneous Disorders								
Galactosialidosis (256540)	β-Galactosidase neuraminidase	+	–	+	–	+	Dwarfism, seizures, coarse facies	AR
Neuronal ceroid lipofuscinosis								
CLN1 Infantile Hagberg-Santavuori disease (256730)	PPT-1	–	+	Macular	+	+	Blindness	AR
CLN2 Late infantile Hagberg-Santavuori (204500)	PPT-1	–	+	Bull's eye	+	+	Blindness	AR
CLN3 Juvenile Batten, Spielmeyer-Vogt disease (204200)	Unknown	–	+	Bull's eye	+	+	Blindness	AR
CLN4 Adult Kufs disease (204300)	Unknown	–	–	–	–	–		AR
Cystinosis (219800)	Unknown	Crystals	–	–	++	–	Conjunctival crystals, renal problems	AR
Galactosemia (230400)	Gal-1-PO$_4$ uridyl transferase	–	–	–	–	–	Cataracts if not treated	AR
Mannosidosis (248500)	α-Mannosidase	++	–	–	+	Pallor, blurred margin	Hurler-like, spokelike cataract	AR
Homocystinuria (236200)	Cystathionine β-synthase	–	–	–	+	–	Dislocated lens, cataract	AR
Refsum disease (266500)	Phytanic acid α-hydrolase	–	–	–	++	–	Cataract, night blindness	AR

* Code numbers refer to the system developed by Victor McKusick and colleagues (McKusick VA, Francomano CA, Antonarakis SE. *Mendelian Inheritance in Man: Catalogs of Autosomal Dominant, Autosomal Recessive, and X-Linked Phenotypes.* 10th ed. Baltimore: The Johns Hopkins University Press; 1992). Table updates from Online Mendelian Inheritance in Man (www.ncbi.nlm.nih.gov/omim).
Plus (+) and minus (–) signs indicate the relative likelihood of occurrence of ocular findings in these systemic disorders. AR = autosomal recessive; ET = constant esotropia; XR = X-linked recessive.

Lens

In many multisystem metabolic diseases, cataracts occur (eg, as a feature of Smith-Lemli-Opitz syndrome and all the galactosemias). In galactokinase deficiency, cataracts may be the sole manifestation of the disease. Lens dislocation occurs in homocystinuria. Lens disorders are discussed in Chapter 23.

Retina

More than 400 inherited diseases involve the retina. The most common, *retinitis pigmentosa (RP)*, may occur as a primary defect in the photoreceptors or as a secondary event arising from sensitivity of the photoreceptors or the pigment epithelium to a generalized metabolic defect. Retinal degeneration is found in peroxisomal disorders (Zellweger disease, Refsum disease), lysosomal disorders (neuronal ceroid lipofuscinosis), and mitochondrial disorders (Kearns-Sayre syndrome).

Fovea

The appearance of a cherry-red spot in the macula is caused by loss of transparency of the perifoveal retina due to edema or deposition of abnormal material in the retinal ganglion cells. The fovea, which is very thin and almost devoid of ganglion cells (the site of abnormal material accumulation in storage disease), normally appears red to brown, depending on the patient's race. With infiltration of the retinal ganglion cells, the thicker perifoveal retina becomes white and its color contrasts with that of the fovea, creating the cherry-red spot. Metabolic diseases that may cause a cherry-red spot include GM_2 gangliosidosis type I (Tay-Sachs disease) and type II (Sandhoff disease), as well as Niemann-Pick disease. The cherry-red spot disappears over time as the intumescent ganglion cells die and optic atrophy develops. Therefore, the absence of a cherry-red spot should not be used to rule out a diagnosis, especially in older children.

Treatment of metabolic disorders

A variety of treatment options now exist for many previously untreatable metabolic disorders. These include enzyme replacement therapy, stem cell transplantation (bone marrow or umbilical cord blood), and dietary changes. Gene therapy is promising, and clinical trials have begun for some disorders. Usually, the earlier a patient is referred to a geneticist, the better the chance will be of a beneficial effect from such treatment.

Examples of treatable metabolic disorders with ocular findings are homocystinuria and cystinosis (see Chapters 20 and 23). Classic homocystinuria is caused by a deficiency of cystathionine β-synthase activity, which is usually detected shortly after birth if neonatal screening measures are employed. Dietary restriction of methionine and supplementation with folate, vitamin B_6, vitamin B_{12}, or betaine or a combination of these can markedly reduce plasma homocysteine levels and prevent disease progression. In most untreated patients with classic homocystinuria, cognitive impairment, ectopia lentis, and thrombotic events develop. The risk of these sequelae is greatly decreased by metabolic control. In patients with cystinosis, systemic cysteamine can ameliorate renal disease, and topical cysteamine eyedrops can prevent or reverse painful crystalline keratopathy.

Familial Oculorenal Syndromes

Lowe syndrome

Lowe syndrome (Lowe oculocerebrorenal syndrome) is an X-linked recessive disorder characterized by renal tubulopathy (Fanconi type) that occurs in the first year of life, leading to aminoaciduria, metabolic acidosis, proteinuria, and rickets. Affected children are severely hypotonic at birth, and cognitive impairment is common.

The most common eye defect is congenital bilateral cataract. The lenses are small, thick, and opaque and may demonstrate posterior lenticonus. Miotic pupils are frequent. Congenital glaucoma often develops. Surgery is frequently difficult, and cyclitic membrane formation and recalcitrant glaucoma are common following surgery. Mothers of affected children may have punctate snowflake opacities, oriented radially within the lens cortex, that indicate their carrier status.

Alport syndrome

Alport syndrome is usually inherited as an X-linked disorder. It is a disease of basement membranes that causes progressive renal failure, deafness, anterior lenticonus or anterior subcapsular cataract, posterior polymorphous dystrophy, and fleck retinopathy. Hematuria begins in childhood. Hypertension and kidney failure occur late in the course of the disease.

Senior-Loken syndrome

Senior-Loken syndrome is an autosomal recessive disease characterized by nephronophthisis, renal failure, and a pigmentary retinal degeneration similar to that of Leber congenital amaurosis (LCA), with a flat electroretinogram (ERG). Children who have received a diagnosis of LCA should undergo renal function studies to rule out Senior-Loken syndrome.

Phakomatoses

The phakomatoses, or *neurocutaneous syndromes,* are a group of disorders characterized by multiple lesions of 1 or more histologic types that are found in 2 or more organ systems, including the skin and central nervous system (CNS). The lesions are commonly multiorgan hamartomas. Ocular involvement is frequent and may constitute an important source of morbidity as well as provide diagnostic information. Four major disorders have traditionally been designated phakomatoses, all of which have important ocular manifestations:

- neurofibromatosis (von Recklinghausen disease)
- tuberous sclerosis (Bourneville disease)
- angiomatosis of the retina and cerebellum (von Hippel–Lindau disease)
- encephalofacial or encephalotrigeminal angiomatosis (Sturge-Weber syndrome)

Other conditions sometimes classified as phakomatoses include

- ataxia-telangiectasia (Louis-Bar syndrome)
- incontinentia pigmenti (Bloch-Sulzberger syndrome)
- racemose angioma (Wyburn-Mason syndrome)
- Klippel-Trénaunay-Weber syndrome

Neurofibromatosis

Patients with neurofibromatosis (NF) manifest characteristic lesions composed of melanocytes or neuroglial cells, both of which are derivatives of neural crest mesenchyme. Although the melanocytic and glial lesions in NF are often called *hamartomas,* this designation is questionable because most lesions do not become evident until years after birth and many are histologically indistinguishable from low-grade neoplasms originating in the same tissues. NF has 2 forms that are distinguished by differences in genetics, diagnostic criteria, morbidity, and treatment.

Neurofibromatosis 1

Neurofibromatosis 1 (NF1) is the most common single-gene disorder affecting the nervous system. It affects 1 in 3000 to 3500 people and has autosomal dominant inheritance with virtually 100% penetrance. Approximately 50% of cases are sporadic, presumably the result of new mutations. The genetic locus of NF1 is on the long arm of chromosome 17 (17q11.2). The *NF1* gene is associated with neurofibromin, which is involved in regulation of cellular proliferation and tumor suppression.

Melanocytic lesions Almost all adults with NF1 have melanocytic lesions involving both the skin and the eye. *Café-au-lait spots,* the most common cutaneous expression, appear clinically as flat, sharply demarcated, uniformly hyperpigmented macules of varying size and shape. At least a few are usually present at birth; their number and size increase during the first decade of life. Many unaffected individuals have 1–3 café-au-lait spots, but greater numbers are rare except in association with NF. Clusters of small café-au-lait spots, or freckling, in the axillary or inguinal regions are particularly characteristic of NF1.

Melanocytic lesions of the uveal tract are common ocular manifestations of NF. Iris lesions are small (usually <1 mm), sharply demarcated, dome-shaped excrescences known as *Lisch nodules* (Fig 28-2). Most Lisch nodules develop between ages 5 and 10 years and are present in nearly all affected adults. An affected adult's eye typically has dozens.

Choroidal lesions occur in one-third to one-half of adults with NF1. These hyperpigmented lesions are flat with indistinct borders. Their number varies from 1 to 20 per eye, and each lesion is typically 1–2 times the size of the optic disc. These lesions may be

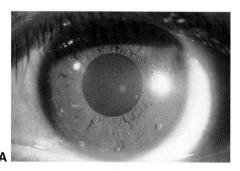
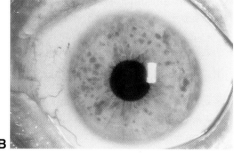

A B

Figure 28-2 Lisch nodules of iris with neurofibromatosis 1 (NF1). **A,** Brown iris has lighter-colored Lisch nodules. **B,** Blue iris has darker-colored Lisch nodules.

difficult to visualize by conventional fundus examination; near-infrared reflectance imaging has a high sensitivity for detection.

Neither the vision nor the health of the eye is affected by these melanocytic lesions, regardless of their extent. Persons with NF1 are thought to be predisposed to uveal melanoma and to several other malignant neoplasms. However, the prevalence of iris (especially choroidal) tumors is still low.

Glial cell lesions The most common neuroglial lesions in NF1 are nodular and subcutaneous neurofibromas, plexiform neurofibromas, and optic pathway gliomas.

NODULAR NEUROFIBROMAS Among lesions of neuroglial origin in NF1, *nodular cutaneous* and *subcutaneous neurofibromas,* or *fibroma molluscum,* are by far the most common. These lesions are soft, often pedunculated, papulonodules. They typically appear in late childhood and increase in number throughout adolescence and adulthood; nearly all adults with NF1 have at least a few. In some cases, hundreds of these lesions are present, causing considerable disfigurement.

PLEXIFORM NEUROFIBROMAS Plexiform neurofibromas occur in approximately 30% of patients with NF1 and appear clinically as extensive soft subcutaneous swellings with indistinct margins. Hyperpigmentation or hypertrichosis of the overlying skin is common, as is hypertrophy of underlying soft tissue and bone (regional gigantism).

Plexiform neurofibromas develop earlier than do nodular lesions, frequently becoming evident in infancy or childhood, and may cause severe disfigurement and functional impairment. Approximately 10% of plexiform neurofibromas involve the face, commonly the upper eyelid and orbit (Fig 28-3). The greater involvement of the upper eyelid's temporal portion gives the eyelid margin an S-shaped configuration. Complete ptosis may result from the increasing bulk and weight of the upper eyelid. Glaucoma in the ipsilateral eye is found in as many as half of cases.

Complete excision of an eyelid plexiform neurofibroma is generally not possible. Treatment is directed toward the relief of specific symptoms. Surgical debulking and frontalis suspension procedures can reduce ptosis sufficiently to permit binocular vision. Clinical trials examining use of biologic agents in the treatment of these lesions are under way.

Jakacki RI, Dombi E, Potter DM, et al. Phase 1 trial of pegylated interferon-α-2b in young patients with plexiform neurofibromas. *Neurology.* 2011;76(3):265–272.

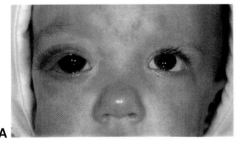 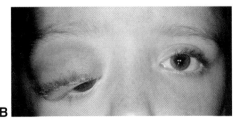

Figure 28-3 Plexiform neurofibroma involving the right upper eyelid, associated with ipsilateral buphthalmos, in a girl with NF1. **A,** Age 8 months. **B,** Age 8 years.

OPTIC PATHWAY GLIOMA This low-grade pilocytic astrocytoma (optic glioma) involves the optic nerve, chiasm, or both and is among the most characteristic and potentially serious complications of NF1. Optic pathway gliomas are present in approximately 15% of patients and are symptomatic (ie, produce significant vision loss, proptosis, or other complications) in 1%–5%.

Magnetic resonance imaging (MRI) is the preferred technique for diagnosis. The orbital portion of an involved optic nerve usually shows cylindrical or fusiform enlargement (Fig 28-4), often with exaggerated sinuousness or kinking, creating an appearance of discontinuity or localized constriction on axial images.

Optic gliomas that become symptomatic in patients with NF1 nearly always do so before age 10 years, often following a brief period of rapid enlargement. Even without treatment, some gliomas enter a phase of stability or slower growth, and spontaneous improvement has been documented in a few cases.

Tumors confined to the optic nerve at the time of clinical presentation infrequently extend into the chiasm. Chemotherapy may be effective in halting their growth. Radiation therapy can be useful, especially in cases of sudden vision loss or rapid growth. However, the efficacy of these treatments is difficult to evaluate, even in large studies, because of the widely variable natural history of this disease. Subtotal orbital excision for relief of disfiguring proptosis in a blind eye can be considered.

In addition to causing bilateral vision loss, tumors involving primarily the chiasm may result in significant morbidity, including hydrocephalus and hypothalamic dysfunction. Chiasmal glioma in patients with NF1 carries a much better prognosis than in individuals without NF.

OTHER NEUROGLIAL ABNORMALITIES There are other, less common neuroglial abnormalities. Abnormal proliferation of peripheral neuroglial or other neural crest–derived cells may occur in deeper tissues and visceral organs as well as in skin (spinal and gastrointestinal

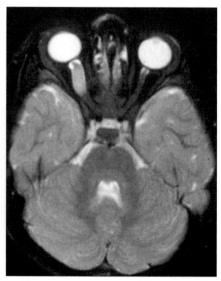

Figure 28-4 Axial magnetic resonance (MR) image of a right optic pathway glioma in a child with NF1. *(Courtesy of Ken K. Nischal, MD.)*

neurofibromas, pheochromocytoma). Prominence of corneal nerves, thought to represent glial hypertrophy, may be observed on slit-lamp examination in as many as 20% of cases. In rare cases, a localized neurofibroma develops within the orbit. Retinal hamartomas that are indistinguishable from those seen in tuberous sclerosis have also been reported.

Other manifestations NF1 is associated with an increased (but still generally low) incidence of several conditions that cannot be explained by abnormal proliferation of neural crest–derived cells. These include various benign tumors that involve the skin or the eye (juvenile xanthogranuloma, retinal capillary hemangioma) and several forms of malignancy (leukemia, rhabdomyosarcoma, pheochromocytoma, Wilms tumor). Also relatively common are bony defects such as scoliosis, pseudarthrosis of the tibia, and hypoplasia of the sphenoid bone (which may cause ocular pulsation). Sphenoid dysplasia may be associated with neurofibromas in the ipsilateral superficial temporal fossa as well as in the deep orbit. Several ill-defined abnormalities of the CNS (macrocephaly, aqueductal stenosis, seizures, and developmental delay) are also seen with greater frequency in patients with NF1.

Diagnosis and monitoring NF1 is diagnosed by genetic testing or based on clinical findings when 2 or more of the following 7 criteria are met:

1. six or more café-au-lait spots that are >5 mm in diameter in prepubescent children or >15 mm in diameter in postpubescent children
2. two or more neurofibromas of any type or 1 plexiform neurofibroma
3. freckling of axillary, inguinal, or other intertriginous areas
4. optic pathway glioma
5. two or more Lisch nodules of the iris
6. a distinctive osseous lesion, such as sphenoid bone dysplasia or thinning of the long-bone cortex, with or without pseudarthrosis
7. a first-degree relative with NF1, according to the above criteria

Lisch nodules may be used to confirm the presence of NF1 in a patient with café-au-lait spots. They may not be present in affected children, but the absence of such nodules in an adult makes the diagnosis unlikely. Some practitioners recommend neuroimaging to look for optic glioma in all children with NF. Others recommend routine examination and reserve the use of neuroimaging for patients who develop abnormalities of vision, pupil function, or optic disc appearance. An appropriate interval for periodic ophthalmic reassessment in childhood is 1–2 years, unless a specific abnormality requires closer observation.

Fisher MJ, Loguidice M, Gutmann DH, et al. Visual outcomes in children with neurofibromatosis type 1-associated optic pathway glioma following chemotherapy: a multicenter retrospective analysis. *Neuro Oncol.* 2012;14(6):790–797. Epub 2012 Apr 3.

Kalamarides M, Acosta MT, Babovic-Vuksanovic D, et al. Neurofibromatosis 2011: a report of the Children's Tumor Foundation annual meeting. *Acta Neuropathol.* 2012;123(3):369–380.

Neurofibromatosis 2

Neurofibromatosis 2 (NF2) is much less common than NF1; it has an incidence of 1:33,000–1:40,000. It is an autosomal dominant condition, and approximately half of all cases show sporadic mutation. The *NF2* gene, neurofibromin 2 (merlin), is located on chromosome 22 (22q12.2) and encodes for a cytoskeletal membrane-linking protein. NF2 is diagnosed clinically by the presence of bilateral acoustic neuromas (eighth cranial nerve tumors) or by a first-degree relative with NF2 and presence of a unilateral acoustic neuroma, neurofibroma, meningioma, schwannoma, glioma, or early-onset posterior subcapsular cataract.

Patients with NF2 typically present in their teens or early adulthood with symptoms related to the eighth nerve tumor(s), including decreased hearing or tinnitus. Ocular findings may predate the onset of symptoms. Therefore, the alert ophthalmologist may be able to help identify the potential for CNS tumors before they become symptomatic. The most characteristic ocular finding in NF2 is lens opacity, especially posterior subcapsular cataract or wedge-shaped cortical cataracts. Up to 80% of patients have epiretinal membranes. Less common findings are retinal hamartoma and combined hamartomas of the retina and retinal pigment epithelium (RPE). Lisch nodules of the iris can occur in NF2 but are infrequent.

Tuberous Sclerosis

Tuberous sclerosis (TS), or *Bourneville disease,* has a reported incidence of approximately 1 in 10,000. Two distinct genes give rise to TS: *TSC1* on 9q34 and *TSC2* on 16p13.3. Their proteins, hamartin and tuberin, respectively, are tumor suppressors. Transmission as an autosomal dominant trait has been documented in numerous pedigrees, but new mutations account for as many as 80% of cases.

The 3 classic findings, known as the *Vogt triad,* are cognitive impairment, seizures, and facial angiofibromas, although all 3 are present in only about 30% of patients with TS. This disease is characterized by benign tumor growth in multiple organs, predominantly the skin, brain, heart, kidney, and eye. Clinical features are divided into major and minor features (Table 28-3). Two major or 1 major and 2 minor features are necessary for a definitive diagnosis.

Table 28-3 Major and Minor Clinical Features of Tuberous Sclerosis

Major Features	Minor Features
Facial angiofibromas	Multiple pits in dental enamel
Ungual fibroma	Hamartomatous rectal polyps
Shagreen patch	Bone cysts
Hypomelanotic macules (>3)	Cerebral white matter radial migration lines
Cortical tuber	Gingival fibromas
Subependymal nodule	Retinal achromatic patch
Subependymal giant cell astrocytoma	Small, white "confetti" skin lesions
Retinal hamartomas	Multiple renal cysts
Cardiac rhabdomyoma	
Lymphangiomyomatosis	

Modified with permission from Roach ES, Gomez MR, Northrup H. Tuberous sclerosis complex consensus conference: revised clinical diagnostic criteria. *J Child Neurol.* 1998;13(12):624–628.

TS is characterized by several distinct skin lesions. The *ash-leaf spot* presents in infancy as a sharply demarcated hypopigmented lesion (Fig 28-5A). Ultraviolet light increases the visibility of these spots in light-skinned people. Facial angiofibromas, often called *adenoma sebaceum* (Fig 28-5B), appear in childhood and are present in three-quarters of adults with TS. These lesions are often mistaken for common acne. Subungual and periungual fibromas are also common after puberty. A thickened plaque of skin known as a *shagreen patch* occurs in approximately one-quarter of cases, typically in the lumbosacral area.

Seizures occur in 80% of patients with TS and may be difficult to control. Severe cognitive impairment is present in 50% of patients, but in others, intelligence may be normal. Characteristic neuroimaging findings include periventricular or basal ganglia calcification (representing benign astrocytomas), and tuberous malformations of the cortex (Fig 28-6). Malignant astrocytomas occur infrequently. Obstruction of the foramen of Munro by tumor may produce hydrocephalus. Cardiac tumors (rhabdomyomas) can lead to early death or severe disability. Bone and kidney lesions are common but usually produce no significant disturbance of function.

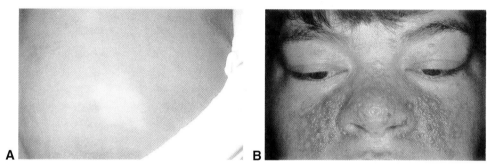

A   **B**

Figure 28-5   Cutaneous lesions of tuberous sclerosis. **A,** Hypopigmented macule. **B,** Adenoma sebaceum of the face.

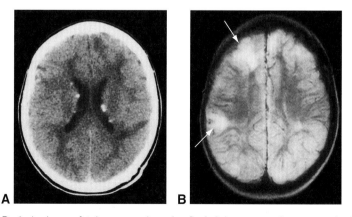

A   **B**

Figure 28-6   Brain lesions of tuberous sclerosis. **A,** Axial computed tomography image showing small periventricular calcifications. **B,** Axial T2-weighted MRI demonstrating tuberous malformations *(arrows).*

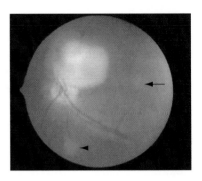

Figure 28-7 Fundus lesions of tuberous sclerosis, left eye. In addition to the large phakoma partially overlying the optic disc, a small hypopigmented lesion *(arrow)* appears in the temporal macula, and a barely visible second phakoma *(arrowhead)* partially obscures a retinal blood vessel near the edge of the photograph, directly below the disc. The lesions of tuberous sclerosis can vary considerably in their opaqueness and visibility.

The most frequent and characteristic ocular manifestation of TS is the retinal phakoma (Fig 28-7). Pathologically, this growth arises from the innermost layer of the retina and is composed of nerve fibers and relatively undifferentiated cells that appear to be of glial origin. The growth is frequently called an *astrocytic hamartoma*. Phakomas are usually found near the posterior pole and involve the retina, the optic disc, or both. They vary in size from approximately half to twice the diameter of the disc. Vision is rarely affected.

Retinal phakomas have 3 distinct appearances. The first is typically found in very young children; the phakomas are relatively flat with a smooth surface, indistinct margins, and a gray-white color that makes them difficult to detect. The second is a sharply demarcated, elevated, yellow-white, calcified lesion with an irregular surface that has been compared to a mulberry. These lesions are more often found in older patients, on or adjacent to the optic disc. The third type is a transitional lesion that combines features of the first 2.

Phakomas are present in 30%–50% of patients with TS. One to several may be found in a single eye, and 40% are bilateral. There is no evidence that the number of lesions increases with age, but individual tumors have been documented to grow over time. Phakomas are not pathognomonic of TS; they occur occasionally in association with neurofibromatosis and in the eyes of unaffected persons. Retinal lesions are more common in individuals with the *TSC2* mutation. Hypopigmented lesions analogous to white spots of the skin are occasionally seen in the iris or choroid.

Management of TS patients by the ophthalmologist includes monitoring of vision and ocular lesions. Difficult-to-control seizures respond to vigabatrin (up to 95% of patients experience significant reduction of seizures). However, patients treated with vigabatrin are at risk for ocular complications, which may be difficult or impossible to monitor in patients with TS.

Aronow ME, Nakagawa JA, Gupta A, Traboulsi EI, Singh AD. Tuberous sclerosis complex: genotype/phenotype correlation of retinal findings. *Ophthalmology.* 2012;119(9): 1917–1923.

Von Hippel–Lindau Disease

Von Hippel–Lindau disease (VHL; retinal angiomatosis, von Hippel–Lindau syndrome) is an autosomal dominant disorder with 95% penetrance that is characterized by the formation of both benign and malignant tumors in multiple organ systems. It is caused by a mutation in the *VHL* gene, a tumor-suppressor gene located on the short arm of chromosome 3, which produces the protein pVHL. A 2-hit model (germline plus somatic mutation similar to that in retinoblastoma) has been suggested for VHL. The incidence of VHL is approximately 1 per 36,000 births. Its most common abnormalities are vascular tumors *(hemangioblastomas)* of the retina and CNS, usually the cerebellum. These tumors have only limited proliferative capacity, but exudation across thin vessel walls leads to fluid accumulations that may attain considerable size and compromise vital structures. Cysts and tumors may also develop in the kidneys *(renal cell carcinoma),* pancreas, liver, epididymis, and adrenal glands *(pheochromocytoma).* Despite its well-accepted classification as a neurocutaneous syndrome, VHL rarely has significant cutaneous manifestations, although café-au-lait spots and port-wine stains *(nevus flammeus)* are seen occasionally. Cognitive impairment is not a feature of this disease. Associated malignant tumors make VHL potentially fatal.

The retinal lesions originally described by von Hippel are capillary hemangioblastomas that usually become visible ophthalmoscopically between ages 10 and 35 years, with an average age of onset of 25 years. Retinal capillary hemangioblastomas are found in up to 85% of patients with the *VHL* mutation. Multiple tumors are present in the same eye in about one-third of cases and bilaterally in as many as one-half of cases. Tumors typically occur in the peripheral fundus, but lesions adjacent to the optic disc have been described.

The hallmark of the mature tumor is a pair of markedly dilated vessels (artery and vein) running between the lesion and the optic disc, indicating significant arteriovenous shunting (Fig 28-8). Characteristic paired or twin retinal vessels of normal caliber may be present before the tumor becomes visible.

Histologically, retinal capillary hemangioblastomas consist of relatively well-formed capillaries; however, fluorescein angiography shows that these vessels are leaky. Transudation of fluid into the subretinal space causes lipid accumulation, retinal detachment, and consequent loss of vision.

Retinal capillary hemangioblastomas can be effectively treated with cryotherapy or laser photocoagulation in two-thirds or more cases, particularly when the lesions are still small. Antiangiogenesis therapy has also shown potential. Early diagnosis increases the likelihood of successful treatment. The ocular lesions of VHL are asymptomatic prior to

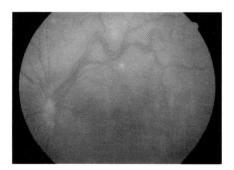
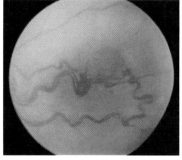

Figure 28-8 Von Hippel–Lindau disease (retinal angiomatosis), left eye.

retinal detachment. Therefore, children at risk for the disease should undergo periodic ophthalmologic evaluation beginning at approximately age 5 years.

Systemically, early tumor diagnosis can significantly reduce morbidity and mortality. The full recommended screening for patients with VHL can be found on the website of the VHL Alliance (www.vhl.org). Molecular genetic testing has been suggested for patients with early-onset (<30 years) cerebellar hemangioblastoma, early-onset retinal capillary hemangioblastomas, or familial clear-cell renal carcinoma.

Maher ER, Neumann HP, Richard S. Von Hippel–Lindau disease: a clinical and scientific review. *Eur J Hum Genet.* 2011;19(6):617–623.

Toy BC, Agrón E, Nigam D, Chew EY, Wong WT. Longitudinal analysis of retinal hemangioblastomatosis and visual function in ocular von Hippel–Lindau disease. *Ophthalmology.* 2012;119(12):2622–2630.

Sturge-Weber Syndrome

Sturge-Weber syndrome (SWS), or *encephalofacial angiomatosis,* consists of a facial cutaneous vascular malformation (port-wine stain) with an ipsilateral leptomeningeal vascular malformation that typically results in the following:

- cerebral calcification
- seizures
- focal neurologic deficits (hemianopia, hemiparesis)
- a highly variable degree of cognitive impairment (with normal intelligence in some affected persons)

SWS is unique among the 4 major neurocutaneous syndromes in that it is not genetically transmitted. However, lesions are always present at birth. The distribution of cutaneous and cerebral involvement suggests a disturbance very early in embryonic development (4–8 weeks' gestation). The incidence is approximately 1 in 50,000.

Calcium deposits that are characteristic of SWS form after birth in brain parenchyma; they usually involve the occipital lobe and varying portions of the parietal, temporal, and occasionally frontal lobes. MRI is less sensitive than computed tomography (CT) for identifying calcification but is preferred for safety reasons and may provide better delineation of other abnormalities (Fig 28-9).

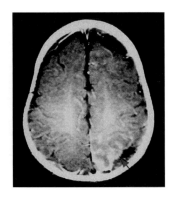

Figure 28-9 Axial gadolinium-enhanced T1-weighted MR image shows vascular malformation with underlying cortical atrophy *(arrow)* in the left occipital lobe of a 4-month-old girl with Sturge-Weber syndrome.

The Sturge-Weber skin lesion, which can be quite disfiguring, consists of numerous dilated, well-formed capillaries in the dermis. The lesion usually involves the forehead and upper eyelid on the same side as the cerebral vascular malformation, with varying extension to the ipsilateral lower eyelid and maxillary and mandibular regions (Fig 28-10). The port-wine stain occasionally does not conform to the distribution of the trigeminal divisions, and the contralateral face, the scalp, and the trunk and extremities may be affected. Hypertrophy of soft tissue and bone underlying the port-wine stain is common, and thickening of the involved skin may develop. Notably, not all children who have a port-wine stain necessarily have SWS.

Ocular involvement

Any portion of the ocular circulation may be anomalous in SWS. When the skin lesion involves the eyelids, increased conjunctival vascularity commonly produces a pinkish discoloration. An abnormal plexus of episcleral vessels is often present.

The retina sometimes shows tortuous vessels and arteriovenous communications. Choroidal hemangioma is the most significant retinal anomaly associated with SWS. The tumor is composed of well-formed choroidal vessels, which give the fundus a uniform deep-red color that has been compared to tomato ketchup (Fig 28-11). Sometimes only the posterior pole is involved; in other cases, the entire fundus is affected. Choroidal hemangiomas are usually asymptomatic in childhood. During adolescence or adulthood, the choroid sometimes becomes markedly thickened. Degeneration or detachment of the overlying retina with severe vision loss may follow. No treatment has been proven to prevent or reverse such deterioration, although scattered application of laser photocoagulation may help.

Glaucoma is the most common and serious ocular complication. It has been reported to occur in up to approximately 70% of patients. Causes of elevated intraocular pressure (IOP)

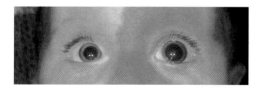

Figure 28-10 Facial port-wine stain involving the left eyelids, associated with ipsilateral buphthalmos in an infant girl with Sturge-Weber syndrome and glaucoma.

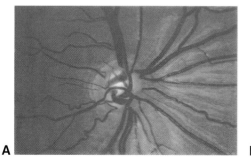
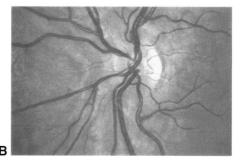

A
B

Figure 28-11 Fundus appearance in an adolescent boy with Sturge-Weber syndrome. **A,** Right eye. Note the glaucomatous disc cupping and deeper red color of surrounding choroid, compared with the healthy fellow eye **(B).**

include elevated episcleral venous pressure, hyperemia of the ciliary body with hypersecretion of aqueous, and developmental anomaly of the anterior chamber angle. Involvement of the upper eyelid skin, choroidal hemangioma, iris heterochromia, and episcleral hemangioma increase the likelihood of glaucoma. Onset of glaucoma can be at birth or later in childhood.

Management

It is essential that patients with SWS undergo a complete ophthalmic evaluation, including measurement of IOP. Sedation or general anesthesia may be necessary for uncooperative children. Patients should be monitored throughout childhood.

SWS glaucoma is difficult to treat. Initial therapy with topical drops can be effective, especially when onset occurs later. Surgery is indicated in early-onset cases and when medical treatment is inadequate. Adequate long-term pressure control can frequently be achieved, although multiple operations are typically necessary. A particular risk of glaucoma surgery in SWS is intraoperative or postoperative exudation or hemorrhage from anomalous choroidal vessels, caused by rapid ocular decompression. The surgeon must exercise special care with implanted drainage devices to prevent excessive early postoperative hypotony. Choroidal or subretinal fluid accumulation after surgery may be dramatic, but spontaneous resorption usually occurs within 1–2 weeks.

Angle surgery (goniotomy and trabeculotomy) has been used successfully in some patients with SWS. Treatment of affected skin with a pulsed-dye laser has been shown to reduce vascularity, considerably improving appearance without causing significant damage to dermal tissue.

> Khaler A, Nischal KK, Espinoza M, Manoj B. Periocular port wine stain: the Great Ormond Street Hospital experience. *Ophthalmology.* 2011;118(11):2274–2278.

Ataxia-Telangiectasia

Ataxia-telangiectasia (AT), or *Louis-Bar syndrome,* is an autosomal recessive disorder that involves primarily the CNS (particularly the cerebellum), the ocular surface, the skin, and the immune system. Though rare (incidence is approximately 1 in 40,000), AT is thought to be the most common cause of progressive ataxia in early childhood. Truncal ataxia is usually noted during the second year of life, with subsequent development of dysarthria, dystonia, and choreoathetosis. Progressive deterioration of motor function leads to serious disability by age 10 years. Intellectual disability may be present along with microcephaly.

Ocular motor abnormalities are found in many patients with AT and are frequently among the earliest manifestations. Characteristically, there is poor initiation of saccades with preservation of vestibulo-ocular movements, similar to congenital ocular motor apraxia. Head thrusts are used to compensate for saccades. Strabismus and nystagmus may also be present.

Telangiectasia of the conjunctiva occurs in 91% of patients and develops between the ages of 3 and 5 years. Involvement is initially interpalpebral but away from the limbus (Fig 28-12); it eventually becomes generalized. Similar vessel changes can appear in the skin of the eyelids and other sun-exposed areas.

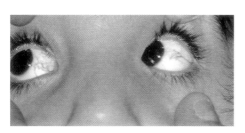
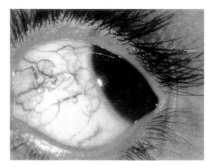

Figure 28-12 Abnormally dilated and tortuous interpalpebral conjunctival vessels in a child with ataxia-telangiectasia, seen only in the interpalpebral fissure.

Individuals with AT show greatly increased sensitivity to the tissue-damaging adverse effects of therapeutic radiation and many chemotherapeutic agents. Defective T-cell function in patients with AT is usually associated with hypoplasia of the thymus and decreased levels of circulating immunoglobulin. Recurrent respiratory tract infections and increased susceptibility to malignancies are frequent causes of mortality.

The causative gene in AT, *ATM* (ataxia-telangiectasia mutated gene), is found on 11q22.3. The protein of ATM is involved in the repair of DNA and the regulation of tumor-suppressor genes. A rapid test from peripheral blood can accurately diagnose AT. AT heterozygosity is present in an estimated 1%–3% of the population. Although gene carriers are generally healthy and cannot be identified except in the context of a known AT pedigree, they are at increased risk for common forms of malignancy and show greater-than-normal sensitivity to radiation.

There is no effective therapy for halting the progression of the ataxia. Several agents (α-lipoic acid, vitamin E, and coenzyme Q_{10}) may slow the deterioration. Neurotoxic chemotherapeutic agents should be avoided, and radiation therapy for malignancy should be reduced to 30% of the usual dosage.

Incontinentia Pigmenti

Incontinentia pigmenti (IP), or *Bloch-Sulzberger syndrome,* involves the skin, brain, and eyes and shows the unusual inheritance pattern of X-linked dominance with a presumed lethal effect on the hemizygous male fetus. Nearly all affected persons are female, with mother-to-daughter transmission in familial cases. IP results from a mutation of the *IKBKG* gene (previously termed the *NEMO* gene) located on band Xq28, which is detected in 80% of affected individuals.

The skin usually appears normal at birth, but erythema and bullae develop during the first few days of life, usually on the extremities, and persist for weeks to months (Fig 28-13A). When healed, the lesions appear as clusters of small hyperpigmented macules in a characteristic "splashed-paint" distribution, most prominently on the trunk (Fig 28-13B).

Approximately one-third of patients with IP have CNS problems that include microcephaly, hydrocephalus, seizures, and varying degrees of cognitive impairment. Missing

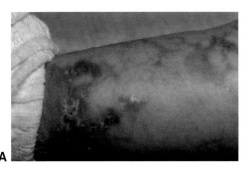 

Figure 28-13 Pigmented skin lesions of incontinentia pigmenti. **A,** Bullous lesions. **B,** Hyperpigmented macules. *(Courtesy of Edward L. Raab, MD.)*

and malformed teeth are found in roughly two-thirds of cases. Less common findings include scoliosis, skull deformities, cleft palate, and dwarfism.

Ocular involvement occurs in 35%–77% of cases and tends to be unilateral or very asymmetric if bilateral, typically in the form of proliferative retinal vasculopathy that closely resembles retinopathy of prematurity. At birth, the only detectable abnormality may be incomplete peripheral retinal vascularization. Abnormal arteriovenous connections, microvascular abnormalities, and neovascular membranes develop at or near the junction of the vascular and avascular retina (Fig 28-14). Rapid progression sometimes leads to total retinal detachment and retrolental membrane formation within the first few months of life. Microphthalmos, cataract, glaucoma, optic atrophy, strabismus, and nystagmus may occur, usually secondary to end-stage retinopathy.

Sequential retinal evaluations for the first 1–2 years of life are necessary to identify eyes that require treatment. The retinopathy of IP has been managed by photocoagulation or cryotherapy with varying degrees of success. Treatment is usually applied primarily to the avascular peripheral retina, similar to the management of retinopathy of prematurity.

O'Doherty M, McCreery K, Green AJ, Tuwir I, Brosnahan D. Incontinentia pigmenti— ophthalmological observation of a series of cases and review of the literature. *Br J Ophthalmol.* 2011;95(1):11–16.

Wyburn-Mason Syndrome

Wyburn-Mason syndrome, also known as *Bonnet-Dechaume-Blanc syndrome* or *racemose angioma,* is a nonhereditary arteriovenous malformation of the eye and brain, especially midbrain, that typically involves the ipsilateral optic disc or retina. Skin lesions are present in approximately half of patients and usually occur on the face. The complete syndrome is considerably less common than an isolated occurrence of similar ocular or intracranial disease. Seizures, mental changes, hemiparesis, and papilledema may result from the brain lesions, which are frequently a source of hemorrhage (unlike the vascular brain lesions of SWS).

Ocular manifestations are unilateral and congenital, and they may progress during childhood. The typical lesion consists of markedly dilated and tortuous vessels that shunt blood directly from arteries to veins. These vessels do not leak fluid (Fig 28-15). Vision

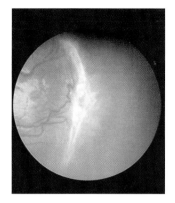

Figure 28-14 Vascular abnormalities of the temporal retina, right eye, in a 2-year-old child with incontinentia pigmenti. Note the avascularity peripheral to the circumferential white vasoproliferative lesion, which showed profuse leakage on fluorescein angioscopy.

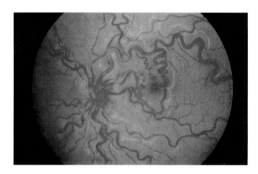

Figure 28-15 Wyburn-Mason syndrome, or racemose angioma of the retina, left eye.

ranges from normal to markedly reduced. Intraocular hemorrhage and secondary neovascular glaucoma are possible complications. More than half of affected eyes are blind, and an additional one-quarter have severe visual impairment. No treatment is indicated for primary lesions. Treatment may be considered for associated complications, such as scatter photocoagulation for ischemic venous occlusive disease, vitrectomy for nonclearing vitreous hemorrhage, and cyclodestructive treatment for neovascular glaucoma.

Klippel-Trénaunay-Weber Syndrome

Klippel-Trénaunay syndrome (KTS) is a neurocutaneous disorder consisting of a vascular nevus involving an extremity, varicosities of that extremity, and hypertrophy of bone and soft tissue. When arteriovenous malformation is also present, the disease is called *Klippel-Trénaunay-Weber syndrome (KTWS)*. Occurrence of KTWS is sporadic, the etiology is unknown, and there is no established incidence. Ophthalmic findings include vascular anomalies of the orbit, iris, retina, choroid, and optic nerve, as well as optic nerve and chiasmal gliomas. KTS is a complex syndrome with no single treatment protocol. Treatment is individualized to the patient. At present, many of the symptoms may be treated, but there is no cure for this syndrome.

Bothun ED, Kao T, Guo Y, Christiansen SP. Bilateral optic nerve drusen and gliomas in Klippel-Trénaunay syndrome. *J AAPOS*. 2011;15(1):77–79.

Intrauterine or Perinatal Infection

Maternally transmitted congenital infections cause ocular damage in 3 ways:

- through direct action of the infecting agent, which damages tissue
- through a teratogenic effect, which causes malformation
- through a delayed reactivation of the agent after birth that damages developed tissue by direct action or inflammation

These infections can cause ongoing tissue damage; long-term evaluation is thus required in order to determine their full impact. Most perinatal disorders have an exceedingly broad spectrum of clinical presentation, ranging from silent disease to life-threatening tissue and organ damage. The common types of congenital infections can be remembered by the acronym TORCH: *toxoplasmosis; rubella; cytomegalovirus;* and *herpes-viruses.* Other infections discussed in this section include syphilis and lymphocytic choriomeningitis virus.

Toxoplasmosis

The etiologic agent of toxoplasmosis, *Toxoplasma gondii,* is an obligate intracellular parasite. Cats are the definitive host, wherein the parasite resides in the intestinal mucosa in the form of an oocyst. Once excreted into the environment, the oocyst can be ingested by many animals, including humans. Humans can also acquire the disease secondarily by ingesting undercooked infected meat or contaminated drinking water. The ingested cyst has a predilection for muscle, including the heart, and neural tissue, including the retina. Encysted organisms can remain dormant indefinitely, or the cyst can rupture, releasing hundreds of thousands of *tachyzoites,* the proliferative phase of the protozoan. The stimulus for local reactivation of an infected cyst is unknown.

Systemic infection in humans is common and usually goes undiagnosed. Symptoms may include fever, lymphadenopathy, and sore throat. The percentage of antibody titer–positive persons in the United States increases with age (<5 years of age, 5%; >80 years of age, 60%).

The incidence of congenital toxoplasmosis ranges from 1 to 10 per 10,000 live births. Toxoplasmosis can be acquired congenitally via transplacental transmission from an infected mother to the fetus. Congenital infection can result in retinitis, hepatosplenomegaly, intracranial calcifications, microcephaly, and developmental delay.

Ocular manifestations besides retinitis include choroiditis, iritis, and anterior uveitis (Fig 28-16). The active area of retinal inflammation is usually thickened and cream colored with an overlying vitritis, frequently in the macular area. This area may be at the edge of an old, flat, atrophic scar (a so-called satellite lesion). Previously, apparently acquired *Toxoplasma* retinitis was thought to represent reactivation of a congenital infection; however, recent evidence suggests that most of these patients are infected postnatally.

The diagnosis of toxoplasmosis is primarily clinical and is based on the characteristic retinal lesions. It can be supported by a positive enzyme-linked immunosorbent assay (ELISA) for *Toxoplasma gondii* antibody. Lack of antibody essentially rules out

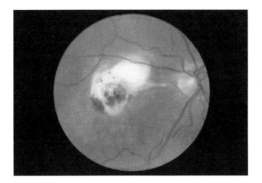

Figure 28-16 Toxoplasmosis chorioretinitis, right eye.

the diagnosis. Because maternal immunoglobulin M (IgM) does not cross the placenta, the presence of *Toxoplasma*-specific IgM in the infant serum is diagnostic of congenital infection.

Ocular inflammation from reactivated toxoplasmosis does not require treatment unless it threatens vision. Vision can be compromised by the location of the reactivation adjacent to the macula or optic nerve or by significant vitritis. Systemic treatment involves the use of 1 or more antimicrobial drugs with or without oral corticosteroids. The most commonly used antimicrobial agents are pyrimethamine and sulfadiazine. Steroids should never be used without antimicrobial coverage. Intravitreal injection of clindamycin and dexamethasone has been reported as a possible alternative treatment.

In the setting of congenital *Toxoplasma* infection, prenatal treatment and treatment during the infant's first year of life appear to decrease the risk of poor visual outcomes. In congenitally infected children, new lesions may occur in the second decade of life; serial monitoring of these patients is thus necessary. For additional details on drug therapy for toxoplasmosis, see BCSC Section 9, *Intraocular Inflammation and Uveitis*.

Soheilian M, Ramezani A, Azimzadeh A, et al. Randomized trial of intravitreal clindamycin and dexamethasone versus pyrimethamine, sulfadiazine, and prednisone in treatment of ocular toxoplasmosis. *Ophthalmology.* 2011;118(1):134–141.

Rubella

Congenital rubella (German measles) syndrome is a well-defined combination of ocular, otologic, and cardiac abnormalities, accompanied by microcephaly and variable developmental delay. Described in 1941 by the ophthalmologist Sir Norman Gregg, the rubella virus was the first virus recognized as a teratogenic agent. The syndrome is caused by transplacental transmission of the rubella virus from an infected mother to the fetus. The incidence has decreased markedly in North America since widespread vaccination of children was instituted in the late 1960s, although rubella remains a cause of infant morbidity and mortality in less-developed countries.

Ocular abnormalities found in congenital rubella syndrome include a peculiar nuclear cataract that is sometimes floating in a liquefied lens cortex, glaucoma, microphthalmos, and retinal abnormalities that vary from a subtle salt-and-pepper retinopathy (most common finding; Fig 28-17) to pseudoretinitis pigmentosa. Diagnosis is based on this

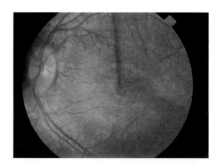

Figure 28-17 Fundus photograph of a 6-year-old patient with rubella syndrome (electroretinogram results normal).

characteristic clinical picture and is supported by serologic testing. The virus itself can be isolated from pharyngeal swabs and from the lens contents at the time of cataract surgery.

Lensectomy is usually required for cataracts. Infected eyes are prone to postoperative inflammation and subsequent secondary membrane formation. Topical steroids and mydriatics should be used aggressively. In adults, rubella virus infection has been identified as a probable cause of Fuchs heterochromic iridocyclitis.

Cytomegalovirus

Cytomegalovirus (CMV), a member of the herpesvirus family, is a ubiquitous virus that can cause a wide range of infection, from asymptomatic acquired infection in immunocompetent individuals to severe infections in newborn infants and immunocompromised patients. Over 80% of adults in developed countries have antibodies to the virus.

Congenital infection with CMV is the most common congenital infection in humans; it occurs in approximately 1% of infants. Clinically apparent disease is present in 10%–15% of infected neonates, and 20%–30% of these cases are fatal. Transmission to the fetus or newborn can occur transplacentally, from contact with an infected birth canal during delivery, or from ingestion of infected breast milk or maternal secretions. Congenital CMV disease is characterized by fever, jaundice, hematologic abnormalities, deafness, microcephaly, and periventricular calcifications.

Ophthalmic manifestations of congenital CMV infection occur primarily in infants with systemic symptoms and include retinochoroiditis (Fig 28-18), optic nerve anomalies, microphthalmos, cataract, and uveitis. The retinochoroiditis usually presents with bilateral focal involvement consisting of areas of RPE atrophy and whitish opacities mixed with retinal hemorrhages. The retinitis can be progressive, or it may present as a quiescent CMV chorioretinal scar that is difficult to differentiate from the scar seen in toxoplasmosis. CMV retinitis can be acquired in children who are immunocompromised (most frequently by infection with HIV/AIDS or following organ transplantation or chemotherapy). The retinitis is a diffuse retinal necrosis with areas of retinal thickening and whitening, hemorrhages, and venous sheathing. Vitritis may also be present.

Diagnosis is based on the clinical presentation in acquired disease and is supplemented by serologic testing for antibodies to CMV in congenital infection. In infected infants, the virus can be recovered from bodily secretions.

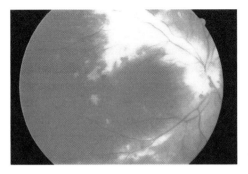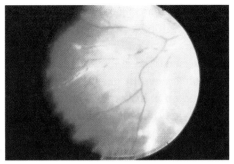

Figure 28-18 Active cytomegalovirus retinochoroiditis in a premature infant, right eye.

Infants with severe systemic or sight-threatening disease are usually treated with ganciclovir. Medications that are available for treatment of older immunocompromised children include ganciclovir, valganciclovir, foscarnet, cidofovir, and fomivirsen. The use of intraocular ganciclovir implants has not been extensively studied in children.

Herpes Simplex Virus

Herpes simplex virus (HSV) is a member of the herpesvirus family, which includes 2 types of simplex virus (HSV-1 and HSV-2), herpes zoster, Epstein-Barr virus, and CMV. Neonatal HSV infection occurs in 1 in 3000 to 20,000 births and is usually secondary to HSV-2. HSV-1 typically affects the eyes, skin, and mouth region and is transmitted by close personal contact. HSV-2 is typically associated with genital infection through venereal transmission.

Congenital HSV infection is usually acquired during passage through an infected birth canal. The neonatal infection is confined to the CNS, skin, oral cavity, and eyes in one-third of cases. It commonly manifests with vesicular skin lesions, ulcerative mouth sores, and keratoconjunctivitis. Disseminated disease occurs in two-thirds of cases and can involve the liver, adrenal glands, and lungs. Eye involvement in congenital infection can include conjunctivitis, keratitis, retinochoroiditis, and cataracts. Keratitis can be epithelial or stromal. Retinal involvement can be severe and may include massive exudates and retinal necrosis. Affected infants are treated with systemic acyclovir. The mortality rate from disseminated disease is significant, and survivors usually have permanent ocular and CNS impairment.

Marquez L, Levy ML, Munoz FM, Palazzi DL. A report of three cases and review of intrauterine herpes simplex virus infection. *Pediatr Infect Dis J.* 2011;30(2):153–157.

Syphilis

Syphilis is caused by the spirochete *Treponema pallidum,* and sexual contact is the usual route of transmission. Fetal infection occurs following maternal spirochetemia. The longer the mother has had syphilis, the lower is the risk of transmitting the disease to her child. If a mother has contracted primary or secondary disease, approximately half of her offspring will be infected. In cases of untreated late maternal syphilis, approximately

70% of infants are healthy. The incidence of congenital syphilis in the United States is 8.5 cases per 100,000 live births.

Signs and symptoms of congenital syphilis include unexplained premature birth, large placenta, persistent rhinitis, intractable rash, unexplained jaundice, hepatosplenomegaly, pneumonia, anemia, generalized lymphadenopathy, and metaphyseal abnormalities or periostitis on radiographs. Congenitally acquired infection can lead to neonatal death. Early eye involvement in congenital syphilis is rare.

In some infants, chorioretinitis appears as a salt-and-pepper granularity of the fundus. Pseudoretinitis pigmentosa may follow. In rare cases, anterior uveitis, glaucoma, or both may develop. In other cases, symptoms may not appear until late childhood or adolescence. Widely spaced, peg-shaped teeth; eighth nerve deafness; and interstitial keratitis constitute the *Hutchinson triad*. Other manifestations include saddle nose, short maxilla, and linear scars around body orifices. Bilateral interstitial keratitis, the classic ophthalmic finding in older children and adults, occurs in approximately 10% of patients.

A diagnosis of congenital syphilis is confirmed by identification of *T pallidum* by dark-field microscopy or fluorescent antibody. The detection of specific IgM is currently the most sensitive serological method.

Congenital syphilis in neonates is treated with intravenous aqueous crystalline penicillin G. Serologic tests are repeated at 2 to 4, 6, and 12 months after the conclusion of treatment, or until results become nonreactive or the titer has decreased fourfold. Persistent positive titers or a positive cerebrospinal fluid VDRL test result at 6 months should prompt retreatment.

Centers for Disease Control and Prevention. Sexually transmitted diseases surveillance, 2011: syphilis. Available from www.cdc.gov/std/stats11/tables/1.htm. Accessed February 19, 2014.

Lymphocytic Choriomeningitis

Lymphocytic choriomeningitis virus (LCMV) is an arenavirus that is transmitted by exposure to infected rodents (including house and lab mice and pet hamsters). Infants with congenital LCMV infection present with CNS abnormalities, including hydrocephaly, microcephaly, intracranial calcifications, and cognitive impairment. Chorioretinal scars, which may involve the entire macula, may occur without neurologic abnormalities. The appearance of these scars is similar to that of scars seen in patients with toxoplasmosis, CMV, and Aicardi syndrome. The diagnosis of LCMV infection should be considered in infants with chorioretinal scars when results of tests for these more common etiologies are negative. Elevated LCMV antibody titers establish the diagnosis. No specific treatment is available apart from exposure prevention.

Malignant Disease

Leukemia

Leukemia in childhood is acute in 95% of cases and is more often lymphocytic than myelocytic. Acute lymphoblastic leukemia is the most common malignant disease of childhood and is responsible for 30% of all cancer cases; there are 4000 new cases per year in the United States. Although the most common ocular manifestation of leukemia is leukemic retinopathy, all ocular structures can be affected. Ocular involvement is highly correlated with CNS involvement.

Leukemic infiltrates in the anterior segment may lead to heterochromia iridis, a change in the architecture of the iris, frank iris infiltrates, spontaneous hyphemas, leukemic cells in the anterior chamber, and pseudohypopyon. Keratic precipitates may be seen, and some affected eyes develop glaucoma from tumor cells clogging the trabecular meshwork. Anterior chamber paracentesis for cytologic studies may be diagnostic in cases involving the anterior segment. Systemic chemotherapy, local radiation therapy, and topical steroids may be effective for anterior segment complications. Leukemic involvement of the iris may be confused with juvenile xanthogranuloma.

The most common ocular findings are retinal hemorrhages, especially flame-shaped lesions in the nerve fiber layer. They involve the posterior fundus and correlate with other aspects of the disease, such as anemia, thrombocytopenia, and coagulation abnormalities. The hemorrhages may have white centers. Retinal hemorrhages in leukemia can resemble those associated with abusive head trauma (see Chapter 27), and they have been reported as the first manifestation of leukemia. Other forms of retinal involvement include localized perivascular infiltrations, microinfarction, and discrete tumor infiltrations. Histologically, the choroid is the most frequently affected ocular tissue, but choroidal involvement is usually not apparent clinically.

Optic nerve involvement occurs if the disc has been infiltrated by leukemic cells (Fig 28-19), which may cause loss of central vision. Translucent swelling of the disc obscures the normal landmarks; with florid involvement, only a white mass is visible in the region of the disc. The presence of disc edema and loss of central vision in a child with leukemia should be considered a medical emergency because permanent loss of central vision is imminent. Such patients should undergo radiation therapy as soon as possible.

Neuroblastoma

Neuroblastoma is one of the most common childhood cancers and is the most frequent source of childhood orbital metastasis (89% of cases). It usually originates in either the adrenal gland or the sympathetic ganglion chain in the retroperitoneum or mediastinum.

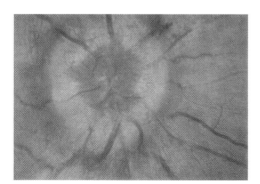

Figure 28-19 Leukemic infiltration of optic nerve.

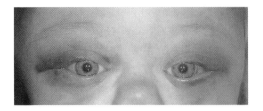

Figure 28-20 Bilateral orbital metastasis from neuroblastoma in a 2-year-old girl, presenting with periorbital ecchymosis.

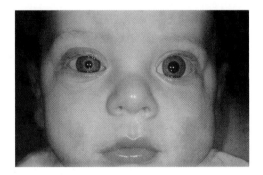

Figure 28-21 Right Horner syndrome, the presenting sign of localized intrathoracic neuroblastoma in a 6-month-old boy.

Approximately 20% of all patients with neuroblastoma show clinical evidence of orbital involvement, which is sometimes the initial manifestation of the tumor.

The mean age at diagnosis of patients with metastatic orbital neuroblastoma is approximately 2 years; 90% are diagnosed by 5 years of age. Unilateral or bilateral proptosis and eyelid ecchymosis are the classic presentations (Fig 28-20). Systemic signs and symptoms may include abdominal fullness and pain, venous obstruction and edema, hypertension caused by renal vascular compromise, and bone pain. Urinalysis for catecholamines is positive in 90%–95% of cases.

Opsoclonus, characterized by rapid, multidirectional saccadic eye movements, is a paraneoplastic syndrome that is associated with neuroblastoma and is not related to orbital involvement. It is associated with a good prognosis for survival, although neurologic deficits may persist. Horner syndrome can occur from a primary cervical or apical thoracic neuroblastoma that involves the sympathetic chain (Fig 28-21). Horner syndrome does not occur from metastatic neuroblastoma.

Treatment modalities include surgery, chemotherapy, and radiation therapy. Neuroblastoma that presents in a child younger than 1 year has a more favorable prognosis than that in older children. Approximately 10% of neuroblastomas undergo spontaneous regression.

Basic Texts

Pediatric Ophthalmology and Strabismus

Brodsky MC. *Pediatric Neuro-Ophthalmology.* 2nd ed. New York: Springer-Verlag; 2010.

Buckley EG, Freedman S, Shields MB. *Atlas of Ophthalmic Surgery, Vol III: Strabismus and Glaucoma.* St Louis: Mosby-Year Book; 1995.

Cibis GW, Tongue AC, Stass-Isern ML. *Decision Making in Pediatric Ophthalmology.* St Louis: Mosby-Year Book; 1993.

Coats DK, Olitsky SE. *Strabismus Surgery and Its Complications.* New York: Springer-Verlag; 2007.

Del Monte MA, Archer SM. *Atlas of Pediatric Ophthalmology and Strabismus Surgery.* New York: Churchill Livingstone; 1993.

Helveston EM. *Surgical Management of Strabismus: An Atlas of Strabismus Surgery.* 4th ed. St Louis: Mosby-Year Book; 1993.

Helveston EM, Ellis FD. *Pediatric Ophthalmology Practice.* 2nd ed. St Louis: Mosby; 1984.

Hoyt CS, Taylor D. *Pediatric Ophthalmology and Strabismus: Expert Consult—Online and Print.* 4th ed. Elsevier/Saunders; 2012.

Isenberg SJ, ed. *The Eye in Infancy.* 2nd ed. St Louis: Mosby-Year Book; 1994.

Jones KL, Jones MD, del Campo M. *Smith's Recognizable Patterns of Human Malformation.* 7th ed. Philadelphia: Elsevier/Saunders; 2013.

Leigh RJ, Zee DS. *The Neurology of Eye Movements.* 4th ed. New York: Oxford; 2006.

Mein J, Harcourt B. *Diagnosis and Management of Ocular Motility Disorders.* Oxford: Blackwell Scientific Publications; 1986.

Miller NR, Newman NJ, Biousse V, Kerrison JB, eds. *Walsh and Hoyt's Clinical Neuro-Ophthalmology.* 6th ed. Philadelphia: Lippincott Williams & Wilkins; 2005.

Nelson LB, Olitsky SE, eds. *Harley's Pediatric Ophthalmology.* 6th ed. Philadelphia: Lippincott Williams & Wilkins; 2014.

Parks MM. *Atlas of Strabismus Surgery.* Philadelphia: Harper & Row; 1983.

Parks MM. *Ocular Motility and Strabismus.* Hagerstown: Harper & Row; 1975.

Pratt-Johnson JA, Tillson G. *Management of Strabismus and Amblyopia: A Practical Guide.* 2nd ed. New York: Thieme; 2001.

Renie WA, ed. *Goldberg's Genetic and Metabolic Eye Disease.* 2nd ed. Boston: Little, Brown & Co; 1986.

Rosenbaum AL, Santiago AP, eds. *Clinical Strabismus Management: Principles and Surgical Techniques.* Philadelphia: Saunders; 1999.

Scott WE, D'Agostino DD, Lennarson LW, eds. *Orthoptics and Ocular Examination Techniques.* Baltimore: Williams & Wilkins; 1983.

Spencer WH, ed. *Ophthalmic Pathology: An Atlas and Textbook.* 4th ed. Philadelphia: Saunders; 1996.

Srodulski K, Katowitz JA, Linton A. *Pediatric Oculoplastic Surgery.* New York: Springer; 2011.

Tasman W, Jaeger EA, eds. *Duane's Ophthalmology on DVD-ROM.* Philadelphia: Lippincott Williams & Wilkins; 2013.

Traboulsi EI. *A Compendium of Inherited Disorders and the Eye.* New York: Oxford University Press; 2006.

von Noorden GK. *Atlas of Strabismus.* 4th ed. St Louis: Mosby; 1983.

von Noorden GK, Campos EC. *Binocular Vision and Ocular Motility: Theory and Management of Strabismus.* 6th ed. St Louis: Mosby; 2002.

von Noorden GK, Helveston EM. *Strabismus: A Decision Making Approach.* St Louis: Mosby; 1994.

Wilson ME, Saunders RA, Trivedi RH, eds. *Pediatric Ophthalmology.* Berlin: Springer; 2009.

Wright KW, ed. *Color Atlas of Strabismus Surgery: Strategies and Techniques.* 3rd ed. New York: Springer; 2007.

Wright KW, Strube YN, eds. *Pediatric Ophthalmology and Strabismus.* 3rd ed. New York: Oxford University Press; 2012.

Related Academy Materials

The Academy is dedicated to providing a wealth of high-quality clinical education resources for ophthalmologists.

Print Publications and Electronic Products

For a complete listing of Academy products related to topics covered in this BCSC Section, visit our online store at http://store.aao.org/clinical-education/topic/pediatric-ophth-strabismus.html. Or call Customer Service at 866-561-8558 (toll free, US only) or +1 415-561-8540, Monday through Friday, between 8:00 AM and 5:00 PM (PST).

Online Resources

Visit the Ophthalmic News and Education (ONE®) Network at www.aao.org/one to find relevant videos, online courses, journal articles, practice guidelines, self-assessment quizzes, images, and more. The ONE Network is a frcc Academy-member benefit.

Access free, trusted articles and content with the Academy's collaborative online encyclopedia, EyeWiki, at www.aao.org/eyewiki.

Requesting Continuing Medical Education Credit

The American Academy of Ophthalmology is accredited by the Accreditation Council for Continuing Medical Education to provide continuing medical education for physicians.

The American Academy of Ophthalmology designates this enduring material for a maximum of 15 *AMA PRA Category 1 Credits™*. Physicians should claim only the credit commensurate with the extent of their participation in the activity.

The American Medical Association requires that all learners participating in activities involving enduring materials complete a formal assessment before claiming continuing medical education (CME) credit. To assess your achievement in this activity and ensure that a specified level of knowledge has been reached, a posttest for this Section of the Basic and Clinical Science Course is provided online. A minimum score of 80% must be obtained to pass the test and claim CME credit.

To take the posttest and request CME credit online:

1. Go to www.aao.org/cme and log in.
2. Click on "Claim CME Credit and View My CME Transcript" and then "Report AAO Credits."
3. Select the appropriate Academy activity. You will be directed to the posttest.
4. Once you have passed the test with a score of 80% or higher, you will be directed to your transcript. *If you are not an Academy member, you will be able to print out a certificate of participation once you have passed the test.*

CME expiration date: June 1, 2017. *AMA PRA Category 1 Credits™* may be claimed only once between June 1, 2014, and the expiration date.

For assistance, contact the Academy's Customer Service department at 866-561-8558 (US only) or +1 415-561-8540 between 8:00 AM and 5:00 PM (PST), Monday through Friday, or send an e-mail to customer_service@aao.org.

Study Questions

Please note that these questions are *not* part of your CME reporting process. They are provided here for your own educational use and identification of any professional practice gaps. The required CME posttest is available online (see "Requesting CME Credit"). Following the questions are a blank answer sheet and answers with discussions. Although a concerted effort has been made to avoid ambiguity and redundancy in these questions, the authors recognize that differences of opinion may occur regarding the "best" answer. The discussions are provided to demonstrate the rationale used to derive the answer. They may also be helpful in confirming that your approach to the problem was correct or, if necessary, in fixing the principle in your memory. The Section 6 faculty thanks the Self-Assessment Committee for reviewing these self-assessment questions.

1. A pediatrician performs the red reflex examination (Brückner test) on a 3-month-old infant. What does this test assess?

    a. accommodation

    b. visual acuity

    c. optic nerve function

    d. ocular alignment

2. In visual acuity testing, what clinical finding is described by the crowding phenomenon?

    a. increase in performance when the patient's family leaves the examination room

    b. increase in performance when reading a single optotype compared to a full line

    c. decrease in performance after repeated testing

    d. decrease in performance when Teller acuity cards are held too close to the patient

3. What is the name of the alignment measurement when the paretic or restricted eye is fixating?

    a. primary deviation

    b. secondary deviation

    c. consecutive deviation

    d. comitant deviation

4. What anatomical feature of the inferior oblique muscle differs from that of the other extraocular muscles?

    a. Its origin is on the medial side on the orbit.

    b. It is innervated by the inferior division of cranial nerve III.

    c. It passes through the trochlea before inserting on the globe.

    d. Its primary action is elevation.

5. What is one of the primary components of the extraocular muscle pulleys?

   a. elastin

   b. striated muscle

   c. hyaluronic acid

   d. chondroitin sulfate

6. Which form of bilateral, symmetric refractive error at a level of 3.5 diopters would place a child at the greatest risk for isoametropic amblyopia?

   a. myopia

   b. hyperopia

   c. astigmatism

   d. no risk of isoametropic amblyopia

7. Which type of amblyopia is most likely to respond to treatment in a teenager who has had no previous amblyopia therapy?

   a. strabismic amblyopia

   b. deprivation amblyopia

   c. anisometropic amblyopia

   d. reverse amblyopia

8. What are the primary synergistic (yoke) muscles that are used for gazing up and to the right?

   a. left inferior oblique and right superior oblique

   b. left superior rectus and right inferior oblique

   c. left inferior oblique and right superior rectus

   d. left superior oblique and right superior rectus

9. What is the term for the positions of gaze in which a single extraocular muscle is the prime mover of each eye?

   a. secondary positions

   b. midline positions

   c. diagnostic positions

   d. cardinal positions

10. What sensory adaptation to manifest strabismus is most commonly seen in patients?

    a. visual confusion

    b. diplopia

    c. stereopsis

    d. peripheral suppression

11. What is the best test for measuring the amount of strabismus in a patient who has an amblyopic eye with visual acuity of 20/400 and eccentric fixation?

    a. simultaneous prism cover test

    b. alternate cover test

    c. Krimsky test

    d. Lancaster red-green test

12. What treatment is most appropriate as initial therapy for high accommodative convergence/accommodation (AC/A) esotropia?

    a. overminused spectacles

    b. alternate occlusion

    c. bifocal spectacles

    d. base-in prism spectacles

13. What eye motility abnormality is commonly associated with infantile esotropia?

    a. manifest vertical nystagmus

    b. dissociated vertical deviation (DVD)

    c. symmetric smooth pursuit in horizontal gaze

    d. ocular flutter

14. What type of exodeviation is most commonly seen in the general population?

    a. pseudoexotropia

    b. infantile exotropia

    c. type 2 Duane retraction syndrome

    d. intermittent exotropia

15. For which type of exodeviation are orthoptic exercises the most appropriate initial therapy?

    a. Duane retraction syndrome

    b. convergence insufficiency

    c. dissociated horizontal deviation

    d. positive angle kappa

16. A patient is found to have A-pattern exotropia with a compensatory head posture. What head posture is the clinician most likely to observe?

    a. chin up

    b. chin down

    c. right head tilt

    d. right head turn

17. What clinical finding accompanies the upward movement of the eye in DVD?
    a. extorsion of the globe
    b. downward movement of the fellow eye on cover testing
    c. upbeat nystagmus
    d. esotropia

18. What clinical finding is most suggestive of a bilateral rather than a unilateral superior oblique muscle palsy?
    a. extorsion of 5° in downgaze
    b. exotropia worse in downgaze
    c. large V pattern
    d. chin-up head posture

19. What finding on examination of an esotropic patient makes the diagnosis of type 1 Duane retraction syndrome more likely than the diagnosis of sixth nerve palsy?
    a. limited adduction of the affected eye
    b. incomitant esodeviation
    c. abnormal head position
    d. limited abduction of the affected eye

20. What clinical finding is most helpful in distinguishing congenital motor nystagmus (infantile nystagmus syndrome) from acquired nystagmus?
    a. abnormal head position
    b. oscillopsia
    c. exponential decrease in velocity of the slow phase
    d. change in direction of the fast phase depending on which eye is fixating

21. Four weeks after bilateral medial rectus muscle recession, a patient presents with a new exotropia of 15 prism diopters. On examination, there is limited adduction of the right eye. What is the most likely diagnosis?
    a. anterior segment ischemia
    b. adherence syndrome
    c. conjunctival scarring
    d. slipped muscle

22. What beneficial effect on the visual field can occur as a result of strabismus surgery?
    a. expansion of the binocular visual field following surgery for exotropia
    b. constriction of an overly wide peripheral field following surgery for exotropia
    c. expansion of the binocular visual field following surgery for esotropia
    d. elimination of monofixation syndrome due to overlapping fields following surgery for infantile esotropia

23. What refractive condition is true for most infants during the first year of life?
    a. relatively flat cornea that steepens over time
    b. hyperopic refractive error that decreases over time
    c. intraocular lens power that increases over time
    d. visual acuity of 20/30, measured by preferential looking (PL), that decreases over time

24. What eye movement abnormality can occur in healthy infants in the first months of life?
    a. intermittent esotropia
    b. constant exotropia
    c. vertical nystagmus
    d. ocular flutter

25. What congenital ocular disorder is most commonly associated with paradoxical pupils?
    a. aniridia
    b. anterior segment dysgenesis
    c. retinal dystrophy
    d. cerebral visual impairment

26. At what age should an infant be able to maintain fixation and react with facial expressions?
    a. at birth
    b. 2–3 weeks
    c. 6–8 weeks
    d. 3 months

27. An 11-month-old girl presents for evaluation and is found to have epiblepharon. The child is playful and asymptomatic, and there is no evidence of corneal involvement. What would be the best initial treatment for this child's condition?
    a. observation
    b. artificial tear eyedrops every 4 hours
    c. surgery to remove a strip of skin and orbicularis muscle from beneath the eyelid margin
    d. Quickert suture repair

28. Which of the following conditions of the affected eye may be associated with pseudoptosis?
    a. hypotropia
    b. DVD
    c. Duane retraction syndrome
    d. infantile esotropia

29. What congenital eyelid malformation would most likely require early repair?

    a. dystopia canthorum

    b. eyelid coloboma

    c. euryblepharon

    d. telecanthus

30. A 2-month-old infant has an enlarging hemangioma of an upper eyelid and orbit, with anisometropic astigmatism and secondary blepharoptosis. What is the preferred primary treatment for this patient?

    a. topical timolol

    b. intralesional corticosteroid injection

    c. oral corticosteroid

    d. oral propranolol

31. Orbital cellulitis can be distinguished from preseptal cellulitis by what clinical finding?

    a. prominent eyelid swelling

    b. presence of sinusitis

    c. chemosis

    d. fever

32. What is the most common location of blockage in congenital nasolacrimal obstruction?

    a. upper canaliculus

    b. valve of Hasner

    c. lower punctum

    d. valve of Rosenmüller

33. Curvilinear tears in Descemet membrane are most often seen in what ocular condition?

    a. congenital hereditary endothelial dystrophy (CHED)

    b. Peters anomaly

    c. primary congenital glaucoma

    d. amniocentesis injury

34. Congenital iris ectropion is most commonly seen in what genetic disorder?

    a. incontinentia pigmenti

    b. neurofibromatosis 1

    c. Marfan syndrome

    d. cystinosis

35. What is the most important associated medical condition to exclude in a patient with sporadic aniridia?

 a. neuroblastoma

 b. neurofibromatosis

 c. Waardenburg syndrome

 d. Wilms tumor

36. Which systemic medication is the most appropriate treatment for an infant with ophthalmia neonatorum secondary to *Chlamydia trachomatis* infection?

 a. erythromycin

 b. doxycycline

 c. ofloxacin

 d. azithromycin

37. What is the most severe ocular complication of Stevens-Johnson syndrome?

 a. conjunctival scarring

 b. panuveitis

 c. acute retinal necrosis

 d. corneal ulcer

38. What finding predisposes a child to glaucoma following surgery for congenital cataract?

 a. small corneal diameter

 b. optic nerve hypoplasia

 c. persistent pupillary membrane

 d. posterior subcapsular lens opacity

39. What is the pattern of genetic inheritance in the majority of patients with primary congenital glaucoma?

 a. autosomal dominant

 b. sporadic

 c. X-linked recessive

 d. autosomal recessive

40. In what genetic disorder is pupillary block glaucoma most likely to occur?

 a. ectopia lentis et pupillae

 b. Marfan syndrome

 c. aniridia

 d. Weill-Marchesani syndrome

41. What type of uveitis is most common in children?

    a. panuveitis

    b. posterior uveitis

    c. intermediate uveitis

    d. anterior uveitis

42. What is the most significant risk factor for developing retinopathy of prematurity (ROP)?

    a. male sex

    b. gestational age

    c. white race

    d. lung disease

43. Why are magnetic resonance imaging (MRI) and ultrasonography the preferred imaging modalities instead of a computed tomography (CT) scan in a pediatric patient with presumed retinoblastoma?

    a. MRI and ultrasonography are better at detecting calcium in the tumor.

    b. CT scan subjects the child to radiation.

    c. MRI and ultrasonography are better at showing bony abnormalities in the orbit.

    d. MRI and ultrasonography are easier to obtain in a child.

44. Moyamoya disease is associated with what ophthalmic disorder?

    a. CHARGE syndrome

    b. morning glory disc anomaly

    c. myelinated retinal nerve fibers

    d. optic nerve hypoplasia

45. A patient is diagnosed with pseudopapilledema. What other ophthalmic finding is frequently seen on examination?

    a. hyperopia

    b. myopia

    c. esotropia

    d. exotropia

46. A 5-mm traumatic hyphema, right eye, is diagnosed in a 12-year-old African American patient. Intraocular pressure is 22 mm Hg OD and 12 mm Hg OS. What laboratory test is indicated?

    a. human leukocyte antigen B27 (HLA-B27)

    b. antinuclear antibody (ANA) titer

    c. sickle cell

    d. β-thalassemia

47. What is the best management of a "white-eyed" blowout fracture in a child?

    a. observation since this injury resolves without treatment

    b. observation for 1 month, then surgical repair of the fracture if the injury does not resolve

    c. observation for 6 months, then strabismus surgery if the child still has diplopia

    d. early surgical repair of the fracture

48. What is the most common cause of visual impairment in children with abusive head trauma?

    a. cortical or cerebral visual impairment

    b. optic atrophy

    c. retinal detachment

    d. vitreous hemorrhage

49. What is the mode of inheritance of incontinentia pigmenti?

    a. autosomal dominant

    b. X-linked recessive

    c. X-linked dominant

    d. mitochondrial DNA defect

50. What is the most common mode of inheritance of neurofibromatosis 1 (NF1)?

    a. autosomal recessive

    b. X-linked recessive

    c. mitochondrial

    d. autosomal dominant

Answer Sheet for Section 6
Study Questions

Question	Answer	Question	Answer
1	a b c d	26	a b c d
2	a b c d	27	a b c d
3	a b c d	28	a b c d
4	a b c d	29	a b c d
5	a b c d	30	a b c d
6	a b c d	31	a b c d
7	a b c d	32	a b c d
8	a b c d	33	a b c d
9	a b c d	34	a b c d
10	a b c d	35	a b c d
11	a b c d	36	a b c d
12	a b c d	37	a b c d
13	a b c d	38	a b c d
14	a b c d	39	a b c d
15	a b c d	40	a b c d
16	a b c d	41	a b c d
17	a b c d	42	a b c d
18	a b c d	43	a b c d
19	a b c d	44	a b c d
20	a b c d	45	a b c d
21	a b c d	46	a b c d
22	a b c d	47	a b c d
23	a b c d	48	a b c d
24	a b c d	49	a b c d
25	a b c d	50	a b c d

Answers

1. **d.** The red reflex examination (Brückner test) evaluates the clarity and symmetry of the red reflex, identifies significant or asymmetric refractive errors, and determines the position of the corneal light reflex, which provides an estimate of ocular misalignment.

2. **b.** The crowding phenomenon is a characteristic feature of amblyopia in which letters or symbols of a given size are more difficult to recognize if they are closely surrounded by similar forms. As a result, the measured "linear" acuity of an amblyopic eye may be worse than visual acuity measured with isolated optotypes. For this reason, for the detection of amblyopia, it is best that isolated letters or pictures not be used to test visual acuity, if possible.

3. **b.** A secondary deviation is the deviation measured when the paretic or restricted eye is fixating. It is larger than a primary deviation, which is the deviation measured when the nonparetic eye is fixating. A consecutive deviation is a strabismus that is in the direction opposite to one that the patient had originally. A comitant deviation is a strabismus that is the same size in all positions of gaze.

4. **a.** The inferior oblique muscle is the only extraocular muscle whose origin is on the medial orbital wall. The inferior division of the third cranial nerve innervates the medial rectus, inferior rectus, and inferior oblique muscles. The superior oblique muscle is the only extraocular muscle that passes through the trochlea. The primary action of the inferior oblique muscle is extorsion. The primary action of the superior rectus muscle is elevation.

5. **a.** Elastin is one component of the pulley; the others are smooth muscle and collagen. Striated muscle, hyaluronic acid, and chondroitin sulfate are not known constituents of the pulleys.

6. **c.** Significant levels of astigmatism can lead to isoametropic amblyopia. Children with moderate degrees of myopia see clearly at near and are not at risk for bilateral amblyopia. Children with moderate levels of hyperopia are capable of accommodating to provide clear vision at distance and at near.

7. **c.** Some cases of anisometropic amblyopia remain responsive to treatment (optical correction, occlusion therapy, pharmacologic penalization) in the teenaged years.

8. **c.** The left inferior oblique and right superior rectus muscles are the prime agonists for gaze into that position. Options *a* and *d* are not correct, because the superior oblique muscle is a depressor of the eye. Option *b* is not correct, as the right inferior oblique muscle has its main elevation action in left gaze.

9. **d.** By having the patient move the eyes to the 6 cardinal positions, the clinician can isolate and evaluate the ability of each of the 6 extraocular muscles to move each eye.

10. **d.** Peripheral suppression is the sensory adaptation that can develop in strabismic patients to eliminate diplopia. Visual confusion and diplopia are the normal consequences of strabismus when there are no sensory adaptations to prevent them. Although some degree of stereopsis may be present in small-angle strabismus with monofixation syndrome, good stereopsis indicates that there is no manifest strabismus and no suppression.

11. **c.** The Krimsky test does not rely on a sensory or motor response from the patient. Motor test results will not be accurate if there is eccentric fixation. The Lancaster test depends on

the patient's subjective localization of the targets, which may not be accurate in the presence of poor vision or anomalous retinal correspondence.

12. **c.** Bifocals reduce the need for accommodation at near and thus allow the potential development of fusion and stereopsis. Overminused glasses increase accommodation. Alternate occlusion theoretically reduces suppression but has no role in the treatment of high AC/A esotropia. Base-in prism would increase the deviation in a patient with high AC/A esotropia.

13. **b.** Dissociated vertical deviation (DVD) is associated with infantile esotropia. Vertical nystagmus and ocular flutter are not. Patients with infantile esotropia have asymmetric smooth pursuit, which is better in the temporal to nasal direction.

14. **d.** Intermittent exotropia is the most common exodeviation. Infantile exotropia and type 2 Duane retraction syndrome are uncommon entities. Pseudoexotropia is the result of certain facial features or a structural abnormality of the retina and is not a true strabismus disorder.

15. **b.** Orthoptic training to stimulate convergence may improve the deviation in patients with convergence insufficiency, a type of convergence weakness exotropia. Patients with Duane retraction syndrome may present with exotropia due to decreased adduction. Dissociated strabismus may manifest with an exodeviation. Both Duane retraction syndrome and dissociated strabismus are treated surgically. Positive angle kappa is a form of pseudostrabismus, in which the eyes appear exotropic, but the visual axes are optically aligned.

16. **b.** Since A and V patterns are variations of a primary position horizontal misalignment, there is no reason for a compensatory head position unless it allows single binocular vision. For a patient with A-pattern exotropia, single binocular vision, if achievable, is attained only with the eyes directed upward; hence, a chin-down head position is most likely. Head tilting or viewing in lateral gaze does not achieve this result.

17. **a.** Patients with dissociated strabismus may have accompanying extorsion and exodeviation (not esodeviation) of the elevating eye. Typically, there is no hypodeviation of the fellow eye on cover testing, due to an apparent violation of Hering's law of motor correspondence. DVD is usually seen in infantile strabismus. In this form of strabismus, any associated nystagmus is of the latent variety, which has a horizontal vector.

18. **c.** Bilateral superior oblique muscle dysfunction causes a large difference in horizontal tropia between downgaze and upgaze. Extorsion in bilateral palsy is usually well over 10° in downgaze. There is usually an esotropic shift in downgaze, and the head posture would be chin down to avoid the cyclodiplopia in downgaze.

19. **a.** Slight limitation of adduction is present in many cases of type 1 Duane retraction syndrome, if looked for carefully. The features listed in options *b, c,* and *d* can be seen in both disorders.

20. **a.** Patients with congenital motor nystagmus (CMN; infantile nystagmus syndrome) often adopt an abnormal head position to take advantage of the better vision that is possible at a null point. Oscillopsia is characteristic of nystagmus acquired in adulthood and is rare in CMN. An exponential decrease in velocity of the slow phase and a fast-phase direction that reverses with a change in fixation are characteristic of latent nystagmus (fusion maldevelopment nystagmus syndrome).

21. **d.** Limited adduction is evidence that the medial rectus muscle has reattached too far posteriorly to be effective as an adductor of the eye. Anterior segment ischemia does not

typically limit rotation and would not be expected after operation on just 1 extraocular muscle per eye. Adherence syndrome causing restriction would arise from adherence created on the opposite aspect of the globe, and the lateral rectus muscle was not included in the procedure. Conjunctival scarring over the medial rectus muscle would, if anything, limit abduction.

22. **c.** Correction of esotropia can expand the binocular visual field. Surgery for exotropia constricts the binocular visual field. Monofixation is not eliminated in patients with infantile strabismus even if the eyes are aligned well.

23. **b.** In general, eyes are hyperopic at birth, becoming more so until age 7 years, when they experience a myopic shift toward plano. The newborn has a steeper cornea and a higher intraocular lens power, both of which decrease over time. Visual acuity of infants aged 3 months is in the 20/120 range when measured by preferential looking (PL). Visually evoked potential (VEP) testing estimates acuity to be 20/20 at 6 months of age.

24. **a.** In the first few months of life, episodes of intermittent strabismus are common. Constant strabismus is not normal, even at this early age. Vertical nystagmus and ocular flutter are also not normal.

25. **c.** Inherited retinal dystrophies are the most common cause of paradoxical pupils. Patients with aniridia and anterior segment dysgenesis have abnormal irises but not paradoxical pupils. Pupillary reactions are normal in cerebral visual impairment.

26. **c.** Although there is some variability, the nervous system is typically mature enough at age 6–8 weeks for an infant to maintain visual fixation and react with facial expressions.

27. **a.** Although epiblepharon may produce an in-turning of the eyelashes, there is often minimal or no irritation of the cornea. If no significant fluorescein staining of the cornea is detected, only observation is required. The epiblepharon often resolves spontaneously with time and seldom requires surgical treatment.

28. **a.** The upper eyelid "follows" the eye in upgaze and downgaze; that is, the eyelid moves in the same direction as the eye. Therefore, the upper eyelid of a hypotropic eye will be lower than that of the fellow eye, producing the false appearance of ptosis. Conditions that cause hypertropia or horizontal strabismus do not cause pseudoptosis.

29. **b.** Eyelid coloboma (eyelid cleft, eyelid notch) carries a risk of exposure keratopathy, and early closure of the eyelid defect is often required.

30. **d.** Although all the listed treatments may be effective for some hemangiomas, oral propranolol is now preferred for the treatment of vision-threatening periocular hemangiomas. Topical timolol may be an effective treatment for superficial hemangiomas but not for orbital lesions.

31. **c.** The presence of chemosis suggests orbital involvement. Eyelid swelling, sinusitis, and fever may be present with both preseptal cellulitis and orbital cellulitis.

32. **b.** Nasolacrimal duct obstruction typically occurs at the most distal portion of the lacrimal duct, because of incomplete canalization at or around full-term gestation (40 weeks) of what was a solid structure in the fetus. This blockage occurs at the valve of Hasner. The canaliculi and puncta and the valve of Rosenmüller, which is in the region of the junction of the canaliculi, are more likely to have canalized normally.

33. **c.** Tears in Descemet membrane (Haab striae) are seen because of a rapid stretching of the cornea in primary congenital glaucoma. They are not seen in congenital hereditary

endothelial dystrophy (CHED) or Peters anomaly. Trauma from amniocentesis may result in a penetrating injury of the cornea. Tears in Descemet membrane may also be seen in a forceps injury sustained during delivery, but these are usually linear, not curvilinear.

34. **b.** Congenital iris ectropion may be an isolated finding, or it may be associated with neurofibromatosis 1, Prader-Willi syndrome, or facial hemihypertrophy. Retinal abnormalities may be seen in incontinentia pigmenti; dislocated lenses, in Marfan syndrome; and corneal crystals, in cystinosis.

35. **d.** In patients with sporadic aniridia, the presence of Wilms tumor must be excluded with a renal ultrasound scan, which must be repeated until molecular genetic analysis rules out an 11p13 deletion and confirms an intragenic *PAX6* mutation. Iris abnormalities that are associated with systemic abnormalities include neuroblastoma in patients with Horner syndrome, Lisch nodules in patients with neurofibromatosis, and heterochromia in patients with Waardenburg syndrome.

36. **a.** Infants with *Chlamydia trachomatis* infection acquired at birth may present with papillary conjunctivitis during the first week of life. Although the eye disease is usually self-limited, *C trachomatis* infection may cause pneumonia and otitis media in neonates. Therefore, systemic treatment with oral erythromycin is indicated.

37. **d.** Conjunctivitis is a common ocular manifestation of Stevens-Johnson syndrome. In severe cases, progressive scarring of the conjunctiva and eyelids may lead to corneal complications, including ulceration and perforation. Panuveitis and acute retinal necrosis are not associated with Stevens-Johnson syndrome.

38. **a.** Microcornea is associated with higher incidences of glaucoma following cataract surgery in children.

39. **b.** Primary congenital glaucoma usually occurs sporadically, but it may be inherited as an autosomal recessive trait. Specific genetic mutations have been identified in some patients.

40. **d.** Weill-Marchesani syndrome is associated with microspherophakia. The microspherophakic lens in this syndrome may dislocate into the anterior chamber, causing pupillary block glaucoma. In the other conditions, dislocation into the anterior chamber does not usually occur.

41. **d.** Anterior uveitis is the most common uveitis seen in children. It is most often idiopathic, related to trauma, or associated with juvenile idiopathic arthritis.

42. **b.** The 2 strongest risk factors for retinopathy of prematurity (ROP) are gestational age and birth weight. Although race and lung disease are also risk factors, they are not as significant as gestational age and birth weight. There is no difference in the risk of ROP between the sexes.

43. **b.** Unlike magnetic resonance imaging (MRI) and ultrasonography, a computed tomography (CT) scan subjects patients to radiation. Children with heritable retinoblastoma are at high risk for secondary radiation-induced tumors, so any additional radiation should be avoided, if possible.

44. **b.** Morning glory disc anomaly has been associated with basal encephalocele in patients with midfacial anomalies, PHACE syndrome (*p*osterior fossa malformations, *h*emangiomas, *a*rterial lesions, *c*ardiac and *e*ye anomalies), and abnormalities of the carotid circulation, including moyamoya disease.

45. **a.** Optic discs with small cup–disc ratios that may resemble papilledema are commonly seen in hyperopic eyes. Optic discs in myopic eyes do not have this appearance. Strabismus is not associated with pseudopapilledema.

46. **c.** Sickle cell testing must be performed in all African American patients with hyphema. Because of sickling of the red blood cells in the anterior chamber, sickle cell trait or disease may result in elevated intraocular pressure, even in the presence of a small hyphema.

47. **d.** "White-eyed" blowout fractures present with marked vertical motility restriction in both directions with minimal soft-tissue findings. Unless there is early surgical repair of the fracture, the inferior rectus muscle and its associated nerve can be permanently damaged.

48. **a.** The most common cause of visual impairment in children with abusive head trauma is from cortical or cerebral visual impairment due to neurologic damage. Optic atrophy and retinal injury may also cause decreased vision, but they are less common causes.

49. **c.** Incontinentia pigmenti shows the unusual inheritance pattern of X-linked dominance with a presumed lethal effect on the hemizygous male fetus.

50. **d.** Neurofibromatosis 1 shows autosomal dominant inheritance. However, approximately 50% of patients do not have a family history of the disease, reflecting the high rate of new mutations in the responsible gene.

Index

(*f* = figure; *t* = table)